|| *The Great American Waistline*

ALSO BY CHRIS CHASE:

How to Be a Movie Star, or A Terrible Beauty Is Born
Life Is a Banquet (with ROSALIND RUSSELL)
The Times of My Life (with BETTY FORD)

The Great American Waistline

PUTTING IT ON AND TAKING IT OFF

by CHRIS CHASE

COWARD, McCANN & GEOGHEGAN • NEW YORK

 Published on the same day in Canada by Academic Press Limited, Toronto.

The author gratefully acknowledges permission to quote from the following materials:
Excerpts from early issues of *Gourmet* magazine reprinted by permission of *Gourmet* magazine.
"Junk Food Junkie," words and music by Larry Groce, © 1974, 1976 Peaceable Kingdom, ASCAP. All rights reserved.
Excerpt from an Ann Landers column reprinted by permission of Field Newspaper Syndicate.
"That Lean and Hungry Look," *My Turn*, by Suzanne Britt Jordan, copyright 1978 by Newsweek, Inc. All rights reserved.
"Want Food Fast? Here's Fast Food," by Paul Gray, reprinted by permission of *Time*, The Weekly Newsmagazine; Copyright Time Inc. 1977.
Fat Is a Feminist Issue by Susie Orbach, copyright 1978 by Paddington Press.
The Thin Game by Edwin Bayrd, copyright 1978 by Newsweek Books.
"Here's to Your Health," KERA TV, copyright 1979 Publication Communication Foundation for North Texas.

LIBRARY OF CONGRESS CATALOGING IN PUBLICATION DATA

Chase, Chris.
The great American waistline.

Includes index.
1. Reducing diets. 2. Food habits—United States.
1. Title
RM222.2.046 1981 613.2'5'0973 80-25564
ISBN 0-698-11069-2 AACRI

DESIGNED BY HELEN BARROW
PRINTED IN THE UNITED STATES OF AMERICA

I WOULD LIKE TO THANK FOR THEIR GENEROUS HELP: Joseph Baum, James Beard, Julia Child, William Rossa Cole, Nancy Devitt, Guy Flatley, Dr. H. Paul Gabriel, Jill Gerston, Larry Goldberg, Lea Gordon Geuyer, Gael Greene, Barbara Haroche, John and Karen Hess, Barbara Kafka, Michi Kakutani, Joe Kanon, Dr. Martin Katz, Elaine Kaufman, Murray Klein, Owen Laster, John McQuiggan, Lou Mercier, William Primavera, Roberta Pryor, Calvin Trillin, Dr. Elizabeth Whelan, Burton Wolf, Joanna Wolper, Helen Worth, William Wright, Frank Zachary, Zanne Zakroff.

CONTENTS

|| *The Great American Waistline*

Introduction

"But wait a bit," the Oysters cried,
"Before we have our chat;
For some of us are out of breath,
And all of us are fat!"
—LEWIS CARROLL

WELL, maybe not all of us. Maybe only 30 million. That's what Mike Wallace said on *60 Minutes*, in December of 1978. "Thirty million Americans are overweight, and 15 million of these are grossly overweight."

Grossly? How come?

"Make the heart of this people fat, and make their ears heavy," cried the prophet Isaiah. But had Isaiah thought things through, or was he just talking silly? Did God, equally careless, pick up the ball and run with it, making heavy not only our ears, but our thighs, our necks, our spirits, none of which could be lightened until Jean Nidetch came along?

These questions are unanswerable, deponents being out of town. Still, certain arguments may be adduced from a look at American, not to mention human, history.

Traditionally, Americans have had scant use for moderation. The pioneers planted hugely, plundered hugely, built hugely, ate hugely, and so did their descendants. "J. P. Morgan's big and plump, forty-eight inches around the rump," runs a line from a ballad that was popular in certain circles (circles my father referred to as "pinko") during World War II.

Until quite recently, fat people were at least respected, the assumption being that they'd made enough money to eat a lot. At the turn of the century, a benign cultural aura still surrounded the overweight. Lillian Russell's hourglass shape, with plump arms, copious bosom, magnanimous hips—its only meagerness a pinched-in waist—caused palpitations in the hearts of men, though the darling (referred to as "airy, fairy Lillian, the American Beauty") weighed 200 pounds.

So thinness has not always been valued. At various stages in history, people who were thin were thought to be poor or ill or eccentric. Tales are told of tribal chieftains whose best wives, like their best pigs, were their fattest ones. In *The White Nile*, Alan Moorehead discusses the African king of Karagwe, one Rumanika, who "had his eccentricities. He kept an extraordinary harem of wives who were so fat they could not stand upright, and instead groveled like seals about the floors of their huts. Their diet was an uninterrupted flow of milk that was sucked from a gourd through a straw, and if the young girls resisted this treatment, they were force-fed like the *pâté de foie gras* ducks of Strasbourg: a man stood over them with a whip."

Brillat-Savarin wouldn't have force-fed anybody, but he did write in *The Anatomy of Taste* (published in 1825; translated in 1949 by M. F. K. Fisher) that while it was all right for a man to be lean, thinness was "a horrible calamity for women: beauty to them is more than life itself, and it consists above all of the roundness of their forms and the graceful curvings of their outlines."

Even in parts of the modern world, corpulence is believed to have its uses. Certain Italian women are said to overfeed their husbands in order to remove them from the sexual sweepstakes and keep the home fires burning.

But the dilemma of present-day America is that it wants to be thin. We are faced with the ironic fact of an overweight nation yearning to breathe svelte, and it is this split in our psyche that this book proposes to examine.

Since America is the land of opportunity, and nothing that interests more than six people fails to generate an industry, food is big business here, and so is dieting. First we glut, then, in a passion of guilt, deny ourselves the joy of our gluttony. Fat is a national obsession. Putting it on and taking it off, we lay waste our days and our money.

Shortly before Christmas of 1978, a *New York Times* book critic, Christopher Lehmann-Haupt, found himself trying to review in a single column Dr. Herman Tarnower's *The Complete Scarsdale Medical Diet* along with Julia Child's most recent opus dedicated to the proposition that the flesh is weak. Lehmann-Haupt admitted that he had lost twenty-five pounds in four and a half months of Dr. Tarnower's protein toast-and-tomatoes, but that he was nonetheless walking around with a copy of *Julia Child and Company* clutched "close to my diminishing frame because, despite Dr. Tarnower's assurances that the renunciation of pasta, dairy products, alcohol, sugar, chocolate, and the rest of the food for which I live, promotes salubrity and serenity, I intend to plunge . . . into Mrs. Child's '*Le Gâteau au Chocolat, Mousseline,* a very tender, moist and delicate and very chocolatey dessert confection.'"

And that guy's an intellectual.

Why are we fat?

We eat too much.

We can also pose other hypotheses and develop them in subsequent chapters:

1. America is a rich country with a vast middle class that has the means to eat as much as it wants.

2. The craze for gourmet cooking that followed World War II creamed us and buttered us and left us *bombe*-d.

3. We have been through a technological revolution that has made eating—or at least preparing—food easier. If a product can be canned, frozen, dried, or boxed, it's right there waiting for us in the supermarkets.

4. Along with the rise of junk and/or fast foods, our gross national waistline has expanded.

5. We consume phenomenal amounts of sugar, since sugar is laced into practically everything, even such unlikely foods as salt. (That children are hooked on sugar is nothing new. Sweets have been offered as a reward since the first cavewoman said to the first cavebaby, "Eat your lion, or you don't get a Hostess Twinkie.")

"She was a butterscotch sundae of a woman," wrote A. J. Liebling, in *Between Meals*, "as beautiful as a tulip of beer with a high white collar. If a Western millionaire . . . could have given an architect carte blanche to design him a woman, she would have looked like Lillian. She was San Simeon in corsets."

Her contours, added Liebling, "did not encourage fasting among her imitators." He considered a dessert that had been named for the actress—"a half cantaloupe holding about a pint and three quarters of ice cream"—and added disapprovingly, "If an actress had a dish named after her now, the recipe would be four phenobarbital tablets and a jigger of Metrecal." (*Between Meals*, by the way, was published back in 1962.)

Lillian had five husbands, a good many more than five lovers, and reigned, a goddess, for thirty-five years. As for her frequent dinner companion, Diamond Jim Brady, that man of substance in both the literal and figurative sense, was viewed with no small awe by lesser mortals. How did he survive all those tons of loaves and fishes? Or was he only doing what any of us might have done if we'd had the chance? And the digestion?

(It turned out poor Jim's digestion wasn't everything it might have been. He died in 1917, at the age of fifty-six, his stomach swollen to six times the size of a normal person's. "Jim Brady is the best twenty-five customers we have," said George Rector, proprietor of a famous restaurant, listing as a typical Brady meal a dinner that had included "oysters, crabs, turtle soup, lobsters, terrapin, canvas back ducks, sirloin steak and vegetables, an entire tray of French pastry, many glasses of orange juice, and two pounds of after-dinner chocolates.")

6. Some of us, particularly those who were overfed infants, develop extralarge fat cells, and lots of them. (When we lose weight, our fat cells shrink in size, but not in number, so the minute we regain the weight, the cells balloon right up again.)

7. Advertising—"Nobody doesn't like Sara Lee"—fills us with lust and midnight longings.

8. Our parents were steatopygous, or—if you can't handle that—lard-assed. (Two skinny parents rarely produce a chunky child.)

9. Our lives are sedentary. And never mind, what about the crazy joggers in the streets. Most of us are still sitting in Barcaloungers sipping beer, watching television, and wishing our flab would fall off. Recent statistics from *Variety*, the show-business newspaper, report the average TV viewer puts in six and a quarter hours a day at the tube, which means if you're a person who doesn't watch at all, then somebody out there is glued to his set for more than twelve hours a day.

The trouble is, our metabolism is genetically wired for greater exertion. Not only don't we have to plow the south forty anymore, but thanks to elevators and escalators we don't even have to climb stairs. A friend of mine admits that he used to drive from his apartment to his bank, four blocks away, and double-park to run in and cash a check.

Instincts have a way of hanging on long after they've served their original purpose. The sociological clock runs faster than the evolutionary clock, and we're saddled with responses that once had survival value but are now inconvenient. The sex drive burns on into old age, even after somebody's had all the babies he or she could possibly use; our aggressive tendencies flourish, even though modern man isn't forced into bloody combat with wild animals.

As for excessive eating, we seem to be stuck, residually, with the appetite for it, even though we've stripped ourselves of the need for so much fuel. Anne Scott Beller, in *Fat and Thin,* suggests that our predatory forebears, living "from one windfall to the next . . . must have 'learned,' anatomically, to store food . . . in times of glut, and to live off that stored subcutaneous surplus when the climate, the season, and the vagaries of the animal species it hunted resulted in scarcities and famine." I've also heard a theory that pleasure was built into sex and food in order that men might not get so busy killing each other they'd forget to eat and make love, thus bringing to an end "the plumeless genus of bipeds," as old Plato described us.

"The very discovery of the New World was the by-product of a dietary quest," wrote Arthur Schlesinger, Sr., pointing out that Columbus came (by inadvertence) to America seeking the spices Europe wanted for its meats.

Throughout history, most cultures that had the wherewithal to do so have feasted. And America has had the wherewithal. What was our first national holiday but a celebration of food? The grim-faced Pilgrim fathers, staggering, apprehensive, off the decks of the *Mayflower* after their fierce sixty-six-day voyage, found bounty.

And if that sounds oversimplified, it is. The *Mayflower*'s passengers had been sustained by a diet of dried beef (which they called salt horse) and hardtack and dried peas and beans. The butter turned rancid, the cheese got moldy, the water went bad, and even the children had to drink beer. If the beer hadn't run out, the ship might have got clear to Virginia, instead of stopping in Massachusetts where, despite friendly Indians and good hunting, half the settlers died between November of

1620 and April of 1621 of what was referred to as "general sickness."

Still, for the fifty or so Pilgrims who made it through the first winter, spring and summer brought marvels. There were nuts in the forests, and deer and elk and moose and rabbits; there were land birds and water birds and every kind of fish in the sea; there were wild fruits and onions and there was the miracle of corn.

So, less than a year after the landing at Plymouth, Governor William Bradford ordered a three-day festival to commemorate the harvest.

Describing the event in a letter, a colonist named Edward Winslow wrote in part, "Our Governor sent four men on fowling, that we might after a more special manner rejoice together, after we had gathered the fruit of our labors."

Three hundred and sixty years later, we're still indulging in the fruit—the corn breads, the turkeys, the geese, the pumpkins, the pies—without partaking of the accompanying labors, and thereby hang some heavy, heavy tails.

I PUTTING IT ON

PUTTING IT ON:
We're fat because the New World's streets were paved with pork chops.

1 A Skimpy Historical Chapter

And ye shall eat the fat of the land.
—GENESIS

DEATHS caused by starvation, says the *Encyclopaedia Britannica*, "occur mainly among the poor."

Got it.

For millennia, much of the world suffered pestilence and famine—starving Romans threw themselves into the Tiber, starving Londoners ate the bark off trees, starving Chinese were gnawed to death by foxes—but America had no famine, so the immigrants kept coming.

In the beginning, English settlers were smug in the conviction that their ways—of worshiping and of boiling beef, to mention just a couple—were God's ways, and far superior to the carryings-on of the natives.

This complacency is taken to task by Waverley Root and Richard de Rochemont (in *Eating in America)* who say, "No Indian was feasting like the members of the privileged classes of Europe, but no Indian was faring as badly as the poorest Europeans either."

By the time Columbus discovered America, declare Root and de

Rochemont, "the Indians were using two thousand different foods derived from plants, a figure Europe could hardly have matched."

There seemed no need for begging at the gates in the New World; it teemed with plenty. "The fruitfull and well watered earth doth glad all hearts . . . And yeelds an hundred fold for one," rhapsodized the Reverend William Morell in 1625. Near the Great Lakes, wild rice grew, and sea turtles thrived along the Atlantic coast, while the rivers that fed into the Pacific were so clotted with salmon at spawning time that one explorer said he could have walked across "on their backs." The sugar maple, a tree unknown to Europeans, provided sap with which to sweeten the New Englanders' cooking (cane sugar didn't arrive from the West Indies until much later), lobsters six feet long were taken from the waters off New Amsterdam (some settlers used lobster as bait to catch codfish), and in the South possums and pigs and sweet potatoes and wild oranges abounded.

Even so, four out of five of the "Gallants" who landed in Jamestown in 1607 were dead by 1610. Historian Samuel Eliot Morison sniffed that the Virginians "seem to have been divided into those who could not and those who would not work," and the *American Heritage Cookbook and Illustrated History of American Eating and Drinking* is equally cutting about "gentlemen who had never worked a day, had no desire to begin, and were among the worst frontiersmen the world has ever known."

(The Virginians who *did* live through the terrible year of 1609 made it because they fed off the oyster beds in the Elizabeth River, laying the foundation for a national oyster passion that did not abate over the next two hundred years. Oysters were the hot dogs and pizzas of their day—whether raw, boiled, broiled, stewed, pickled, creamed, scalloped, or added to soups and omelets, early Americans could not get enough of them.)

To give the Jamestowners their due, had they been good frontiersmen, they'd still have seen trouble. Half the cattle they'd brought from home were killed off by Indians (although, to be sure, the improvident settlers ate the other half without waiting for calves to be born and replenish the stock). Indians also attacked the Virginians while they were planting grain, and a whole year's crop was never sown at all. One starving Jamestown citizen went mad, killed his wife, "powdered" (salted) her, "and had eaten part of her before it was knowne."

The cannibal was duly hanged, but his malfeasance plagued the minds of his fellows. "Now whether she was better roasted, boyled or carbonado'd, I know not, but such a dish as powdered wife I never heard of," said Captain John Smith, good friend of Pocahontas.

(Eating one's relatives and acquaintances has never been looked on kindly in the Western world. Fiji kings may have found the roasted noses of victims succulent, but Europeans and Americans, reading about the diet, were not amused. Two hundred and sixty-five years after the ravenous Virginian polished off a slab of lady, a man named Alferd [*sic*] Packer was lost with five buddies in the sparsely populated and hard-frozen mountains of Colorado near Lake San Cristóbal some time in January of 1874. Alferd passed the time until spring by making a light lunch of his companions, and the following April, he showed up—alone—at the Los Piñios Indian Agency. He was fat, had plenty of money, "and his conduct invited suspicion." In due time, he confessed his misdeed, and there's a lovely though apocryphal story that has the judge at his trial saying sternly, "Alferd Packer, not only are you guilty of the heinous crime of cannibalism, but you have eaten the Democratic majority of Hinsdale County!")

If the 1600s were tough on the Virginians, by the 1700s existence in the Colonial South was easy, for the big plantation owners anyway. (My husband's little girl once handed in a school paper on feudalism that I find still full of wisdom. "The lord's life was a good life," she wrote, "but the serf's life was a hard life.")

Slavery (there were only a few slaves in 1619; by 1776, there were half a million) provided the labor that permitted one Colonial governor to describe the South as "the land of good eating, good drinking, stout men and pretty women."

Perusal of their breakfast menus explains the stoutness of the men. One visitor to a plantation in 1774 described the planters' 10:00 A.M. repast as "cold turkey, cold meat, fried hominy, toast and cider, ham, bread and butter, tea, coffee and chocolate."

(For a look at a more spartan Southern aristocrat, here's an excerpt from the diary of William Byrd, in the year 1709: "I rose at five o'clock in the morning and read a chapter in Hebrew and 200 verses in Homer's *Odyssey*. I ate milk for breakfast. I said my prayers. Jerry and Eugene [servants] were whipped. I danced my dance. I read law in the morning and Italian in the afternoon. I ate tough chicken for dinner.")

Up North, people were chomping down pie for breakfast, and cider was replacing beer (which in 1634 had cost only a penny a quart) as the drink of choice. This was logical, since grain didn't grow in New England, but apples did. "Cider was to early Americans what drinking water, milk, orange juice, soft drinks and martinis are to us," says Stuart Berg Flexner in *I Hear America Talking*.

(Some two hundred years later, Horace Greeley, like a reformer railing against marijuana as a step on the way to heroin, began editorializing in his newspaper against the "cider swilling" that, he said, led to more potent stimulants "so that whole families died drunkards and vagabond paupers." Numbers of citizens, inflamed by Greeley's words, went forth with hatchets and attacked apple trees.)

For the most part, the colonists ate meat and dough (cookies, cakes, pies, breads, rolls, biscuits, cobblers, tarts), shunning vegetables, although John Adams once wrote home to his wife Abigail, "Pray how does your asparagus perform?" and Thomas Jefferson's garden grew all kinds of produce, plain and fancy. Jefferson was one of the rare Americans who would eat tomatoes, which were widely believed to be a poisonous form of apple.

When Jefferson went to Paris as United States envoy, he became fascinated with French cooking (this caused an infuriated Patrick Henry to accuse his old friend of abjuring "his native victuals"), and eventually brought a French chef to the White House. He was the first, but certainly not the last, president to do so.

In the backwoods, repasts were far from French. Frontiersmen along the Carolina-Virginia border sometimes fried bacon, left it sitting in its rendered grease, poured rum on the whole business, and served it "at once for meat and drink." And certain other settlers (living in a fort built west of the Mississippi) who developed diarrhea from eating too much buffalo meat nonetheless persisted in the habit until they had conquered the problem and each man could down ten pounds of buffalo a day. "It made us quite fat, and there were no more sick among us," testified one of their number.

The 1800s saw pioneers crossing the wilderness, cooking anything that would stay in the pot—beaver tails, marrow bones, buffalo tongues.

James Fenimore Cooper called Americans "gross feeders" who liked their food heavy and indigestible. "The predominance of grease in the American kitchen, coupled with the habits of hearty eating, and of constant expectoration, are the causes of the diseases of the stomach which are so common in America," Cooper said, but a British novelist named Frederick Marryat came up with an explanation, if not an excuse, for American gulosity. "The cookery in the United States is exactly what it is and must be everywhere else," wrote Captain Marryat. "In ration with the degree of refinement of the population."

In 1856, the periodical *Harper's Monthly* also took up the subject of American coarseness, commenting disdainfully on workingmen at their lunches: "They swallow, but don't eat; and, like the boa constrictor, bolt everything, whether it be a blanket or a rabbit."

The workingmen continued to arrive on these shores in droves. Between 1846 and 1852, a million Irish came to America, driven from home by the failure of the potato crop. One man I know describes his Irish grandfather's journey through the gates of Ellis Island: "He was a tiny little skinny thing, he was only thirteen years old, and his intention was to marry a very stout German lady, which act he believed would make him feel secure. He did it, too. She made him do his drinking in the cellar, but they didn't starve."

They didn't starve. Even though the reality was often different from the dream (in Boston, laborers worked fifteen hours a day for fifty cents, a fact which, when he discovered it, caused Ralph Waldo Emerson some surprise), most newcomers to the promised land were better off than they'd been elsewhere.

"Tell Thomas Arran to come to America; and tell him to leave his strap what he wears when he has nothing to eat in England for some other half-starved slave," one immigrant wrote home, according to Dale Brown in his book *American Cooking*. And: "Tell Miriam there's no sending children to bed without supper, or husbands to work without dinners in their bags."

(Of course, in the early days of America, the rich were fat and the poor were thin because when the rich were being carried through the muddy streets in sedan chairs—this happened not in Asia, but in Annapolis, Maryland—it was the poor who were doing the carrying, and building muscles for their trouble. Nowadays, the picture is reversed; the poor are paunchy from too much starch and sugar. There's a poster in the New York City subways showing a fat smiling group above a legend that asks, "Do you know this family is undernourished?" And the skinny rich—"You can't be too thin or too rich," Babe Paley is credited with having taught us—are showing off their dieted and exercised close-to-the-bone bodies in *Town & Country* magazine.)

Between 1820 and 1960, thirty-four million Europeans emigrated to the United States and fathered and grandfathered the American middle class to which most of us belong. In Mexico, they say you've joined the middle class when you buy your first pair of shoes. Americans were luckier, but, in the process of homogenizing ourselves, we became, increasingly, a nation of white-collar workers and white bread eaters.

New foods came over with each new wave of immigrants—hamburgers, sauerkraut, frankfurters with the Germans, waffles with the Dutch, pastas, salamis, cheeses, olive oil with the Italians. The Greeks made a soup of lemons and knew things to do with eggplant and lamb, the Russians and Poles brought borscht and blinis, the Hungarians goulash, the Scandinavians the pastries called Danish, and it was a Chinese cook on a work gang in San Francisco who invented the western sandwich by making egg foo yong (an Oriental omelet filled with chopped meat and vegetables) and putting it between two slices of bread.

Sometimes, it was a question of lend-lease completing its cycle. Early Spanish explorers, finding in America tomatoes, peppers, chocolate, paprika, and potatoes, had borne these wonders home to Europe, and when later Spaniards returned to the New World as immigrants, they demonstrated special uses for chilies and coriander and for the chocolate the Aztecs had served only to kings.

Unfortunately, it took a long time for Americans to put much value on these riches that had arrived with the poor, so anxious were the sons and daughters of immigrants to turn their backs on their roots and become true Yankees.

". . . We are made up of a lot of different nationalities mainly brought from the lower classes, and in almost any decent-sized village of our country there is a baker from Hungary or Poland or France who can and does still make his round, odorous healthful loaves," wrote M. F. K. Fisher in *How to Cook a Wolf*, a book which first appeared in 1942. Yet, she went on, in spite of this, "we continue everywhere to buy the packaged monstrosities that lie, all slicked and tasteless, on the bread counters of our nation."

The American enthusiasm for falling to in somebody's else's dining room began in the 1830s when, say Root and de Rochemont, "the first real restaurants appeared in major American cities, and along with hotels, country inns and local taverns, they too began to persuade American housewives that keeping up with one's neighbors meant staying abreast of the French."

(It didn't always work. In 1838, the mayor of New York complained to

his diary about the pernicious French influence of serving only one course at a time, rather than laying all your viands on the table. "Your conversation is interrupted every minute by greasy dishes thrust between your head and that of your next neighbor, and it is more expensive than the old mode of showing a handsome dinner to your guests and leaving them free to choose. It will not do.")

Eating out. Citizens who could afford it took to it happily, greedily. If you were a working-class New Yorker in the year 1838, you could go to a place called The Rainbow, at 49 Howard Street, where the "Bill of Fare" offered beefsteak for twenty-five cents, or mutton chops for eighteen and three quarter cents—and the price included ale! (A note on The Rainbow's menu specified that the tavern would soon start charging for the ale, which would be "supplied to families at eight cents a quart. This ale is brewed expressly for The Rainbow, consequently there can be no doubt as to its purity and quality.")

If you were higher on the scale of New York society, you might have been bidden to a Union Club feast such as the breakfast tendered Mr. Wilkie Collins by Mr. William Seaver on the morning of October 22, 1873. William Cullen Bryant attended, so did the Austrian minister, Baron Lederer, the Spanish minister, Admiral Polo, and Governor Ingersoll of Connecticut, and this is what they ate:

OYSTERS

FILET OF BASS, A LA NORMANDE   SMELTS, TARTARE SAUCE

LAMB CHOPS WITH GREEN PEAS

CASSEROLE OF LOBSTER

BAKED OYSTERS IN THE SILVER SHELL

OMELETTE WITH KIDNEYS AND TOMATOES

CHICKEN, MARYLAND STYLE

PATE OF GOOSE LIVER WITH TRUFFLES

BASTION OF EELS IN JELLY

▶

STUFFED PEPPERS EGGPLANT STRING BEANS CAULIFLOWER

CANVASBACK DUCK WOODCOCK

SALAD

TUTTI FRUTTI FRUITS ICE CREAM

COFFEE ETC.

Doesn't your mind reel trying to figure out what the "etc." could have been?

But no need to go on about it. After a breakfast like that, the gents were probably able to discuss international affairs until lunchtime without taking a break for a snack.

(Dismayed by all this gadding about, a Virginia lady named Marion Cabell Tyree compiled a book on housekeeping—it was published in 1877—saying she would consider her labors worthwhile if she could disseminate enough knowledge of domestic arts to make "American homes more attractive to American husbands, and spare them a resort to hotels and saloons for those simple luxuries which their wives know not how to provide . . .")

At the turn of the century, roof-garden dining became a popular pastime, and Reisenweber's, on New York's Columbus Circle, was a fashionable place to be seen. Reisenweber's offered "a frog dinner, country style, $1.25, served in the Gardenia Grill every evening," and featured, besides, "The Poinciana Quintet—Best Negro Entertainers."

If you weren't invited to the Union Club, and you couldn't afford Reisenweber's, or even The Rainbow, you could turn to a book that listed *Receipts for the Poor* and find: "Take a sheep's head, a pound and a half of Scotch barley, three pounds of potatoes, ½ pound of onions, some pepper and salt, with cabbages, turnips and carrots, boil them in two gallons of water. It will make six quarts of good soup."

Take a sheep's head. Right.

Rummaging through our past, we begin to find auguries of our present. For instance:

Always, some Americans have been entrepreneurs of the fast buck. When food processing first took hold, one critic accused technology of beginning to "run ahead of conscience," and documented his case. Herring from Maine was widely sold as "imported French sardines," and in a single year the state of North Dakota consumed ten times as much "pure Vermont maple syrup" as the state of Vermont produced.

Always, some Americans had a sweet tooth. Cakes were among the glories of the Colonial wives. ("The Pilgrim Fathers must have come over to the country with the Cooking book under one arm and the Bible under the other," wrote Charles Joseph Latrobe in 1836, marveling at the variety of desserts available in New England.) And George Washington, during the summer of 1790, spent $200 on ice cream.

Always, some Americans advocated what we now think of as health food. The Shakers—a religious sect dedicated to celibacy, which may be why there aren't more Shakers around—ate fruits, vegetables, and made their bread from whole wheat flour. So did a Presbyterian minister named Sylvester Graham who put out a *Journal of Health and Longevity*, and inveighed against "pork, condiments and hot mince pie."

Dr. Graham said men needed bran as horses needed hay, and Bronson Alcott, Louisa May's daddy, was even more ferocious. In Fruitlands, his Utopia (established with Charles Lane), believers were permitted to drink nothing but spring water, eat nothing but grains, fruits, and roots; one woman was expelled for admitting she had squirreled away a fish head.

And always, some Americans (whether for snobbish reasons, or for the sheer wonder of its tastes) flirted with French cuisine, while other Americans disdained the influence of a country whose citizens were believed by many to live exclusively on frogs and salad.

"Democratic enthusiasm . . . made a virtue of crude and tasteless food," says Daniel Boorstin (now the Librarian of Congress), "and obsession with the delights of the palate was considered a symptom of Old World decadence."

Many foreign visitors agreed that Americans set a rough table. In the 1830s, an English lady named Harriet Martineau complained about a meal she had been served in Tennessee. "The dish from which I ate," she wrote later, "was, according to some, mutton, to others, pork. My own idea is that it was dog."

Mrs. Martineau notwithstanding, most early American cookbooks were solidly against foreign infiltration. "To our disgrace," scolded Eliza Smith, compiler of a famous cooking manual, "we have admired the French tongue and French messes." Mrs. Hannah Glasse agreed, railing against "the blind folly of this age, that would rather be imposed upon by a French booby, than give encouragement to a good English cook!"

If you could find a good English cook, that is.

(Pro- and anti-French discourse abided into modern times, with authors such as Gerald Carson hinting that Francophiles could take their duck *bigarade* and stuff it. "To the Yankee race, from Maine to California, there are dearer glories—blueberry slump and the small-mouthed pot of baked beans.")

The heaviness of the American diet led directly to the heaviness of the American people. They didn't take it to heart, they were too busy taking it to mouth.

Novelist Charles Dickens described an American breakfast at which he was a guest as having been composed of "tea, coffee, bread, butter, salmon, shad, liver, steak, potatoes, pickles, ham, chops, black-puddings, and sausages." And, said he, "Dinner was breakfast again without the tea and coffee."

Once more, testimony from Waverley Root and Richard de Rochemont:

"Dickens' suspicion that the American diet was unhealthy echoed the opinion of the Count of Volney, who had written that Americans deserved first prize for a diet sure to destroy teeth, stomach and health. But if many Europeans thought Americans ate the wrong foods, none of them reported that Americans did not get enough food."

Enough and too much. Still, an occasional foreign visitor, far from being put off by the feeding habits of the American native, found them charming. "Rudyard Kipling, at the end of the nineteenth century, was enchanted by Pennsylvania Dutch farmers and their 'fat cattle, fat women,'" writes Evan Jones, while another chronicler of the omnivores who settled around Lancaster, Pennsylvania, says, "Probably it is the superabundance of pork and pie the Dutch have been eating for generations that turns so many of them into walking mountains of flesh."

Okay, when did walking mountains of flesh start looking bad to their fellow creatures? Particularly, when did fat women stop being sex symbols and skinny women elbow them—with elbows honed to razor sharpness by caloric denial—aside?

Consider the paintings of Peter Paul Rubens. *The Judgment of Paris* dates back to 1638. There they stand, Juno, Venus, Minerva, three fleshy goddesses, waiting for Paris to choose the fairest. Bert Parks wouldn't have looked at any of them. Out of Juno's thighs alone, half a dozen modern fashion models could be carved.

As for Pierre Auguste Renoir, born in 1841, he was still painting ripely voluptuous nudes right up until he died, in 1919.

Which is just about the time it all started changing.

"Prohibition, and the flapper's concern for a trimmer figure put an end to plentiful and leisurely dining, as elegant restaurants lost out in popularity to the speakeasy," reads a sign in a case at the New-York Historical Society.

Gloria Swanson, the movie queen, remembers that everything began to be different after World War I: "Women raised their skirts from their ankles to just around their knees. It really came as quite a shock, considering the way it had been."

Girls hacked inches off their hair, and pounds off their hides; if you were going to powder your suddenly visible knees, you needed to be able to find them.

"Pet and die young," cried the college daredevils who smoked and fooled around in the backs of cars. Girls wore hot-water bottles filled with bootleg gin hanging from their necks, and while bathing beauties of the day—dressed in stockings, as well as skirted suits—look a bit lumpy by modern standards, compared to the buxom lovelies who'd come before, they were positively scraggy.

Boyish, that was the image the flappers fancied. They strapped down their chests, and worked to make themselves birdlike (trying to be ortolans instead of pigeons), they flamed their youth instead of their crepes suzettes, they were jazz babies.

By the 1920s, mourned A. J. Liebling, "It was no longer any use taking a woman to a great restaurant except to show her off. She would not eat, and out of ill temper disguised as solicitude for her escort's health, she would put him off his feed as well."

That "brilliancy" of the eyes and "freshness" of the skin noted by Brillat-Savarin in those members of the fair sex who "leaned toward gourmandism" gone, all gone, and with them, contentment. Since skinniness became the mode, few American women with robust appetites have known a happy day or drawn an unguilty breath.

PUTTING IT ON:
We're fat because we discovered chocolate mousse.

2 Gourmet *Magazine* and the Beginnings of Sauces for the Lower Classes

Sweep on, you fat and greasy citizens.
—WILLIAM SHAKESPEARE

IT ISN'T TRUE that we're the fattest people in history. We're not even the fattest people in *our* history.

"Probably this country will never again see so many fat, rich men as were prevalent at the end of the last century, copper kings and railroad millionaires and suchlike literally stuffing themselves to death," wrote M. F. K. Fisher in *An Alphabet for Gourmets*.

It isn't true, either, that in the 1940s Americans started eating on a more gargantuan scale. As previously noted, twenty-course sit-down meals were more popular a hundred years ago. But what did come with the 40s was the birth—among ordinary, grass-roots, non-robber-baron, servantless Americans—of a great gourmet craze that took thirty-five years to reach its apogee: a *poulet* in every pot, and Cuisinarts nuzzling espresso machines in every kitchen.

It wasn't until after World War II, food expert James Beard has said, "that Americans began to think of eating as pleasurable." Because our soldiers had come home, and they had been everywhere, and they "had tasted the real thing."

The world was tired of austerity. During the war, America had been isolated, no fashions from Paris, no fabrics available, so when Christian Dior came along with his New Look, he made history. Here was a man using tons of material, saying that shape was important again, giving women waistlines, telling them to take off their Rosie the Riveter overalls and look pretty rather than useful.

It was the same with food. Even in this country, there had been shortages and ration coupons. If the butcher gave a mother one lamb chop, it was apt to be cooked and cut up to feed the baby, while the other children sulked.

One American who had seen the future coming was Earle MacAusland, who in 1941 (before we got into the war) started *Gourmet, the Magazine of Good Living*.

An early MacAusland editorial informed his readers that the art of being a gourmet could be found "in a thrifty French housewife with her *pot-au-feu* or in a white-capped chef in a skyscraper hotel. But wherever it exists, the practitioner of this art will have the eye of an artist, the imagination of a poet, the rhythm of a musician, and the breadth of a sculptor."

Not one word about the hips of a hippopotamus.

Mr. MacAusland deplored "the mad hurly-burly of our modern daily existence" and said a wise person who cultivated his palate would feel a whole lot better.

Some of *Gourmet*'s first readers felt a whole lot worse. "I must admit that the contents of *Gourmet* shocked me and led me to believe that we may again be in the dark ages if food worship—admired and cultivated by the Roman sensualists—is again to grip the world at a time when it is bleeding," complained Edith L. Wile in a letter. "While Rome burns, would you have the palate catered to in the western hemisphere? The menu . . . was most revolting. Could anyone dare to attempt such orgies at a time like this? Perhaps it is an unfortunate moment to start such a journal. Imagine what a British soldier might feel on reading this!"

Mr. MacAusland was not confounded; he stuck to his guns. And his butter. "We feel that there is as much a place for a magazine dealing with fine foods as there is a place for fine automobiles, clothes, or any other quality merchandise . . . we think that more thought should be given both to the preparation of foods and to the manner of eating them, attempting to eliminate the attitude, fairly prevalent, of eating merely to satisfy one's hunger. . . . The cultivation of taste should be encouraged in all lines . . ."

Would you believe it? Edith L. Wile backed down. "Perhaps my intense feeling over the situation in the world led me to make too hasty a judgment. I do wish, however, that thrift and economy could be injected into the American way. Nowhere is waste greater than in the American kitchen."

MacAusland concurred. He said a true gourmet never wasted anything, and during the first years of his magazine, he strenuously supported America's war effort, urging cooks to fight Hitler and Hirohito by returning to their butchers animal fat, which fat would then be collected by the government and used to make TNT. (Although the crudity of the signs in certain New York meat markets—"Ladies, please do not bring your fat cans here on Saturdays"—would not have amused the proper publisher.)

In the beginning, rich folks took to *Gourmet* like Brillat-Savarin took to truffles. One reader wrote that the magazine would be "of interest to my staff," another that *Gourmet* was spreading gracious living throughout America, "making homes more desirable—something to be protected—even worth fighting for."

What Earle MacAusland had joined together—feeder and reader—no man has yet put asunder. When he died at the age of ninety, his widow Jean took over as publisher. Mr. Mac, as the *Gourmet* staff called him, remained to the end a handsome chap, a staunch Republican, and an avid fisher of salmon. Every summer he went fishing, and sometimes sent the salmon to Brooklyn to have it smoked, then to the staff at the magazine to slice up and divide among themselves.

Zanne Zakroff, a willowy brunette who in 1978, at age thirty, was delighted, astonished, and terrified (in that order) to find herself food editor of the prestigious magazine, spoke of her employer with affection and amusement when I talked with her a year before his death. "He is a gentleman. His brother-in-law once told me he had never seen Mr. Mac mowing his lawn without a jacket on."

In his later years, MacAusland no longer wrote editorials, but, said

Miss Zakroff, "he certainly dictates all of the business. And he refuses ads. He won't take an ad just because it represents money. It has to be quality. The advertiser has to be addressing himself to Mr. Mac's audience, and nobody who's a cut below. I don't think Mr. Mac realizes people don't have servants anymore; he leads a somewhat sheltered existence."

The staff at *Gourmet* is dedicated, but not highly paid. "Most of the people who work here have trust funds and wealthy husbands," says Miss Zakroff, admitting ruefully that she has neither. "Just a beagle pup."

If MacAusland was careful when it came to salaries, he spared no expense on behalf of his readers. "The paper is the best quality paper and the printer is the top printer in the country," Zanne Zakroff points out, adding that *Gourmet,* at $1.25 per issue, is less expensive to buy than a much newer magazine called *Food and Wine* that goes for $1.50 a copy.

"Mr. Mac just balks at raising the price, he doesn't like to penalize *Gourmet*'s fans." *Gourmet* does, in fact, provide its readers with services on which the company loses money, or at best breaks even. Binders for storing old copies of the magazine are offered at cost, no markup. On the other hand, the *Gourmet* cookbooks and travel books turn a tidy profit.

But *Gourmet* has been a success right from the start. By 1967, its circulation was 300,000. In 1978, it was up to 665,000, and all achieved without trial offers, cut rates, or promotions. *Gourmet* now calculates its carry-over audience (those who see it, even if they don't buy it) to be more than two million people, with the heaviest distribution in the Northeast.

Its appeal, say the editors simply, is to snobbery and sophistication. It's a fantasy magazine for food the way *Vogue* is a fantasy magazine for clothes.

"Most of us can't have Porthault linens and Waterford crystal and dine on *foie gras* and drink champagne," says Zanne Zakroff, "so *Gourmet* is, certainly, escapist, but we're also trying to carry on tradition, to represent the best of all possible worlds. I remember getting a letter saying, 'I've been a subscriber since the 40s, and *Gourmet* is not only beautiful, it's the only magazine I receive which contains no bad news.'"

Occasionally, a subscriber will take his business elsewhere. "We lost some who said, 'I'm going to *Bon Appétit,*'" says Miss Zakroff, "but then *Bon Appétit* went through a period of flux which our readers didn't care for, so they came back to us." *(Bon Appétit,* which started life in 1955 as a promotional giveaway brochure, was bought in 1975 by an entrepreneur named Cleon Knapp, whose base of operations is Los Angeles and who, unlike Earle MacAusland, is prodigal with cash for his top employees. "I pay them outlandish salaries," he says cheerily. Unwilling to compete with *Gourmet,* Knapp went for lower income readers; no recipe may be printed in *Bon Appétit* unless every one of its ingredients can be found in any supermarket.) *Bon Appétit*'s circulation is now one and one half million, but *Gourmet* is still said to be the most profitable food magazine.

Why would a subscriber leave *Gourmet,* even for a short time? "Too complicated recipes," says Miss Zakroff frankly. "We used to have a heavy tendency toward French restaurant food which was rich, difficult to prepare, and needed a lot of exotic ingredients.

"We will *always* print some intricate recipes which are never meant to be made by a housewife. They're meant to be read, they're for the armchair cook. But recently we've made an effort to become more international, partly because international cuisine is so interesting, and also because French restaurant cuisine is not healthful, and today Americans are very concerned with health."

And with fat. Fat. Fat.

Despite *Gourmet*'s recent interest in moderating its readers' load, you could gain weight just by gazing at, say, the Toffee Ice-Cream Cake in the March 1979 issue. "Combine two sticks of butter and two cups of sugar," the recipe begins, and that's before you get to the chocolate or the ice cream.

"Our menu section is probably a little extravagant," Zanne Zakroff says, "but we don't expect our readers to dine from those menus every night of the month until the next issue. They are special occasion menus, to fill special needs."

Home cooks who come to grief with a *Gourmet* recipe, and who phone or write to complain, find the magazine deals courteously with their problems. "We'll always talk them through a recipe," Miss Zakroff says.

The staff, like the magazine's founder, puts a value on manners, and you won't find the receptionist chewing gum or filing her fingernails. As for the two associate editors, Marjorie Webb and Nancy Purdum, who track down the props—the silver, the tablecloths, the china—for the spectacular color photographs, they are both blessed with a highly developed sense of aesthetics.

Zanne Zakroff offers an example of the two women's skill. "We were shooting a menu that was very casual. August. Verandah luncheons. We wanted to capture a lot of what we associate with the word 'verandah,' a kind of grandmother's house feeling. We used white wicker, and Marjorie and Nancy were able to get some beautiful old Vaseline glass for the platters."

Those platters, heaped with chicken salad, and surrounded by homemade strawberry-ice-cream sodas, were pretty enough to stir up nostalgia even in people with grandmothers like the old lady who ran the Barkis gang.

Luis Lemus, Mexican-born and in his sixties, shoots all the magazine's photographs that aren't done abroad, and is himself a bona fide eccentric. Nobody is permitted into his studio—a cluttered, smallish room, hung with a rubber chicken (Lemus loves practical jokes) and featuring piles of discarded forks, mugs, pieces of fabric—while he is shooting. His camera is venerable (decrepit might be a better word) and he doesn't own a light meter, but uses a metronome.

"With the metronome beating, he's able to gauge how much time he's going to take on a certain shot," Zanne Zakroff says, admitting she has no idea what she's talking about. But Lemus's pictures are splendid, so nobody is going to fuss about the way he gets them.

"He won't even show us his lighting," Miss Zakroff says. "He says that's his business. We're allowed to look through the camera at the setup before he starts, but if we fuss too much with the food, he gets disgusted, and cries, 'Oh, you girls—'"

Unlike the cooks who have to prepare food for television commercials, roasting half a dozen turkeys in order to get one perfect golden bird, *Gourmet*'s cooks (Miss Zakroff and three assistants) don't protect themselves against emergencies. If a soufflé is to be shot, a soufflé is baked, and it sits there until Lemus shoots it. Should it collapse while he's shooting, another soufflé is baked and the picture is reshot. "We don't play with the food either," says Miss Zakroff. "There's no shellac on the string beans to make them shine. Only thing is, if Marjorie and Nancy bring back a soup tureen the size of a bathtub, and I've made a small amount of soup, we put tin cans, or marbles, in the bottom of the bowl, just to fill up the space so the soup will float on the surface."

The *Gourmet* staff gets to eat the results of the cooks' efforts, and there is plenty of good stuff around, because even the recipes printed in the letters column (entitled Sugar and Spice) have to be tested. If a garlic mayonnaise is whipped up, it isn't thrown out. "We just cruise the office," says Miss Zakroff, "and find out if somebody is having cold poached bass, or would like to make some."

That most of the world outside her world—on the 28th floor of a big Third Avenue office building—may not be acquainted with cold poached bass doesn't seem to occur to Zanne Zakroff who's up there elevating our taste and doing it in the merriest way possible.

Nothing that is cooked goes begging. The managing editor "loves anything with a bone, and oysters and clams, so she gets those things. Other people love chocolate. Other people love Chinese food. Other people love garlic."

The *Gourmet* kitchens—there are two of them—are more than adequately furnished, but not with anything particularly flossy. The kitchens have tiled floors, plenty of copper pots, and plenty of ordinary pots, because *Gourmet*'s cooks believe they ought to face much the same problems as the home cook faces. "We have some pretty ratty equipment," Miss Zakroff says. "To replace a pan nowadays can cost $45, so you keep the crummy pot, even though you know it's always going to scorch on that one side."

Miss Zakroff contends that at least 25 percent of the recipes that go into the magazine are developed right on the spot. "All of us cooks work together, and then anyone else who happens to be meandering through the kitchen can say, 'Oh, my aunt used to do something like that, only I think she put tomato in it,' and if that sounds okay to us, we try tomato."

The only dissatisfaction Miss Zakroff expresses is that she has to use electric stoves. "Some building ordinance prohibits our having a live flame."

A born cook, Zanne Zakroff put her first dinner on the table when she was seven years old. "I made meat loaf, which was fun, because I mixed it with my fingers. When I was ten, I gave a surprise anniversary party for my parents, and invited their friends. I did a macaroni salad, and a green salad, and shish kebabs, because I didn't know how to cook anything fancy, but I thought that the grown-ups could barbecue the meat. My parents and their friends were flabbergasted."

Miss Zakroff, who grew up in the suburbs of Chicago, on the North Shore, came to New York with a burning ambition to work at *Gourmet,* and was told by Maurice Moore-Betty, a food writer and operator of a cooking school, that she didn't have a prayer. "There's no turnover," he said. "People don't quit, they die. Frank E. Campbell just comes and picks them up."

Nevertheless, Maurice Moore-Betty made a telephone call on her behalf, and next thing Miss Zakroff knew, she was at *Gourmet* typing invoices. "I would have washed dishes, swept floors, anything," she says.

As she moved up the ladder to associate editor, Miss Zakroff discovered that she "didn't want to do any more editorial work. I didn't care anymore whether "drawbridge" was one word, two words, or hyphenated. I didn't want to look it up ever again. What I loved was cooking, so I left, and went to Paris, to a cooking school called La Varenne. The magazine was nice, and offered me a leave of absence, but I quit, to be fair to everyone. 'Look,' I said, 'a Rothschild might ask me to run away with him over there, anything could happen.'"

What happened was that *Gourmet* asked Miss Zakroff to return, not to the typewriter but to the kitchen. Which she did.

When the food editor left, she became food editor. It frightened her. "I went to my boss [executive editor Jane Montant] and said, 'If I can't do it, please don't be kind to me and keep me on, because it would not be a kindness, it would be a cruelty.'"

So far, so good.

Miss Zakroff plans menus, tries to balance them, tries to figure out whether or not they're practical—are the people in Iowa going to be able to replicate the dishes?—and all this while working out of season, because the magazine has a four-month lead time.

She listens to her assistants or to anyone else who has an idea—"I take it under advisement, and if it sounds like it makes sense, we do it"—but on the day when one of her menus is to be photographed, she herself goes shopping. "I tell the butcher, 'I want that chicken breast and that chicken breast and that chicken breast.' I pick everything, down to the parsley, because there's so much at stake."

Occasionally, the editorial staff gives Miss Zakroff a hard time. Like with the tuna fish. "There's a section of the magazine called Gastronomie sans Argent," she says. "It's about how to eat well but not expensively. And we're very careful, because we used to get complaints. 'Gastronomie sans Argent, my elbow! You had *crème fraîche* in there, and that's not cheap if you have to buy it!' So one month I proposed tuna fish. The French and the Italians use tuna fish like crazy. But some of the editorial staff resisted. 'Oh,' they said, 'tuna is *so* women's magazine.'

"'You don't eat tuna fish?' I asked one of the editors.

"'Yes,' she said, '*I* do, but—'

"'Well,' I said, 'you work at *Gourmet* magazine, and you live in a nice home—'

"'That isn't what I mean,' she said. 'You know what I mean.'

"'Listen,' I said, 'we're not going to have Tuna Noodle Bake with Potato Chips on Top. I'm not a subversive person, I've been here for eight years, I'm reasonably aware of what the magazine stands for—'"

Miss Zakroff won. *Gourmet* offered a tuna fish sauce for pasta, a tuna fish spread—"We called it a pâté, but it was really a spread"—and a *Salade Niçoise*, not because it was so unusual, but because it would make a nice picture—"and tuna fish is not really very photogenic."

One time, the Gastronomie sans Argent section was devoted to old bread, the end of the loaf, the crumbs you're left holding after a dinner party and, says Zanne Zakroff, "Kemp Miles [an associate editor] came up with this wonderful ice cream that was made from leftover Boston brown bread. In addition to the normal components of cream and milk and egg yolk. The brown bread gave it its flavoring; it was just terrific."

Chacun à son goo.

Anyway, Zanne Zakroff's in her kitchen, all's right with *Gourmet*, and Mr. Mac's attempt to initiate "a healthy curiosity in those who have heretofore thought of eating as merely the satisfying of hunger" is heading into its fifth decade.

If *Gourmet* addressed itself to the upper crust (and I'm not talking about Boston brown bread), *Holiday*, begun some years later (and now defunct) was a manual for up-scale living that encouraged the more rank and vile of us to spread our wings.

A lot of the original staff of *Holiday* had worked during World War II in the Office of War Information, and on *Yank*, the Army weekly. Harry Sions, the articles editor, was a *Yank* alumnus, while Frank Zachary, the art director, and Lou Mercier, the picture editor, came from OWI. Bill Wright, one of Harry Sions's protégés, recalls the *Holiday* enterprise as having involved some bravado. "There they were, this fraternity of ex-GIs, none of whom had ever been on a pleasure trip to Europe—they'd only traveled as enlisted men—telling the public where to go and what to do when it got there."

Fortunately, says Wright, Slim Aarons, the photographer, could be trusted to piece out the holes in his confreres' knowledge. "He had some money, he was a kind of gadfly, he knew what was going on everywhere. If he found a new ski resort in Switzerland, he'd come back, sit on the corner of somebody's desk, tell us about it, and we'd feature it in the magazine."

Frank Zachary, now editor of *Town & Country*, gives some of the credit for the epicurean boom to the World's Fair of 1939, where he worked as a publicity man. "Before the war, there was only one great French restaurant in New York. That was Chambord. There were a few good Italian restaurants like Tony's, which grew out of a speakeasy. But the World's Fair had Henri Soulé at the French Pavilion, and it had the Polish Pavilion, the Czech Pavilion, the Italian Pavilion, the Brussels. And once the war started, all those chefs were stranded here, and they opened restaurants."

"And after the war," adds Lou Mercier, "when *Holiday* got into the business of sending people around to different places, and worrying about where the hell those people would eat, and it was discovered that Lock-Ober in Boston, for instance, had been great in the old days, and was still great in the new days, we did something about it."

One of the things they did was to start giving awards to Best Restaurants. "*Holiday* pioneered the idea of the Best Restaurant list," says Frank Zachary. "People would call up from towns all over the country and say, 'Listen, there's a great restaurant here,' and we'd check it out, we'd send Silas Spitzer to sample the place. I don't think there was another restaurant critic in a magazine at that time."

"I don't even think there was a restaurant critic in a newspaper at that time," says Mercier.

Silas Spitzer, *Holiday*'s main eater, was a fat man. "He loved his food," says Zachary, and Mercier shakes his head in agreement. "There's no way that the pursuit of good food is going to make you thin."

On the other hand, Ted Patrick, onetime editor-in-chief of *Holiday*, and the spirit behind the magazine's involvement with cuisine, happened to be built very sparely. "Patrick once opened a restaurant called

Hapsburg House with Ludwig Bemelmans, who'd been a waiter, an innkeeper and was a superb writer and artist," Zachary recounts. "This goes back to the 30s. They were both always interested in food. To the extent that they opened a goddamn restaurant!"

Bemelmans later became one of *Holiday*'s featured writers on food, as did Joseph Wechsberg, but Zachary calls Lucius Beebe "the greatest of them all. We'd give him five thousand dollars, see if he could spend it in a week eating and drinking in London. With the traveling, the hotel, the clothes, he spent it easily. Lucius was a gourmet, and a professional newspaperman. He met his deadlines, gave you fine pieces. He approached the work from the point of view of a dandy, that was his act, but he did it in a good-humored way that was fun.

"Nowadays, the trouble with these cats, these food experts, is that they don't have any fun. They're so goddamn serious it's a bore. Wine-ophiles are so silly. And describing a dish as 'brilliant'! Come on—"

Frank Zachary believes today's restaurants don't measure up to the great restaurants of twenty years ago. He mentions Soulé, Roger Chauveron. "The restaurateurs were great cooks, for chrissake. And there aren't any more like them. Grenouille? Le Cirque? There isn't a restaurant I can think of that compares in quality to Chauveron."

Zachary and Mercier echo Jim Beard's notion that the new interest in food coincided with our postwar prosperity. "The minute the lid was off, everybody flew in all directions," says Mercier. "Everything exploded, food, travel, and in a general sense it was *Holiday*'s function to tell about it."

"Up until then, there were damn few good restaurants in America," Zachary says. "San Francisco had a couple, New Orleans had Antoine's, Galatoire's, Arnaud's, there was maybe a good steak house in Kansas City. But American boys who'd gone abroad had discovered there was a big wide world out there, and that big wide world contained a lot of good food."

It's possible to view the whole gourmet phenomenon of the past thirty-five years as a function of class-jumping. We were going to get away from roast chicken on Sunday afternoon, and plain meat and potatoes every other night. We were going to experiment, we were going to be Continental, we were going to eat—ugh—snails.

The rich had always known about pheasants dressed in their tail feathers; now it was the turn of the middle class. After the war, not only military personnel but American civilians began traveling fervently. Soon three and a half million of them were going to Europe every year, while 350,000 more ventured to the Pacific and the Orient.

They came home, as the soldiers had, with a new appreciation for foreign flavors and began what *Time* referred to as "the great American love affair with the kitchen."

One of the first chefs to seize the day was the late Dione Lucas who, like Earle MacAusland, had somewhat anticipated the fever for puff pastry and, in 1941, opened a Manhattan branch of the Cordon Bleu Cooking School. (The mother école in Paris had been founded in the 1800s to help orphans learn to cook and "make their way in life.")

By 1947, Dione had her own television show, and she was a wonder. Not just for the way she cooked, but for the way she talked. She called a chicken a "chicking." "Take the chicking," she would begin, and viewers would roll around on the floor, helpless with mirth and adoration.

But it wasn't until Julia Child heaved onto the small screen in 1962 that the wit hit the pan, and the fit really hit the fans.

PUTTING IT ON:
We're fat because we fell in love with Julia and the high-priced spread.

3 *Julia...*

A feast of fat things . . .
—ISAIAH

"LOOK, Finnegan," says an indignant mustached gentleman (one of two couples in a *New Yorker* cartoon by William Hamilton) as he leans over his brandy and into the face of the cigar smoker across the table. "The great meals you've had are no greater than the great meals we've had."

Great meals was the name of her game, and Julia Child brought the American public a message: It's easy to cook fantastic French food.

Julia wasn't intimidating, Julia was earthy, Julia was friendly. Millions came to know French food through Julia. She demonstrated complicated dishes that anyone—not just rich folks with servants—could put together, and her followers sniffed the air after having wrought Julia's *coq au vin,* unable to believe the magic they had accomplished with their unpracticed American fingers.

Nobody was more surprised by her raging success than Julia herself.

"Surprised and pleased, I may say. I think people were just

interested in cooking, and I happened to be the right woman at the right time."

The fever to stew, poach, blanch, coddle was in the air, and Julia was the catalyst, Julia brought it home. In 1977, looking back, *Time* magazine said: "Julia Child's 1961 book, *Mastering the Art of French Cooking*, and her superbly low-key, artfully maladroit TV demonstrations were immensely influential in persuading her fellow citizens that serious cuisine is not some kind of Gallic voodoo but rather the art of the eminently possible."

Maladroit like a fox.

As a girl, Julia McWilliams of Pasadena, California, would rather have been a basketball player than a chef. (She, her sister, and her brother were all six-footers, which induced her mother to tell one interviewer, "I have produced eighteen feet of children.") Julia was a total dud in the kitchen, but it didn't matter—the McWilliamses had a cook.

At Smith College (class of '34), Julia dreamed of being an important novelist, and afterward, she spent a few years in New York working for W & J Sloane in the advertising deparment, and a few more years back home in Pasadena doing "virtually nothing," and enjoying it hugely. When World War II came, she joined the Office of Strategic Services, volunteered for duty in the Far East, and, in Ceylon, met Paul Child, himself an OSS official, and ten years her senior. Although he considered himself a devout bachelor, Paul found that his single days were numbered. Julia, he explained to the *New Yorker*'s Calvin Tomkins, "seemed like a pretty great woman to me."

In 1946, at the age of forty-four, Paul Child married Julia McWilliams. In 1948, on a job for the United States Information Service, he was assigned to Paris.

Julia, whose girlhood diet of choice had been jelly doughnuts, and who'd been known to set the stove on fire (she once roasted a duck without first putting it in a pan), now decided to go to the Cordon Bleu and learn the secrets of three great chefs—Max Bugnard, Claude Thillmont, Pierre Mangelatte—who were teaching there. Bugnard, by then in his seventies, had worked as a young man under Escoffier, and Julia "adored" him. In the first flush of enthusiasm, she nearly killed herself and Paul by rushing home to whip up richly sauced lunches. "We both got terribly bilious," she said later.

But she had found her métier, and her future.

Along with two Frenchwomen named Simone Beck and Louisette Bertholle, she opened a cooking school (they called it the Ecole des Trois Gourmandes) in the kitchen of the Childs's Left Bank apartment.

"We would cook all morning, then sit down and eat it, with Paul at the head of the table to pour the wine," Julia told Calvin Tomkins.

The same three ladies were responsible for *Mastering the Art of French Cooking*. The Frenchwomen had been working on it before they met Julia, but welcomed her as a collaborator and interpreter because the book was being written for the American market.

It took ten years from inception to publication. Their first American publisher, Houghton Mifflin, paid the women a $250 advance, then rejected the manuscript when it was turned in. In defense of Houghton Mifflin, Julia says the 800 pages consisted entirely of recipes for poultry and sauces.

So it was back to the chopping board. Cut, test, add, rewrite, change. In 1961, Alfred Knopf finally brought out Volume One, partly because two Knopf editors, William Koshland and Judith Jones, had recognized the revolutionary properties of the copy. "It was like having a teacher right there beside you in the kitchen, and everything really worked," said Mrs. Jones.

Exactly what the collaborators had intended. "We felt the book should break down into something intellectually reasonable, so you could see the connection between things," Julia said. "The idea was to take French cooking out of cuckoo land and bring it down to where everybody is. You can't turn a sow's ear into Veal Orloff, but you can do something very good with a sow's ear."

By the time Volume One of *Mastering the Art of French Cooking* came out, Paul Child had resigned from the Foreign Service, and he and Julia had moved back to America and were living in a house (once owned by philosopher Josiah Royce) in Cambridge, Massachusetts. There Paul designed a kitchen for his wife, a kitchen complete with restaurant stove and hooks on the walls for seemingly numberless pots and pans. Julia was planning to give cooking lessons while Paul (an accomplished artist, engraver, and photographer) was going to spend his time painting and taking pictures.

Julia went on an interview program at Boston's educational TV station, WGBH, to help push her cookbook, took along a bowl and wire whisk to demonstrate the French way of beating egg whites, and so charmed the viewers that twenty-seven of them wrote in.

For WGBH, that was a horde.

The station asked Julia to do a cooking show, and the rest is writ in heavy cream. Julia became "The French Chef," and our Prima Boilerina Assoluta. You couldn't go to anyone's house for dinner without having somebody ask the hostess, "Are these Julia's *Pears Hélène?*"

Noncommercial stations all over the country picked up the WGBH shows and Julia reached people who'd never before cooked with wine, and who thought *turbot* was some kind of airplane.

In 1979, seventeen years after the first *French Chef* segment had been shot in the basement of the Boston Gas Company, Julia was still at it, concocting a brand-new batch of shows. She had better quarters now, more staff, she was photographed in living color, but she was the same Julia, holding up a great big ugly monkfish by its tail, remarking to her audience on the wonders of the fish's "skin that moves around" and "its marvelous teeth."

The 1979 series was particularly tough because Julia was not only doing complete menus, appetizer through dessert, in half an hour, but when she wasn't at the studio rehearsing or taping, she was working at home, readying the new recipe book that would feature all the dishes prepared on the air.

"It's a lot of work," she acknowledged at 8:30 one Monday morning, before rushing out to shop for her ingredients of the day. Among the things on her mind at that early hour was a *savarin* to be featured on next week's show. "It's a yeast dough rich with eggs and butter. You know what a *baba* is? A *savarin* is just a great big *baba*. Baked in a ring mold and soaked in a rum syrup." Her voice dropped. "Very nice," she growled happily.

But Julia, we have to get to the hard part. The fat part. For almost twenty years, you've kept us eating not wisely but too well. I mean, Julia, you're still talking "rich with eggs and butter." Do you feel responsible for some of our pussle-gutted (that's right, pussle-gutted, I got it right out of the thesaurus) shapes?

"Phooey," trumpets Julia, who takes care of her own calorie counting, and expects the rest of us to do the same. "I have to diet practically all the time, or I'd be Mrs. Six-by-Six."

Moderation is the ticket to a reasonable life, Julia declares. "If I'm dieting, I try to keep down to 1200 calories. I find the best way to do that is to eat very little breakfast, just some fruit, practically no lunch, and then have a normal dinner. And rarely a dessert."

Or at least very little dessert. Because, adds Julia wistfully, "I would rather have one spoonful of Chocolate Malakoff than two bowls of Jell-O. Wouldn't you? You have to think that food is your life, and the sensible diet is a varied diet. Use moderation, exercise, watch your weight, and pick your grandparents. Mine on my father's side lived to be about ninety-five. I'm lucky."

Over the years, the recipes Julia has presented in her books and television shows have somewhat diminished in opulence, as the public fear of fats and sugar has increased, but Mrs. Child is never going to be a Calvinist. "If you're careful with your diet and your weight, you can certainly permit yourself an orgy now and then. What's life about if you can't have fun?" she demands.

Denying the accuracy of a magazine piece that described her arriving to test-bake brioche bearing "six kinds of margarine" ("I have never mentioned the name of that other spread publicly, and I never shall"). Julia blames many of today's food phobias on what she calls "nuttery."

"I mean, there's just a lot of nuttery going on without any scientific basis. I'm not a nutritionist, but I know you have to have some cholesterol. If you don't have it naturally in your blood serum, your body will leach it out of your liver, or anything else that's available.

"As for natural and organic, they don't mean anything. Chemicals are natural. People go on about natural and organic food, and they haven't any idea what they're talking about. All they really mean is, 'I don't want to be poisoned by insect spray.'

"I think it's been useful to make us aware that you have to be careful what kind of insecticides you use, but when you consider that we have 220 million people to feed in this country, I think it's just remarkable how well we do it."

Because everybody wants a good story, says Julia, the press is inclined to go off half-cocked. (Half-cooked? Half-baked?) She recalls the case of a woman who'd been taking mercury pills and eating half a pound of swordfish twice a day, and attributed her mercury poisoning to the swordfish. "That was a big scare."

As for the current sugar scare, "That's another thing I think people go off the deep end about. If you follow that dictum of moderation in all things, you won't eat too much sugar. If you're going to eat a lot of processed food, you're probably in trouble, but if you eat fresh food, you should be all right. You constantly hear you're being poisoned with one thing or another, but what the hell, if you listened to all that, you wouldn't eat anything."

These days, talk of "gourmet" food may also raise Julia's ire. "I think the word 'gourmet' has become so bastardized that it doesn't mean anything at all. I just use the term good cooking. You have good cooking, and you have elaborate cooking. Elaborate cooking can be good too. I think some people, when they're really feeling their oats, decide they'd like to be really elaborate, so why not? If it's good, and it's fun? I think as a hobby it's a great deal of fun to try out some elaborate things."

Julia sees hope for the future of epicurism in the number of students who are presently willing to work hard at becoming good chefs. In 1974, she'd mourned that fewer and fewer young people—even in France—were willing to spend the hours required to turn them into first-rate cooks, but all this "has changed a lot in the last few years. Like the two young women who worked with me [on the television show *Julia Child and More Company*]. One of them is the mother of two children, and in the summertime she goes over to Nantucket and is chef in a restaurant there. And the other, who went to the Culinary Institute in Hyde Park, is now chef at a restaurant here in Boston. Both of them work just like Trojans."

(Julia needed help with her TV cooking because she herself could do only two or three dishes in half an hour, and since every dish on the menu had to be shown in its finished state, there was a good deal of backstage preparation.)

In 1980, Julia announced that she was finished with twelve-hour workdays, and would take a rest. *Julia Child and More Company* would be her last TV series. "I'm sixty-six years old," she said. "I want to spend more time with Paul."

This didn't mean television audiences needed to go Child-less; commercial broadcasting finally seduced Julia. These days, she contributes cooking tips to ABC's *Good Morning, America*.

At home, Julia and Paul Child say they have no favorite foods. "We don't care, as long as it's good and fresh," Julia says. "I think when you run into people who say everything is awful, they just don't know how to shop properly. If you have your mind set on getting fresh beets, say, and beets aren't in season, you're not going to get any fresh beets. You have to find out what is in season, and you have to know where to shop. I do most of my shopping in supermarkets because I don't want to do specialized foods that people can't find. One supermarket's good for meat, another one's better for vegetables. If you take your food seriously, you find out where the good places are, and you take the time to go to them."

The Childs own a little house in France, and Julia notes that French cooks "are getting more like us, more adventurous. They're breaking out of the old straitjacket. I think it's high time, because they worked in a very rigid tradition; everything had to be classically done."

As for the American fascination with, not to mention confusion about, recent French contributions to gastronomy, Julia clears everything up with a few words. "*Minceur* is just diet cooking. *Nouvelle cuisine* just means 1970 French cooking."

Having learned all she knew about the French from *Vogue* and *Harper's Bazaar*, Julia remembers her astonishment when she and Paul first arrived in Le Havre, in 1948. "I expected everybody to be little tiny petite creatures. I was delighted to see great big hearty ones."

But isn't there such a thing as too big? Too hearty? Isn't the ordinary middle American killing himself through his mouth?

"I don't know if you can make any kind of generalization," Julia says. "I think it depends on how people were brought up, how their families taught them to eat."

Or how Julia Child taught them to eat, if it comes to that.

We followed where Julia led. We laughed at her jokes, we applauded when she patted back into shape some not quite perfect pudding. Her courage gave us courage. Julia refused to get rattled when the butter was frozen, or the knife wouldn't slice the pig. "Never apologize," she advised us, and we took her to our hearts; she was our heroine.

She was also our first national food celebrity.

After her, the deluge.

PUTTING IT ON:
We're fat because we swallow food authorities whole.

4 The Experts: Mimi and Craig and John and Karen and Gael and Bud...

Jeshurun waxed fat, and kicked . . .
—DEUTERONOMY

JULIA and her heirs. Amateur and professional, inspired she them. In the spring of 1979, Lauren Kaye, the twenty-four-year-old chef to New York City's Mayor Koch, faced with the necessity of whipping up a banquet "for 120 people, plus a dog," could find tranquillity only in thoughts of Julia Child. Because Julia "lets you know that if you make a mistake, you can cover it with parsley or whipped cream."

What Julia had been to Lauren Kaye, in the way of encouragement, James Beard had been to Julia Child. "I'll never forget how kind he was to Simca [Simone Beck] and Paul and me when our first book was published," Julia told Evan Jones. "We were nobodies from nowhere, yet he took us right in hand, introduced us everywhere, and really gave us our start in the New York food world."

Beard, now seventy-six, a giant of a man who fancies showy clothes—one observer testifies to having seen him standing outside his brownstone in a powder-blue Ultrasuede suit—and food and people and writing and lecturing and traveling, is probably the most beloved member of the food establishment.

He grew up in Portland, Oregon, and went to London when he was nineteen with the idea of studying opera. His mother had given him advice: "A sandwich at the Ritz is worth three meals in any other restaurant, no matter how poor you may be or how hungry!"

Beard's interests in drama and food converged in 1946 when, having come to New York to be an actor, he was hired to head up a TV cooking show called *I Love To Eat*. By 1955, he had established his own cooking school (to attend which there is now a two-year waiting list). Classes are conducted in Beard's kitchen, and a less pedantic teacher is hard to imagine. Students are taught to use their hands. "I can't stand prissy people who think there's something dirty about sticking fingers in food," Beard has said.

Still, it wasn't Jim Beard, despite the two-season run of *I Love To Eat*, who decisively cracked the television barrier—it was Julia, whom everyone in the country referred to by her first name. Until Julia made cooking look like fun, vast segments of America hadn't been paying much attention, but by 1973, Horace Sutton was able to write in *Saturday Review/World* of the new fascination with gastronomy as having created "a food fraternity" that not only served the public and "pandered to its needs, but also coached it, tutored it, and led it on explorations into gastronomic lands that only the experts and a small circle of native practicing gourmets had hitherto charted. The food fraternity has become a vast craft that includes wine and food editors (every newspaper has to have one), restaurant critics, food ferrets (who uncover hard-to-find comestibles in hard-to-find markets), underground gourmets (who uncover little-known, inexpensive restaurants), cookbook assemblers . . . newsletter writers, syndicated columnists, food and restaurant consultants, cutesy-pie radio commentators and TV personalities . . ."

Most of these colleagues, competitors, fellow travelers of Julia's had been lavish with praise for Beck, Bertholle, and Child when Volume One of *Mastering the Art of French Cooking* appeared, and this was news in itself because, kindly Jim Beard aside, the New York food establishment, as Calvin Tomkins observed, was "not known for its generosity of spirit."

You can say that again, and not limit your food establishment to New York, either.

Take the case of Robert Courtine, a famous French food authority and writer for *Le Monde*. Asked to appraise a Time-Life volume called *La Cuisine des Provinces de France*, Courtine read the manuscript and, according to Horace Sutton, "added his comments, frequently acerbic, in the margins. Somehow the marginal commentary was set in type and appeared in the first printing. The book is now a collector's item."

John Hess, a journalist who has written widely on food, wryly refers to the 1969 Time-Life-Courtine collaboration (unintended though it was) as "the first self-roasting cook book."

That compendium of French provincial recipes, masterminded by the late Michael Field, was also savaged in print by Craig Claiborne, who called Field "a former piano player," and said that he, Craig, had compiled "a stack of notes thicker than the book itself on the errors in it."

(Michael Field was never a Claiborne favorite. In 1965, when Field was running an East Hampton restaurant, Claiborne came, ate, and gave the place a one-star rating.)

After the Claiborne attack on his Time-Life efforts, Field wrote an article for *McCall's* entitled "New York's Ten Most Overrated Restaurants." They were almost all restaurants Claiborne favored.

Nora Ephron, in those days identified by *New York* magazine as someone "who has written for the *New York Post*," did a piece on the food establishment's involvement with Time-Life cookbooks—half a million subscribers had signed up for all eighteen volumes, so there would be work enough for everybody—and the food establishment's involvement with itself.

The food establishment, Michael Field told Miss Ephron, was "mindless, inarticulate, and not very cultivated."

The food establishment, Nika Hazelton told Miss Ephron, was "a world of self-generating hysteria."

Ephron quoted Claiborne on Beef Wellington ("I hate the stuff"), she quoted Mimi Sheraton on Craig Claiborne ("He is his own man and there is no way to be a friend of his"), and she quoted James Beard on the terrors of a recent party with other food people ("You could hardly move around for fear someone would bite you in the back"). *Plus ça change, plus c'est la même chose*.

Ephron herself offered a lighthearted theory for the rise of the food establishment. Never mind the traveling fighting men of World War II, the postwar travel boom, and the shortage of domestic help that drove housewives into the kitchen, she said. The real rise of the food establishment began with curry.

"In the beginning," she wrote, "just about the time the Food Establishment began to earn money and fight with each other and review each other's cookbooks and say nasty things about each other's recipes and feel rotten about each other's good fortune, just about that time, came curry. Some think it was beef stroganoff, but in fact, beef stroganoff had nothing to do with it . . . The year of the curry is an elusive one to pinpoint, but this much is clear: it was before the year of *quiche lorraine*, the year of *paella*, the year of *vitello tonnato*, the year of *boeuf bourguignon*, the year of *blanquette de veau*, and the year of beef Wellington. It was before Michael stopped playing the piano, before Julia opened L'Ecole des Trois Gourmandes, and before Craig had left his job as a bartender in Nyack, New York. It was the beginning, and in the beginning, there was James Beard and there was curry and that was about all."

Now there's more.

In the old days, theater critics had the authority to say which plays lived and which died. Today, restaurant critics have the authority to say which restaurants succeed and which fail. "Restaurant reviewing," wrote Lawrence Van Gelder in the *New York Times*, "next to the destruction of subway car doors, is New York's principal industry." Once food became entertainment, food writers became stars. Mimi Sheraton is read in the *Times* the way movie critic Pauline Kael is read in the *New Yorker*.

Curtiss Anderson, writer, editor, and high liver, offers two examples of the Sheraton clout:

"On 58th Street, between Second and Third Avenues, there was a sweet little French restaurant called Rive Gauche. It was owned by a Mom and Pop couple, and Mimi reviewed it and gave it two stars. After that, it was full at both lunch and dinner. About a month later, Mimi went back, the restaurant had changed chefs, and she knocked off a star. Next day, it was a sea of white tablecloths. The French couple sold out.

"You can see the opposite of that with a restaurant in the same block called Tre Scalini. Mimi's review of Tre Scalini came out on a Friday. Three stars. At about ten-thirty that morning, I called to make a reservation, and I said to the owner, 'You're going to have a terrible time today,' and he said, 'Why do you say that?' I said, 'Didn't you read the review?' He said yes, but he didn't think it was all that important. Normally the place would have been 30, 40 percent filled for lunch, but when I arrived at 12:30 that day, there was a line out in front of the door.

"I think Mimi is very honest and straightforward, and one of the better writers among the food people, and I think she would agree that it isn't her intention to ruin a place or make a place, but that's the power of her column."

When food reviewers began to get hot, they found themselves not only competing with theater and movie reviewers for attention, but also edging out fashion writers as a source of amusement.

"Having developed its own personalities and its own audience," wrote Horace Sutton, "the food fraternity has stolen some of the glitter that once surrounded that other inbred and sharpnail breed, the arbiters of haute couture. The members of the food fraternity watch each other with eagle-eyed acuity, talons at the ready."

Sutton quoted Craig Claiborne (who started assessing restaurants for the *New York Times* in 1957, quit some years later, then returned) on his onetime opposite number, Clementine Paddleford, of the *Herald Tribune*. "Clem knew not one thing about food. She would sample a dish and ask the chef what was in it. If you pander to the chef, you can't be objective in what you say."

(Paddleford good-naturedly agreed. She said if Claiborne was the *foie gras* of food writing, she was the liverwurst.)

Leaping to Paddleford's defense, John Hess and his wife Karen declared that at least Clem's recipe for New England clam chowder was authentic, which Claiborne's was not. "Imagine not using salt pork!"

The Hesses (authors of *The Taste of America)* talk freely and acidly about food experts in America, referring to "the gourmet plague."

Here, from their book, a few of the accusations they level at the most famous of our native food stars.

Craig Claiborne:

He uses too much flour, turning otherwise palatable mixtures into "library paste."

He finds canned bouillon acceptable as soup stock.

He says milk and cream freeze well, but "they do not. Frozen cream 'kernels' on thawing, and milk acquires a flat taste."

He can't make a *beurre blanc*, despite his pride in "knowing all the sauces."

He promotes brand names, i.e., Fluffo, Pepperidge Farm, Medaglia d'Oro, and General Foods Rock Cornish game hens ("Flabby midgets with no more taste of game than a wad of cotton," say the Hesses).

James Beard:

He suggests topping a pie with "gelatinized whipped cream."

He puts sugar in his bread recipes.

He's taken fees from Pillsbury, Nestlé-Stouffers, Planters.

He believes Fannie Farmer to have been a gastronomic deity, when in fact "the lady was a very poor cook."

Julia Child:

She pines for American chicken breasts, even when she is in Grasse, France.

She calls herself The French Chef, "although she is neither French nor chef."

She sweetens her brioche crust.

She adds flour to lentils, although "they are quite farinaceous enough."

She serves French bread with lasagna.

There's a lot more, and you don't have to read between the lines to get the idea that the Hesses lay about them with tongues as sharp as Julia's cleavers.

John Hess also does commentaries for a news program shown on New York's public television station, Channel 13. In one of these, he talked about the American obsession with fat. Pondering the information that the state of Wisconsin had refused to let an overweight couple adopt a child, Hess called attention to the further fact that "stout young Christians" were being turned away from Oral Roberts University in Tulsa. "Cross my heart and hope to diet," Hess said.

In person, John and Karen Hess turn out to be charming, gentle people, but they have no antipathy whatever to going on record with their fierce opinions.

John Hess reads aloud from a yellowed French newspaper clipping (translating as he goes) giving a Frenchwoman's impression of ugly Americans. "Everywhere you see men and women . . . of an enormity you rarely see in Europe . . . arms like hams, triple chins and jowls, monstrous stomachs, prodigious thighs, and all covered with a fantastic layer of fat."

But Julia Child tells us the French get pretty big too. The Hesses disagree. "Julia doesn't see France, she doesn't see what's in front of her eyes," John Hess says. "Go to a French school and look at the children. Go to a French park and look at the people."

"They're tiny," contributes Karen Hess. "It's not to say you don't sometimes see an enormously fat person, but it's rare, it's something you remark on."

The Hesses spent nine years abroad, while he worked as a foreign correspondent for the *New York Times*. When they came home, he put in a year as the *Times* restaurant critic, which duty he enjoys more in retrospect than he did in the observance. "To have it behind me is interesting, but I ate so many bad meals. And Karen ate so many bad meals, and I didn't see why she should have to when she wasn't getting paid for it."

Karen Hess (*Newsweek* once called her the best American cook in Paris) says her husband's job reviewing restaurants was "a burden. But we both learned a lot. It was tremendously instructive."

Since their book came out in 1977, have the Hesses softened on the food establishment? Don't think it. They've got peeves they haven't even petted yet.

Gael Greene, *New York* magazine's resident trencherperson, earns low Hess marks. "Did you see that movie about people who eat themselves to death?" demands John Hess. "Greene went on a trip to France that sounded like that, she was eating these enormous meals twice a day, and all she talked about was shoveling food in her face, which is after all antigastronomic. And disgusting. A person who really likes food for its flavor doesn't want a meal with eight courses."

As for Craig Claiborne, Hess accuses him of going after "the snob vote. He actually wrote that an untrimmed sandwich was 'vulgar, crude and uncouth.' His pitch for the *nouveaux riches* of New York's East Side is revolting. I mean he did a piece in the *Times*—it dominated the section—about what to do with leftover caviar!"

Mrs. Hess laughs. "You put it into scrambled eggs. Fourteen ounces of it, if you have that much left over. At $200 a pound."

"Claiborne talks to these great chefs," says Mr. Hess, "and he asks them, 'If you had only one more meal to eat, what would you choose?' but he never understands it when they say, 'Oh, maybe a *cassoulet*, a bean dish, or *tête de veau*.' What they eat themselves they don't serve to their customers because the customers won't think those things are elegant enough. 'Nobody's going to travel 200 miles to my restaurant to eat a roast chicken or blood sausage or rabbit stew,' these cooks say.

But if you're lucky enough to eat with a chef's family and the help, you get these wonderful things."

John Hess faults the food establishment for the American accent on fanciness. "The chief disservice of the gourmet crowd is offering a hard-working woman a recipe which has got to take twelve hours to prepare. They see Julia on a half hour show, and they try to duplicate what they see, and then it comes out badly and they're disappointed when they eat it and they think they did something wrong. The gourmet crowd gives you a choice between twelve hours of preparation, or junk food. The whole thing is out of proportion. People could learn to be pleased with a stew, with a soup."

Karen Hess nods. "French home cooking is unknown in this country."

That approval can be bought and sold is much on the Hesses' minds. "In most of the country—not just New York, to be fair—food writers are puffs for industry," says Mr. Hess. "Recipes come from Madison Avenue, and are put right into the newspapers, printed as they're received, often to plug trade names."

Celebrity cookbooks are another of John Hess's grievances. "The overwhelming majority of cookbooks aren't worth feeding to your furnace. All scissors and paste jobs. Anybody can write one. Nobody in the publishing trade ever asks, 'Can this person cook?' It's just, 'Can they sell this book?'"

Are any food writers good influences on consumers?

"Mimi Sheraton was wonderful when she was writing as a consumer-shopper for *New York* magazine," says Karen Hess. "Her diatribes on Big Macs and Howard Johnson's, that was fabulous material."

(Sheraton once upbraided Jim Beard for his approval of McDonald's secret sauce. The sauce was "not to be thrown overboard," Beard had said, to which Sheraton retorted that the stuff should be thrown "if not overboard, then down the toilet." She also compared the texture of McDonald's hamburgers to that of "baloney sausage," said the shakes were "like aerated Kaopectate," and that McDonald's was guilty of "perverting the taste of children." The Hesses not only agreed, but added a postscript of their own. "The gourmets are guilty of perverting the taste of grown-ups.")

Karen Hess has kind words for Marcella Hazan *(The Classic Italian Cook Book)*, Diana Kennedy *(The Cuisines of Mexico)*, and Madeleine Kamman (a French lady who ran a cooking school in Massachusetts, until she returned to France this January) but says that most of the food writers she can tolerate are not Americans.

"Let me tell you about an interview we had with the food editor of one of this country's major newspapers. We met her in the restaurant of this very fancy hotel. And she was having two desserts, but she put saccharin in her coffee. She was gross."

So we're back down to it. Fat.

"I think that finally it's the lack of flavor in our food that makes us eat too much," says Karen Hess. "We are dissatisfied without knowing why. Flavor tells you you've had enough, it turns off a kind of appestat. Without flavor, you don't feel satisfied, you keep stuffing your face."

Where have all the flavors gone?

"With the good wheat germ in our flour, with Jersey milk and barnyard fowl and fresh farm produce and Grandma's cooking," says John Hess.

The problem begins with the children. "A properly raised kid would eat mashed vegetables and soft meats and bread soaked in milk and see sugar rarely," says John Hess, "but we start them on sugared baby food and then they're propped up in front of a TV set, and TV hammers away at them about junk food and candies, and at school, there's a vending machine in the corner.

"Nibbling is a habit, like smoking, and it grows with the child. Go to an office in midtown at eleven o'clock in the morning, and on every desk you see this junk. People come in carrying their coffee and cakes. Or the coffee wagon comes around just before lunch. Then they go out to lunch.

"All day long, they're eating on the sly. You go to someone's house and there are bowls of this and that on the coffee table. People are never satisfied. It isn't even that they enjoy the eating, it's just habit. So that's why they're fat. And being fat makes them neurotic.

"My theory is that this society, and the world, in fact, is somewhat bonkers. And one of the forms it takes is this super self-consciousness. People are fat, and they keep eating because eating is a function of being tense, and one of the things they're tense about is that they're overweight."

The Hesses say it's getting worse, too. "Cookbook writers dump wheat germ into something, and call it natural," says Karen Hess. "They add soy sauce or zucchini to bread, do horrible recipes and call them health food. And you find ridiculous 'diet' products like Lite beer and Lite whiskey."

For years, says Mr. Hess, "people managed all right as far as food was concerned, provided they weren't so poor as to be starving, or so rich and ignorant as to stuff themselves." Now, not only is there sugar and saccharin in everything, but poor quality oil inhabits our mayonnaise, and we gorge on fat-fried snacks and petroleum-based protein extenders. "You're eating," John Hess declares, "a lot of pre-chewed, digested, reconstituted foods that don't have any body to them, and of course you're not full. In a diet of greens, fruit, whole cereals, there's roughage which is good for you and also fills you up."

He pulls at his belt, displaying newly pierced holes to prove his point. "Karen has just finished editing the American edition of *Elizabeth David's Bread Book*. She baked more than four hundred pounds of bread, and we ate most of it, and I've lost fourteen pounds. None of my pants fit."

Gael Greene tends to agree with the Hesses that we eat too much sugar and salt, but she has a disagreement with the Hesses on another subject, namely herself. She does not, she says, eat two enormous meals a day, even in France. "Except in cases of serious emergency—feeling faint, trying to indulge a greedy companion, or a pressing deadline for *New York* magazine. Even on my most excessive gastronomical binge—it became a piece called 'Nobody Knows the Truffles I've Seen'—where we had three-star dinners every night, most of us just nibbled at lunch."

She thinks a bit, then confesses to a trip during which she did justice to both lunches and dinners. "Outside Lausanne, at the most exciting French restaurant in the world. I couldn't bear not to taste as many of Frédy Girardet's dishes as possible, so after lunch, we ran around a lot, jumping and leaping, trying to make room for dinner. But the point of Girardet's cooking is you don't feel stuffed, the portions are tiny, and at his place, it would be hard, even criminal, not to eat.

"When you have access to five or six three-star meals in one week, you pace yourself. I almost always lose weight in France, even though dinner is elaborate, with four or five courses and all kinds of enticements at the end, glacéed fruits, incredible pastries, cheeses that make you think, 'Oh, God, I'd better eat this now, I may never see it again.' So you taste and you taste, but the end result is you don't eat a single piece of junk food, you're not eating anything that isn't worth eating.

"I think when the food is glorious, you tend to eat much less of it."

This sounds suspiciously like Karen Hess's good-flavor-turning-off-our-appestats-by-satisfying-us-sooner theory, so the Hesses and Greene may have more in common than is apparent at first blush.

Speaking of blushing, Gael Greene has been accused of writing about food as though she were writing about sex, which accusation doesn't daunt her. "The passion for cooking and eating is part of the sensuality explosion America is experiencing. It's another expression of hedonism. What Tom Wolfe calls 'the Me Generation.' It has to do with the pursuit of pure pleasure. Perhaps we have finally overcome our puritanical restraint and can let ourselves enjoy more than a mean little lamb chop and a rice custard for dinner without feeling vulgar. When you get to be sensitive about food, and very discriminating, all your senses—eyes, ears, nose, taste buds—are working, and these are the same senses that are involved in making love. There is even a chemical, norepinephrine, that acts as a neural transmitter in both eating and sex.

"One outgrowth of the women's movement, which is certainly not frivolous, has been an investigation of why many women fail to respond sexually, and that discussion has led to men and women making greater efforts to get in touch with their senses. You expand your sensory awareness by smelling perfume, by burying your face in a flower, by licking whipped cream off the back of your hand, by swirling and sipping a great wine."

Gael Greene came to food writing as a reporter, not a home economist, and Clay Felker, *New York*'s master builder, boasted that she was his invention. "You never had a hot meal until I made you a critic!" he cried, and Greene thought the crack was so funny she spread it all over town.

Felker had phoned her about the critic's job a few months after he'd started the magazine, and she'd said no. "I couldn't possibly afford to write at the prices you're paying."

An indignant Felker fought back. "People are begging to be our restaurant critic without pay, if we'll just pick up the tab for their meals."

It made Greene reconsider. "I thought, 'How wonderful to order from the left side of the menu instead of the right.' I had just written a profile of Craig Claiborne for *Look*, and I adopted Craig's rules for reviewing restaurants. 'Always go three times, always pay your own way, be anonymous.' I learned on the job."

Gael Greene denies that food critics have contributed to the bulging of America. "Food writers don't make anybody fat. But I do think Julia Child's ability to convey a message that anyone can cook, that it's fun, that food is wonderful, and Jim Beard writing with the joy and imagination that inspired us all, and Craig Claiborne making ethnic food seem accessible and simple, has certainly helped people—especially men—become more interested in cooking. And the emergence of certain powerful restaurant critics or influential cookbook writers has played a crucial part in making food a fashionable obsession."

Greene can't exactly put a date to the instant when her own interest in food burgeoned into passion, though "the discovery of eggplant and the first taste of sweetbreads were seminal. Then, one innocent September, my husband and I were in France, and we went five hundred miles out of our way to eat at Pyramide. We lurched home giggling and blissed out on great food. That was the beginning. I took cooking lessons. I went to Dione Lucas. My friends and I were very competitive, cooking for each other and against each other. We were getting very serious about what we put into our mouths. And our cooking became better all the time. In recent years I've had a chance to cook with some of France's greatest chefs and everything is easier, clearer, less complicated. To criticize food, you must cook, or you lose touch."

Losing touch is bad, losing weight is good, right? (It is necessary always to reintroduce the subject of fat, keeping one's eye on, if not the sparrow, at least the marrow, of this book.) "I've always been voluptuous and I can eat well without gaining weight," says Greene, explaining that being five feet nine inches tall is a decided advantage to a woman who eats for a living. "But often, just before the bathing suit season, I'll take off ten or fifteen pounds."

She takes off ten or fifteen pounds the same way anybody else does: She stops eating. "Or I eat very little, mostly protein, for a week or ten days."

When she's working, Gael Greene rarely finishes what's put before her. "I have to taste at least a little bit of everybody's dish. I always go to a restaurant with at least one other person, and sometimes with two or three people. All those tastes add up quickly." Recently, Greene noticed that she had almost stopped drinking before dinner "unless the wine is really extraordinary. And I try to dance after dinner. I dance until I can't dance another step, and then dance for half an hour more. That provides an exhilaration and exertion similar to jogging.

"The last two trips to France, we danced after almost every meal. And there were times when that was agony. There was a dinner at Alain Chapel's restaurant near Lyons, a glorious exercise in excess. To get up after that and drive seventeen miles to Lyons to dance, you really had to be determined. But after about fifteen minutes of pain and despair on the dance floor, you suddenly start to feel very good."

Like Julia Child, Gael Greene comes out in favor of the occasional orgy. "I think most of us suspect cholesterol can be a problem, and surely everyone knows that obesity is dangerous, so people who care about what they put in their mouths indulge extravagantly when they're eating great food, and are careful at other times. I have friends who casually use a pound or two of butter to cook a great meal; then, for the next two or three days, they'll have fish and cottage cheese. A great fish, properly poached or broiled, is a beautiful thing, but too few people have ever eaten a great fish because most fish is overcooked."

Some food experts are fat, some are thin. "Craig Claiborne," reports Gael Greene, "eats very little. And if somebody puts too much on his plate, he's disturbed."

In Greene's mind, the American problem with obesity is really two problems. "One is imaginary. There are many women who diet constantly and talk endlessly about how fat they are, and they're not fat. The other problem is real. A lot of Americas *are* overweight. Partly because of the old theory that a fat baby was a healthy baby, we've created grown-ups with excessive fat cells. Fat babies become fat grown-ups. Even when they diet, they regain the weight too easily."

While Greene refuses credit for adding a single pound to a single citizen, she acknowledges that she does have the power to make us try a new beanery, or abandon an inept one.

"I worry about it. When I'm going to do a review that is critical, I see the faces of the people who are going to be devastated. Most of my critical reviews have been of restaurants that were dying, or truly outrageous, or of places that will live forever because they're not there for the great food. Thousands of tourists come to New York every year, tourists who care nothing about food, and they may always be charmed by Mamma Leone's.

"Or take '21.' '21' is virtually a club. A table downstairs means you're accepted. What they do to the food between the purveyor and the table is not terribly important. I've learned a lot about what goes on behind the scenes, so I understand the problems of the restaurateur, but I can't let that make me any less tough as a critic because if the customer is paying a hundred dollars for dinner, it must be absolutely glorious."

As she files through restaurant after restaurant on her ceaseless quest for "glorious" food, led by respectful maître d's, Greene knows she's lucky.

"When I was growing up, I used to go to double bills and see Rosalind Russell in all those movies where she was the career girl in those Adrian suits. Roz and her man would have dinner in the Barberry Room, and come home in a carriage through Central Park.

"My life is exactly like that, it's the way I dreamed it. Of course there's the dreariness of having to sit down and write an article against a deadline, and there are men who turn out to be wounded and not loving, and sometimes the cleaner ruins your best dress, but mostly, it's all like my fantasy, if not better. I dreamed it would be this way, and isn't it incredible? It really is."

Unlike Gael Greene and other members of the food establishment, the *New Yorker*'s Calvin Trillin, known to friends, family, and name-droppers as Bud, doesn't take his reputation in the world of eats seriously. (He does take his eating seriously.)

Trillin has written two books, *American Fried* and *Alice, Let's Eat*, about food and where to find it in North America, and when the first one came out, he waited with trepidation for the reviews. "I thought, my God, what if it's reviewed by one of the grown-up food writers. They'll go crazy, they'll rip it apart. They're so competitive, they're obsessed with the subject of food, each of them has the feeling he's the only person who actually knows what's going on.

"Well, they were very nice to me. They're smart enough to know you can't go around dismissing *everybody*, so to show some magnanimity of spirit, they said, 'Oh, Trillin's okay. He writes about hamburgers and things, but he's funny.' Two of the nicest reviews of *Alice, Let's Eat* were by two grown-up food writers in the process of vicious attacks on each other."

Restaurant reviewing, says Trillin, "is a necessary function, I suppose. I like the idea that people will argue about where the best pastrami is, but I would never want to get involved in actually finding out. Same with hamburgers, same with anything."

Trillin, who was brought up in Kansas City, believes that food critics are more important in New York than they are anyplace else. Important in the sense that hordes of people follow them. "There are critics in other places, but there are very few cities in the country where a good restaurant can remain unknown to people who care about eating. Basically, you're talking about New York and New Orleans and maybe Chicago. The number of places that are worth eating in in, say, Knoxville, is six or eight. And everybody knows 'em. In Cleveland, even if it's a little place with no sign, everyone knows about it. And that's true in Kansas City too. New Orleans is a little different. In New Orleans, everybody's interested in eating, so people there take on food critics. The guy who's doing the plastering in your house is arguing about where the best Poor Boys are.

"A friend of mine is obsessed with New Orleans food, he has three- and four-hour meals. 'It's funny,' he says, 'as much of this food as I eat, I only gain about five pounds a year. The problem is, I've been here nine years.' It's true. He weighs forty-five pounds more than he did when he came.

"In New Orleans, people don't understand how anybody from someplace else could live that far from fresh oysters. But as far as attracting crowds, we're talking about New York. Partly because the communications industry is here, and partly because there are so damn many restaurants—I think there are something like 60,000 restaurants in New York—that you really can find previously undiscovered places, and you can move people this way or that way."

It was a visit to fellow journalist John McPhee that started Trillin on the road to stalking food for thought and profit. "Alice [Mrs. Trillin] and I were at McPhee's house in Princeton, and he had one of these big country kitchens, and on one wall he had framed some menus from meals he'd liked when he'd gone eating in France. I said, 'Well, gee, McPhee, you're not the only one that's been around.' And I got a Winstead's hamburger menu next time I was in Kansas City. It had a couple of good things on it, like their motto, which is, 'Your drinks are served in sanitized glasses,' and I framed it and hung it on my kitchen wall so I could tell McPhee I was a sophisticate like he was.

"Then another thing happened. I was coming back from Europe once, and I was reading *Life* magazine, and they had a food review in the front of the book, and at that time they were also running a series like 'Sophia Loren's Rome,' and I thought, why don't I do 'Buddy Trillin's Kansas

City,' with me sitting at Arthur Bryant's up to my elbows in barbecue sauce. So I did a gourmet tour of Kansas City for *Playboy*, and a couple of U.S. Journal pieces for the *New Yorker*, things like the Crawfish Festival at Breaux Bridge, Louisiana, and suddenly I was a food writer, but it was really an accident.

"From my point of view, I started using the food writing as comic relief from writing about murders or race problems. I think of it as a way to make jokes. But food people are crazed. Not just the food writers, the people in every town in the country. I have a whole file of letters from people who write to say, 'Next time you get to such and such a town, you have to eat at this place.' No matter what city I go to, there's almost always one or two crazy food people who accost me to tell me about a little Mexican restaurant.

"I get phone calls at odd hours too. Still, I rarely hear from anyone saying you should do a story on this or that. Except about food. Food, my God, they'll call and say, 'Listen, I've driven all the way to Kansas City from Columbus, and Bryant's is closed, and I'm standing on 58th and Second, what am I supposed to do?' None of them starts by saying, 'You may think it's odd that I'm calling,' they just get right into it.

"Eating is totally personal to people. A guy will phone and say, 'What are you talking about barbecue? You've never been to Joe's in Jacksonville,' and I have to promise him next time I'll go there.

"Yesterday, I got a long letter from some lawyer. I often get long letters from lawyers, and I think, who's paying for this? Whose time is this? I hope it's the local utility instead of some aged widow trying to hire this guy to sue the city for something. Because I get 8- or 10-page single-spaced letters discussing food. This one yesterday was about catfish."

In the course of his research for *American Fried*, Trillin met an investment banker who had access to a computer that could offer advice about four hundred different restaurants. "He would say to the computer, 'It's Tuesday night, and I want to go to an Italian restaurant on the East Side, medium priced.' But of course he had all the wrong information fed into the computer, stuff like whether or not the restaurant had a garden, nothing interesting like whether or not the food was good."

The phenomenon of "the grown-up food writers" and their hold on the public interests Trillin—"Julia, Craig. I've heard people in Columbus call him Craig, the way peasants call Fidel, Fidel"—but he, like Gael Greene, absolves the food establishment of responsibility for making Americans mountainous.

"If you go to a town where you can't get anything good to eat, where nobody writes about food, and nobody cares about food, and you're at the restaurant where the high school graduating class is coming for their prom, and they all look great, you think, gee, aren't these wonderful-looking American kids? They're fresh and nice and trim, maybe two fatties in the whole class. And then you see their parents coming in, and their parents are *fat,* really fat, fatter than most Europeans, fatter than most anybody. And it isn't from gourmet food. As my friend Fats Goldberg, the pizza baron, always says, 'I didn't get fat on *coq au vin.'*

"I don't know if the food people are innocent, exactly, but they aren't the reason everybody's getting fat. Because when you think about the whole gourmet thing, I would guess demographically it's rather narrow; there are whole classes of the country it doesn't really affect.

"And to a great extent, it's tied to kitchen gadgets and kitchen machinery. I once offended a food person in Los Angeles. I was on her radio show and she said, 'Isn't food life?' Some crap like that. And I said, 'No, I think a lot of this stuff is tied to industry. You know, get the husband interested in being a *sous-chef,* and you can sell him the Cuisinart next Christmas.

"Look at where those stores are that sell the wire whisks and stuff; they're in restored shopping centers that used to be warehouses, and they've all got cutesy names, they're middle-class shopping places."

Trillin rejects the theory postulated at the beginning of this book of a vast middle class with enough money to eat itself rotund. "It's your cleaning lady who's fat," he says. "Fat from eating starches.

"Furthermore, per capita income in the United States is something like fifth in the world, not anywhere near first. Even if you don't count Arabs, which is not a fair per capita income because only seven people have it.

"Where the United States *is* number one is in energy consumption. A couple of weeks ago, I asked a waitress in Disneyland about the gas shortage. 'Well,' she said, 'I only live four blocks from here, so I *could* walk.' It was clear that the Germans would have to be threatening the walls of the city and all the civilian cars comandeered by the Defense Board before she *would* walk; it had just never occurred to her.

"I wrote a little Talk of the Town piece [in the *New Yorker*] about the gas shortage, and I touched on the jogging craze in California. I said a lot of people in Beverly Hills who are running have never walked. They never took that intermediate step. They went straight from Jaguars to running."

Like other food experts polled here, Trillin comes out in favor of a diet of moderation, but scorns carrot and raisin salad. Alice has "some kind of brown rice tendencies, no question, and when I'm out of town, natural food fanatics sort of nibble away at her," but, says Trillin, as soon as he gets home, he sets her straight. Alice tries to give him and their two little girls sensible meals—broiled fish, asparagus—but when the Trillins travel, she makes no trouble for her husband. "I think if you don't eat two really good meals a day in Italy, you're crazy," Trillin observes. "I mean, anybody who actually went over there and said, 'Better not have pasta for lunch because I just had it last night' is crazy."

Anyhow, he adds, almost wistfully, "I've never been thin. Nobody in my family's ever been thin. There's a family joke about peasant thickness. I could lose fifty pounds and not be thin, I'm just not built that way."

After *Alice, Let's Eat* came out, Trillin appeared on several talk shows and during the course of one of them, the host asked why the author-eater wasn't fatter. Trillin credited Alice with shaping him up. "I said," he recalls, "that Alice's method was so complicated and subtle that I probably couldn't go into the whole thing, but I could sum it up with the word nagging. Nagging, and occasionally, for a change of pace, ridicule, and general verbal abuse. That's how she's been able to do it."

PUTTING IT ON:
We're fat because we dream of spending $4,000 for dinner.

5 *Scandal(s) in the Haute Meal(s)*

The fat is in the fire.
—WISE OLD FOLK SAYING

WARNING: This chapter has absolutely nothing to do with fat. Or very little. I just thought it might amuse you, and cure you of a misapprehension or two. For instance, do you think being a food star automatically guarantees the life of Cindy Lou? A ton of pleasurable freeloading, while your arteries slowly harden to the sound of violin music and the smell of fresh-baked chocolate roll? Guess again.

In 1975, poor Craig Claiborne discovered that working at the gourmet's trade could lash back at a guy, causing him to be prayed for by the sanctimonious, and excoriated by Third World enthusiasts and everybody's mother who ever said, "Eat your vegetables, children are starving in Europe."

The way it began was with the Channel 13 auction. The Channel 13 auction is an annual fundraiser perpetrated by a New York City public television station. Viewers get the chance to bid for various goods and services that have been donated by various charitable and/or publicity-seeking individuals and organizations.

Among these organizations, in 1975, was the American Express Company. They offered a dinner for two at any restaurant in the world that would accept their credit card. American Express set no limit on the cost of the dinner, expecting, according to a company spokesman, that the winner of the feast might "run up a bill as high as $500."

Craig Claiborne's top bid of $300 earned him the chance to eat and drink himself silly at no cost (except to his liver), though I guess we have to figure his $300 bid in there someplace, kind of like $50 deductible insurance.

Anyhow, Claiborne spent the next several weeks fantasizing about where and when he and a companion of his choice might best debauch themselves. Then, in the fullness of time—and looking forward to the fullness of tum—he chose a little Parisian restaurant called Chez Denis, owned by a man named Denis Lahana.

First, though, a trial run for Craig and two friends, an "investigatory dinner." Claiborne pronounced it "sumptuous." Lobster, *foie gras*, sweetbreads, roast quail, and like that. The plastic flowers offended the Claiborne eye, but the Claiborne taste buds reeled with ecstasy.

So Mr. C. parleyed with Monsieur Lahana. "We told him we were about to celebrate a birthday and that money was no obstacle in ordering the finest dinner in Europe," Clairborne later revealed in the *New York Times*.

M. Lahana rose to the occasion, and so did the check. To $4,000. "This, we must hasten to add," said Claiborne, "included service and taxes."

Thank God for small favors.

M. Lahana had told Claiborne there would be enough food to serve ten people, and enough wine for four, but Claiborne stuck by American Express rules, which "called for dinner for two. The dinner party would be made up of me and my colleague, Pierre Franey. Anything left over, we knew, would not go to waste."

It was to be, promised Denis Lahana, "a dinner *à la française*, in the classic tradition." Thirty-one dishes, and nine great wines, plus Calvados and cognac drunk out of Baccarat crystal.

Among the delicacies Claiborne and Franey ultimately tasted:

Fresh Beluga caviar, three soups, broiled oysters, lobster in a truffled sauce, a pie made with red mullet, chicken in a cream sauce. Also, partridge "nested in a bed of cooked cabbage," a fillet of beef, and three kinds of sherbet. The sherbet was to clear their palates so the diners could come back, fresh-mouthed, to ortolans "cooked whole, with the head on, and without cleaning except for removing the feathers," and wild duck, and roasted veal "wrapped in puff pastry with fresh black truffles about the size of golf balls."

There followed vegetables, and cold meats, and three kinds of sweets.

Claiborne gave the meal a mixed review. Some of the wines were "extraordinary," "ageless and beautiful," "magnificent," but, he said, the overall display of the food was "undistinguished, not to say shabby." And while he found most of the concoctions exemplary, the lobster had been too chewy, the pheasant had been "presented on a most ordinary dish," and some of the rations that should have been hot were lukewarm.

If it was heat he was looking for, Claiborne soon found it. Upon his return to America, he discovered that while a $4,000 dinner might not upset your stomach, it could give you a terrible headache.

At home and abroad, the bad reviews rolled in. Claiborne didn't get a much better press than King Atreus, the legendary Greek who killed his nephews, had them baked up in a pie, and served them to their father. The French were so incensed by the Claiborne orgy (reporters pointed out that $4,000 was a year's wages for many a French worker) that Denis Lahana's restaurant was forced out of business, the Vatican newspaper deplored conspicuous consumption "while millions are starving," and American columnist Harriet Van Horne dubbed the Claiborne-Franey evening wrong "morally, esthetically and in every other way."

Civilians got into the act too. In less than a week, the *New York Times* received 250 letters, "virtually all condemnatory." One New Yorker wrote that the account of the $4,000 dinner "was one of the most disgusting things recently published in a news organ." A Jersey City letter writer wanted to know how anyone could "reconcile this smugly decadent story and almost daily reports of worldwide hunger and starvation," and a Yonkers woman called the article "an insult to the sensibilities of your readers."

Stung and apparently surprised by the public outrage, Claiborne replied to his critics in three brief paragraphs. This is what he wrote:

"I view with enormous regret the emotions of those who feel that the meal on which I dined in Paris for $4000 was obscene or decadent or a symbol of contempt for the hunger that exists in the world today.

"I would like to ask those who were not amused if they seriously believe that as a result of that evening I have deprived one human being of one mouthful of food. To put it another way, if the meal had not occurred, would one more mouth have been fed, one more body nourished?

"I feel enormously privileged to have participated in that meal and have no intention of putting an onus on American Express. It was my enthusiasm and excess that caused the total bill. But I do not think it represents contempt for world hunger any more than if I had won the Mercedes-Benz that was put up for auction."

Fair enough? It wasn't an "onus" Craig put on American Express, it was the bite. By the time another week had passed, the *Times* had received 225 more letters, and a few hardy souls had actually come to Claiborne's defense.

"I was appalled by the degree of appalledness indicated by the letters you ran," wrote a woman from Albany. "It indicates unfortunately that we have lost our sense of humor." And a woman from Lakewood, New Jersey, wanted to know how many of the indignant Claiborne critics "would hand over winnings to the poor and hungry if they were to win at the lottery, if they were to hit it big in the stock market, if they were to inherit $4,000 from their great-aunts?" Then she answered herself. "Not a one."

Oddly enough, seven months before the Claiborne contretemps, in an article in the *New York Times Magazine*, Waverley Root had addressed the subject of "enjoying food while millions starve," and the "hair-shirt mentality" of people who "protest at the simultaneous existence of gastronomy and famine in the world." To be sure it was unjust, he said, for some populations to have too much food, while others starved, but he could not see why "because some people have to eat badly, we should all eat badly."

Root held macho sentiments—steak and potatoes are manly, more imaginative cuisine is sissy stuff—and residual puritanism responsible for much of the American attitude toward food. "The Puritan eats to maintain strength in order to get on with the serious business of earning his bread by the sweat of his brow, the only permissible seasoning; to take pains to make his food tasty would be abandonment to sensual self-indulgence . . . The Puritan . . . distrusts food, an insidious tempter, leading the weak down the primrose path to eternal damnation. Obviously, only tempting food can do this. Therefore, a proper concern for our salvation demands that we avoid tastiness. Bad food is good food—or at least, virtuous food."

Protesting against those who demanded "not that the underprivileged should eat better but that the privileged should eat worse," Root concluded: "As for the ill-fed, from whom may they expect the most sympathy—from those who like to eat or from those who don't?"

Craig Claiborne pigged his way into trouble several years before John McPhee came a cropper on the great meal scene. In Claiborne's case, it was ordinary John and Jane Doe looking to make a citizen's arrest, but McPhee drew the fire of the formidable Mimi Sheraton.

The McPhee squall was born in the February 19, 1979, issue of the *New Yorker*, and grew into a typhoon almost overnight. John McPhee, who can describe the game of tennis, or the state of Alaska, or truck farming in upstate New York with equal and miraculous clarity, turned his attention to the culinary prowess of a friend who ran a restaurant within a hundred miles of New York City. The friend, a chef who had been trained on the Continent, and treasured his privacy, said McPhee could chronicle him, but only if his identity was disguised. "Why don't you call me Otto?" he suggested.

So the saga of Otto (who liked to cook for the few who could find him, who worked in worn-out trousers with patched knees, and a sailor hat drawn down over his ears) was born, and ran for more than fifty pages and twenty-five thousand words.

McPhee wrote about "emanations of flavor expressed in pork and coriander, hazelnut breadings, smoked-roe mousses and aïoli." He wrote about "fresh rainbow trout," and lobster with green eggs "clinging like burrs to its ventral plates . . . so crunchy and so fresh-tasting with lemon juice" and "sauteed squares of lemon sole, with Swiss chard and anchovies," and "Swedish-fried potatoes, which are cut in ganglion strings and cooked in very hot fat, where they enmesh in a filament mass that comes up golden and crisp."

He wrote about the chef's wife, responsible for the restaurant's sweets. "There is a nurse," he said, "from Bellevue who goes berserk in the presence of Anne's meringue tortes and ultra-chocolate steamed mousse cakes, orders every dessert available, and has to be carted back to Bellevue." He wrote about mocha meringues, *gâteau victoire au chocolat*, and trifle made of slices of *génoise* covered with peaches, strawberries, brandy, wine, and custard cream. McPhee's descriptions of the menus at Otto's and Anne's could have got saliva from a stone.

En passant, however, Otto had tendered McPhee some very tough opinions about establishments other than his own. He called New York's most famous French dining rooms "the frog pond restaurants," he said he'd had Maine mussels at Le Cygne, and they were "awfully tough," he said he'd found ice crystals in his meat at La Caravelle, he said the *sole farcie Elzévir* at Lutèce wasn't fresh—"It isn't pristine. It has a fishy taste"—and worst of all, he conjectured that the *turbot de Dieppe poché* at the same restaurant was frozen, "which is the only kind you can buy, unless it's flown over."

Soon the cry of wounded chefs was heard in the land. Michel Crouzillat of Le Cygne said his mussels were "excellent. I taste them all the time. I think the whole article is made up." Roger Fessaguet, chef at La Caravelle, rejected both the ice crystals story and the frog pond nickname. "I am very upset," said M. Fessaguet. "I am the chef here for nineteen years, and I never saw frozen meat. This is an insult." Furthermore: "The name frog should never be used. I fought for this country in the Korean War, and this is pure crap. I would never call a Japanese a Jap." Roger took a swipe at Otto's raiment, too. "If he is respectable, he should dress properly. And they are even in violation of the Board of Health when they wash the dishes by hand. He is the lowest kind of chef."

André Soltner, owner-chef of Lutèce, fought back even harder, firing off a telegram to William Shawn, editor of the *New Yorker*, demanding an apology. "To allow an anonymous source to hide behind the great prestige of the *New Yorker* and accuse Lutèce of using frozen sole and turbot is irresponsible," he fumed.

Delighted gossip columnists asked if Soltner might sue the magazine, and Soltner said no. "I haven't the time or the money." Even so, he was gathering evidence against Otto, pulling together bills from his fish suppliers that would show that Lutèce did not now "nor have we ever, served frozen turbot or frozen sole."

The beleaguered William Shawn said he'd been trying without success to reach McPhee. Half the food writers in town were having the same trouble.

"Anyone who was interested in food was determined to find Otto," Gael Greene remembers. "I'd been in Mexico, and when I came home, there were all these messages on my machine, one from Craig Claiborne, saying, 'Who is Otto? What do you think?'

"Everybody wanted to know, who was this glorious cook? And how could it be that we had not discovered the best restaurant in America? We felt we had to taste this glorious food. And if it wasn't glorious, then how dare Otto criticize the chefs of New York, and who is John McPhee and what does he know about food anyway?"

Greene undoubtedly reflects the gourmet establishment's position. "In the world of culinary journalism," said a reporter in *Time* magazine, "the great Otto flap caused almost as much consternation as the 1926 disappearance of Agatha Christie did in London. None of the professional eaters-out knew who Otto might be or where. Reporters pumped other reporters, chefs, food authors, anyone who might draw a bead on the wayward *cuisinier*."

It was Mimi Sheraton who dug Otto up, only to bury him again under a very bad notice. Tracking the elusive chef, she used deduction, induction, and a stringer who telephoned politicians around McPhee's home in Princeton, New Jersey, because politicians eat out a lot, and besides they have to know everything that goes on in their wards. Sheraton, reported *Newsweek*, "went after Otto as if he were the perfect béchamel sauce."

Sheraton said she'd had to. "When you're in the news business, and everybody is trying to find something out, then it's your job to tell them."

Tell them she did. Otto's place turned out to be the Bullhead Inn, in Shohola, Pennsylvania, Otto himself turned out to be a man named Alan Lieb, and the food, according to Sheraton, turned out to be pretty sad stuff.

Mimi called the pâté "soft and bland," described a "truly awful first course composed of briny, pale-yellow artichoke bottoms of the type usually canned, topped by large chewy gray snails that tasted dank and musty. Covered with a heavy brown sauce that formed a film instantly, the dish bordered on the inedible."

Sheraton also suggested that the duck might have been frozen, and that the veal birds didn't fly. They were, she grieved, "roll-ups of dry tough veal wrapped around almost raw bacon, which in turn enclosed clumps of wet bread."

The cakes were good, the wine was fine, the check was reasonable, but the trip wasn't worth the taking. "While it is true," said the *Times* critic, "that one cannot make a definitive evaluation of any restaurant on the basis of a single meal, it is equally true that there is a minimal level of quality below which a great and experienced cook cannot sink even on his worst day."

Alan Lieb, sniffed Mimi, had "a long way to go in developing his own palate for seasoning and combining ingredients, and in mastering basic cooking techniques."

Pleading that he had promised his subject the boon of namelessness, McPhee had tried to stop Sheraton from publishing her piece, but Mimi could not be moved. "You were in no position to promise for anybody else," she said. "Besides, you didn't break your promise, you didn't tell me his name."

At first, the Liebs insisted that Sheraton's broadside was of little moment to them. "Poor Mimi Sheraton, she mistook prosciutto for raw bacon," sympathized Mrs. Lieb, and said that she and her husband would have had to sell their fifty-seat restaurant if they'd got a three-star review in the *New York Times*. "We just don't have the energy or capacity to deal with crowds."

Alan Lieb did offer an apology to Lutèce. "We love eating there. It's just that I have never seen fresh turbot in the Fulton Fish Market, and I assumed none was available."

Still, the fracas wasn't over. Mimi Sheraton got mad because *Newsweek* had printed her picture, and a couple of columnists for the *Village Voice* got mad because Mimi Sheraton had savaged the Liebs. Columnist A, Joel Oppenheimer, said the Bullhead Inn was a "fantastic little French restaurant," and he hoped that "quiet, private people who appreciate care and can make their own judgments will find their way to Shohola and enjoy." Columnist B, Geoffrey Stokes, suggested that Mimi Sheraton had been "determined" not to like the food.

"And I wondered why. There were a couple of possibilities. One is that John McPhee, who had waxed symphonic over the Liebs' food in his *New Yorker* piece, has a tin palate, and that Sheraton was genuinely enraged at the thought of people—her people—being sent off to Pennsylvania . . . on a wild goose chase. If the food was as poisonous as she described it to be—if indeed it 'bordered on the inedible'—that would be reason enough.

"The other is that she was carrying a contract."

Stokes went on to explain that a contract was "a favor, a bribe, a fix," and tried to reason out why Mimi Sheraton would want to do in the Bullhead Inn.

Although an attack on the Liebs seemed "of no direct benefit" to any of Sheraton's "cronies," Stokes finally decided that it was the discovery of the restaurant by McPhee that posed the "threat to the New York City food establishment . . . If 'Otto' were really as wonderful as McPhee claimed, why didn't anybody know about him?

"'Anybody' in this case doesn't mean just anybody; it means the swirl of stars and groupies in the New York restaurant world . . . Everybody knew when Claude left the Palace, and just who was going to bring what (and whom) to the covered-dish celebration for Joe Baum. And everybody, in that circle, cares about such things. Passionately. Therefore, they were affronted when McPhee came riding into town . . ."

(Certainly Gael Greene's question—"How could it be that we had not discovered the best restaurant in America?"—supports Stokes's proposition.)

Calvin Trillin says Sheraton had no choice but to pursue Otto. "The thing about Mimi is, she really does her job, and whether you agree with her or not, she doesn't do it casually. In the case of the McPhee piece, it was her job to find the place, because John really did kind of taunt the grown-up food writers by saying, 'This restaurant is on your turf, and you don't know about it.' He didn't just leave out the name, he made a thing about it."

On the other hand, says Trillin, "What Mimi did to that restaurant, she's never done before. She's always very careful, she goes two or three times, she orders a lot of different things, she goes different times of day. I don't think she's a mean-spirited person, but that piece read like a grown-up food writer saying, 'Ha, we'll show this McPhee, who the hell *is* he?'

"There's McPhee, probably the single best writer of nonfiction prose in the country, a marvelous reporter, but to the food people, it really is, who's this pisherkeh?"

John Hess told Trillin the same thing had happened to him when he, Hess, came back from France. "I had covered a number of wars. But the gourmets were saying, 'Who is he? Is he up to this?'"

Trillin explains that the "grown-up food writers" are forced to approach their calling with gravity. "In order to go from restaurant to restaurant, test all the pastramis, worry about whether or not the Cygne is overrated or underrated, you really have to believe in what you're doing. If you said to the grown-up food writers, 'Look, is it more important to have peace in the Middle East or to be right about whether the third-ranking restaurant in New York really should be fifth?' they're all intelligent people and they would all say it's more important to have peace. But they don't believe it. They're crossing their fingers behind their backs."

In Shohola, Pennsylvania, peace was shaky too, and the Liebs put the Bullhead up for sale.

"Friends tried to talk them out of moving, but the pressure got to them," says writer-editor Guy Flatley, who has a summer house near the Inn. "Alan is one of the most sensitive, civilized men I've ever met, and the food he turns out is extraordinary, but people were telephoning from the Middle West and saying, 'We're going to be in your area, and we want to come by and decide for ourselves if your food is good or bad.' And Mrs. Lieb had to handle all these calls, and the whole thing was just too hard on both of them."

Three months after the McPhee piece appeared, authorities at the *New Yorker* were still being questioned about the magazine's checking department, which is famous for its infallibility. How was it that nobody had found out if Lutèce served frozen turbot before permitting McPhee to suggest that it might?

"Special circumstances," said editor Shawn. "Nobody here including the checking department knew who Otto was. I can't think of another instance of that. I would not even have asked because I have utter confidence in McPhee."

Alan Lieb, on the other hand, may never have confidence in anyone again. In the only photograph I ever saw of him, he was sprinting away from a news photographer. He was wearing a brown paper bag on his head.

PUTTING IT ON:
We're fat because we can travel first-class while staying at home (and everyone knows how they stuff you on luxury liners).

6 The Theme-ing of America

Peace ye, fat guttes, lye downe
—WILLIAM SHAKESPEARE

HAVE A statistic. The average American eats seven meals a week away from home.*

More women are working, more families have two incomes and are willing to spend a larger part of these incomes on grub served up by a stranger. A 1979 Gallup Poll asked diners-out (accosting them, I guess, somewhere between the check and the parking lot) if they thought the meal they'd just chomped down was a good value. Seventy-three percent of the women said yes indeed, but only fifty-four percent of the men agreed, leaving us to conjecture about the disgruntled males who wanted to be home watching football.

Anyway, more people are going to restaurants. But tracking down great chefs and four-star cuisine isn't the only game in town. Food has become entertainment.

Enter theme dining. You don't just have a meal, you're wafted away

* *Restaurant Business* magazine.

on a fantasy trip to Old Napoli or New Delhi. I have a friend who's convinced there isn't an ordinary restaurant in the city of Los Angeles. "If you go to a place that has Polynesian food," he says morosely, "there's model canoes hanging out over the highway, and inside there's black magic masks and weirdness."

Certain restaurateurs who have heard getting there is half the fun, make trips, rather than destinations, their theme. In New York City, you can hop a car (there's something called the Autopub, where little kids and their divorced daddies line up for the thrill of climbing into an imitation automobile in order to be served a hamburger) or a ship (Dr. George Schwarz who, when he isn't running a restaurant, is head of radiology at St. Vincent's Hospital, equipped the dining room at One Fifth [Avenue] with furnishings from the old ocean liner *Caronia*) or a train (if you're wandering through Bloomingdale's department store).

Le Train Bleu is named for a gone-but-not-forgotten first-class choo choo that once chuffed its way from Paris to the Riviera. The original Train Bleu had a blue engine, but its dining car was mostly green, which is just how Bloomingdale's has reproduced it. The store opened the mahogany-paneled, velvet-lined, brass-trimmed facsimile in July of 1979 and discovered an amazing number of shoppers willing to pay in the neighborhood of fourteen dollars apiece (to be sure, that's with a glass of wine and a dessert) for the privilege of lunching in back of the housewares department.

As you stand in a long, plush corridor, waiting to be seated, a man's disembodied voice wafts over you. "*En voiture, attention, passagers pour Lyons et Marseilles,*" he calls. When he's not talking, a radio plays music, along with commercials. The day I was there, Frank Perdue came on the air, chatting up his chickens, and the lady in front of me, half-distressed by this intrusion into her daydream, turned to her companion. "Well, at least he's French," she said. *A la recherche de Frank Perdue*.

Theme restaurants don't charm everybody, in fact they infuriate an English writer named Philippa Pullar who declares that "Eating out has become an experience, but not one for the palate. . . . When there are monsoons splashing into crocodile-infested lakes, one does not notice the crowd of waiters giggling in the tropical plants handing around the plate of whitebait that is about to be served to you; when there is a naked woman to watch, the wine waiter is a chimpanzee and the pudding comes in a bed-pan, you might not notice the disgusting salad of beetroot, hard-boiled eggs, tired lettuce and dreadful dressing, the pale dead meat."

Oddly enough, Joseph Baum, the original—and maybe the only—genius in the world of theme restaurants, agrees to some extent with Miss Pullar. Sitting at a prime table in Windows on the World, the restaurant he created 107 stories above the city, he's a little like God looking over his handiwork and finding it good. Baum doesn't especially like to talk about himself, but he's too much of a gentleman to disappoint a journalist, once the journalist has run him to ground.

"In Windows on the World, I let you know you're up in the air," he says. "There is a feeling about the place that's exciting. But I am not telling you I am doing this inside of a railroad car. I do not believe in creating restaurants in washtubs or in urinals."

Baum was born into the food business—"I worked in my parents' hotel in a small town in upstate New York. I learned about life, and waitresses. I liked it."

After college and the Navy, he became an accountant. "When I involved myself in kitchens again, people said, 'What do you know about kitchens? You're an accountant.' And when I started doing accounting procedures in the restaurants, people said, 'What do you know about accounting? Go back to the kitchen.'"

Journeying to Florida, Baum started food operations for the Boca Raton Club and the Roney Plaza, but after a few years headed North again. "I was in love with New York, and I was in love with ladders, wherever they reached."

First rung in the New York area was a restaurant at Newark Airport. Baum brought Albert Stockli (the great chef with whom he later started The Four Seasons) to Newark. He also introduced the sparkler snowball, a ball of ice cream covered with syrup and coconut, and studded with lighted sparklers.

"I maybe wouldn't do that again," he says cheerfully, admitting that some of his early ideas were pretty flashy. "I'd been influenced by a showman who'd come long before me, a man named Ernie Byfield, who'd run the old Pump Room in Chicago."

In 1956, Baum, by then a member of Restaurant Associates, was working with a man named Jerry Brody of whom he speaks admiringly. "Jerry was the boss, and he was the one who dug up all the opportunities."

One of the opportunities was a location in Rockefeller Center. "It was the communications center of the world; what we needed was a senate, a caucus club, a place where people came to exchange ideas—a forum."

Thus was born The Forum of the Twelve Caesars. Twelve, because Bill Pahlman, who was going to design the restaurant, happened to own twelve paintings of Roman emperors. "Then we began doing research," Baum says. "The Museo Nazionale in Naples, Suetonius, Robert Graves, Morris Kaplan, Gilbert Highet, Milan, Rome, the Cornell library. I'm a nut, I like to reach beyond. I felt New York needed a flamboyant restaurant of quality, but I always had my tongue somewhat in my cheek. I couldn't believe anyone would really take some of it seriously. We had a Tarte Messalina on the menu, and giant oysters we called the Oysters of Hercules. Forum was a not too subtle joke, but it was a good joke."

It was also a joke with a twenty-year run. "A classic restaurant," says Joe Baum sardonically, "is one which lasts the length of its lease."

Although Fonda del Sol didn't last that long, Joe Baum loved it. "The restaurant was ahead of its time. Based on its investments and costs, we had to charge more than people were willing to pay for Latin-American food. In 1960, that is. Also, nobody knew whether it was formal or informal, a woman didn't know exactly how to dress when she went there—"

He stops. "Still, if it had been good enough, goddammit, it would have worked."

The Four Seasons worked. It's still working, two decades later. Paul Goldberger wrote that any good restaurant "must cater at least somewhat to an element of fantasy. The fantasy that The Four Seasons represents—beyond those its kitchen attempts to purvey—is the fantasy of grand scale and pure order, all combined with modern design."

That must have pleased Joe Baum. Eager to cede credit to others, he speaks of Samuel Bronfman (who provided the Seagram Building that houses The Four Seasons, and who hired as architect Mies van der Rohe, assisted by Philip Johnson) and of Garth and Ada Louise Huxtable, who designed the china and silver, and of Antonucci, who did the graphics. "Do you know what it means to have the opportunity to work with all those people?" Baum says.

One room of The Four Seasons is built around a reflecting pool, and in that room the curtains are made of fragile metal chains, so the very air seems to shiver with light. Each season of the year, the plantings are changed, the uniforms of the help are changed, the kinds of foods served are changed. "Refreshment and change," says Joe Baum. "That's what the seasons bring. I had the opportunity to build a great restaurant, something soaring and glittering. I worked with authorities like Virginia Zabriskie on the anthropology of the seasons.

"And I had some idealistic notions. I thought, for instance, that we could make it so Mrs. Astor would feel comfortable if Mrs. Yifniff from Wisconsin was sitting at the next table. Well, I was wrong. Mrs. Yifniff may go to The Four Seasons, but Mrs. Astor isn't completely comfortable beside her. People still want to know there's a Siberia they don't have to go to, though I swear to you there isn't a bad table at the Seasons."

Joe Baum sighs. "I'm not a good snob."

People don't go to restaurants only because they're hungry, so with each restaurant he works on, Baum considers "how the place is going to live, once it's started. Who's going to come there? Lots of people think you can take a restaurant and reproduce it in another city, but a restaurant is not like a play that can travel to another town, it is related to everything that happens around it. I don't go around with a satchel full of funny ideas looking for a place to put them. I say, what's here? What are the elements?

"There was a place called Holland House in Rockefeller Center. It wasn't doing very well. Rockefeller Center asked Restaurant Associates to look at it. I had an idea. Do an Irish restaurant which would be a little bit different, where the wood would look old, secondhand, but shine like hell. Where you could go in, have a drink, buy oysters by the piece, shrimp by the piece, have a great sandwich and not have to sit down. I thought I could legitimize lunchtime boozing. If you wanted a couple of fingers of Scotch at lunch, you'd be having a sandwich at the same time. Not cute food, simple food.

"I figured this would work because it was in Rockefeller Center. It wouldn't have worked on Tenth Avenue because on Tenth Avenue they've got the real thing. I wanted to call it Lovely Houlihan's, make a play on the Hawaiian song, 'Lovely Hula Hands,' but nobody liked that joke. Then George Lois, with whom I was working, said, 'No, we're going to call it The Bloody Nose,' but nobody liked that either. Finally, since my son's name is Charley, we called it Charley O's."

Baum's biggest challenge had to be the job he masterminded for the New York–New Jersey Port Authority, in the World Trade Center near

Wall Street—twenty-two restaurants, of which Windows on the World is only one. (By then, he'd left Restaurant Associates, and was president of Inhilco, a subsidiary of Hilton International, which he's also left.)

"We were working with public agencies, public funds, so it was 1 percent inspiration, 9 percent perspiration, and 90 percent justification. But that's only fair. Somebody has to take responsibility and somebody has to take criticism."

Referring to a show he'd seen at the Museum of Modern Art, a show featuring plans for architecture that was never built, Baum says, "The trick is to do it. You not only have to create the concept, you have to create the vehicle by which the concept can be carried out. You have an obligation, whatever the problems, to see that the job gets done."

There are close to a thousand people working in the restaurants at the Trade Center, and they feed 25,000 customers a day, so Joe Baum must be considered to have got the job done.

Windows on the World, with its eagle's-eye views of rivers, bridges, boroughs, skyline, is an example of a Baum triumph over skeptics. "They told me, 'You're crazy, out of your mind. Nobody's ever going to come down to the lower end of Manhattan at night.'"

Windows has turned into the single largest grossing restaurant in the world (sixteen million dollars in 1978), it sells more wine than any other restaurant in the world, and its luncheon club has four thousand members and collects a million dollars in annual dues. (At night, the restaurant is open to the public, at noon it's a private club, although by law, 120 of us great unwashed lunchers have to be admitted every day.) "And now," chortles Joe Baum, "everybody says, 'Well, what did you expect? Look at the location!'"

Because Windows' theme is the view, Baum demonstrates that there's never more than one table between the eater and the panorama of sea and clouds and buildings. "You're sitting in an acre of space, yet you have no such feeling. You never see more than one section of the room. You have the sense of being in an exciting restaurant, rather than a small bistro, the sense of food, people, the rhythm of service, activity going on all around you. The tables are designed a quarter of an inch lower than usual, so you feel good resting your elbows on them, there's double padding underneath the tablecloths. We've tried to take eating, a human need, and elevate it to a civilized pleasure."

If you mention that people who don't give a damn about food come to

Windows just for the cityscape, he will agree. "But people who don't give a damn about food always want to know where the best restaurants are."

Joe Baum says eating and dining are not the same. His own record shows that he's hired the best cooks he could entice into his establishments. But what about the growing fear of butter and cream and cholesterol? Are diners more watchful, less amenable to delight than they used to be?

"There's no question there's a new consciousness of calories," Baum says. "When you consider the chocolate cake now, you ask yourself, 'Do I think it's worth it?' I have no concern about that. It just requires that I be more seductive, create more need for you to buy."

With Sesame Place, a new amusement park that opened in July of 1980, in Langhorne, Pennsylvania, Joe Baum got another chance to practice his food seductions, this time on children. Sesame Place was conceived by the people who produce *Sesame Street;* they hope it will be the first of many small theme parks all around the country.

For the park's Sesame Food Factory, Milton Glaser designed a restaurant with a green floor ("It feels like you're in the middle of a salad bowl," says Baum) and he made all the kitchens—where pizzas and bread are baked, and salads are tossed, and desserts are composed—with transparent windows and transparent ovens, so a visiting child feels he's part of a theatrical event.

Fascinated by the idea of teaching good nutrition—"We had a chance to do something with food for children at the age when their tastes are being formed"—Baum still wanted the lessons to be fun. So far, he's had no complaints, though french fries and Devil Dogs are conspicuously missing from the menu.

At Windows on the World and The Four Seasons, Baum may have been willing to tempt adults with sinful chocolate cakes, but the kids at Sesame Place get zucchini cookies called "gadzuchs!" and peanut butter brownies. Sesame Place pizza is made with whole grain flour, and less salt and fat than ordinary pizzas. Sesame Place barbecued chicken legs are baked, not fried. And potato snuffles are potatoes and cheese shaped into rounds and baked. And hot dogs have no nitrites.

"No frying," says Joe Baum. "No sugar. No hamburgers. We're not trying to be kooky, but I have a belief that familiar food drives out unfamiliar. When you have a hamburger on the menu, lots of youngsters don't give the other things a chance."

Although Baum never runs out of enterprises—he recently designed a Scandinavian Food Center in Tokyo and created a food arcade for the Fisher Brothers Manhattan skyscraper, Park Avenue Plaza—he hasn't yet created the theme restaurant of his dreams, where he can play at being the star of old Bing Crosby movies. "I want to have an in-town roadhouse, wear a wing collar, blow smoke through the air-conditioning system, tap-dance on the tables, and serve chicken and ribs."

To make good things pay is Baum's stated credo, and toward that end "I work my ass off. It's just the restaurant world, nothing earthshaking, but it gives me a great deal of satisfaction."

Joe Baum believes in what he calls "essences" (for instance, The Big Kitchen, in the World Trade Center, isn't a converted kitchen, it's eight food shops interconnected and decorated with tiles and wooden tables), but there are plenty of restaurateurs who simply go out and buy a stable or an abandoned swimming pool into which they can move tables, chairs, and waiters wearing horse collars or water wings.

In Los Angeles, a man named John Wilson runs nostalgia auctions, providing such objects as complete English bars, knocked down in the mother country, packed up in boxes, and shipped to the USA to be bought by anybody who has the cash. Wilson sold a "paneled room with baronial fireplace" from Barclay's Bank in London to an Oklahoman for $32,500.

His auctions, says Wilson, are attended by "the Who's Who of the theme restaurant business."

Forget about Who's Who. Some theme restaurant hustlers belong in What's That. A hapless feeder can visit a fake monastery (where fake monks wait on table, their sneakered feet peeking out from under long robes) or a pseudosubmarine (where a guy with no money and a lease on a windowless cellar has painted the place green, exposed the pipes, and serves lousy seafood, hoping patrons will feel as though they're underwater).

American ingenuity thrives. In Lincoln, Nebraska, a restaurant called Barrymore's was started in the back of a theater that once was home to touring companies. Nobody knows if any Barrymore ever set foot in the place, although Sarah Bernhardt is reputed to have done so. After the touring and the vaudeville died, the theater was converted to a movie house, by dint of dropping a movie screen in front of the stage. Since none of the backstage space, upstage space, or wings were any longer in use, an enterprising restaurant person built a wall between the screen and the backstage area and started serving food on the boards where once song-and-dance men crooned and shuffled. The waiters are called stagehands, and customers enter through the old stage door.

In the port city of Savannah, Georgia, a restaurant called The Pirates' House advertises itself on postcards as having been "a rendezvous for bloodthirsty pirates and sailors." According to the restaurant's literature, unsuspecting seamen were shanghaied from The Pirates' House, and "stories still persist of a tunnel, extending from the old Rum Cellar beneath the Captain's Room to the river, through which these men were carried, drugged and unconscious, to ships waiting in the harbor."

The underground tunnel may be a myth, but there's a nice hole in the restaurant's floor (a hole with a fence around it) that is reputed to be the way into a cavern where pirates once hid, and if you go to The Pirates' House with little children, they're given pirates' masks to wear, and mommies have to poke food through the mouth slots.

Gregg's Greenhouse, a restaurant in Sarasota, Florida, thrives in the midst of three acres of natural jungle. Diners are given a "landscape index" that helps them to identify Confederate Jasmine, or a Monkey Puzzle Tree, as they sit looking out of a mostly glass house. And in La Jolla, California, there's a place called The Torrey Club that has taken for its theme New Money. The *nouveaux riches* are welcome there. The Torrey Club probably doesn't think of itself as having a theme, but *Restaurant Business* magazine says the establishment's brochure "boasts that millionaires-at-30 can mingle in the sauna with Nobel laureates, that Rolls-Royces park next to Porsches," and that "the newspapers lying around are most likely to be the *Wall Street Journal* and *Barron's*."

A feeling of security, even a false feeling, is lovely while it lasts, or so many people wouldn't still be taking tea in the Scott Fitzgerald-haunted Palm Court of the Plaza Hotel. (For those who require a more hard-edged sense of safety, there's an eating place in Houston, Texas, that was converted from a bank. And "the most sought-after tables at the Ballatori Italian Restaurant," a news dispatch from Houston tells us, "are actually positioned inside an enormous steel vault.")

The smell of money—new or old—may sharpen the appetite, but if we separate hunger for riches from simple, fat-forming greed, we raise a question: Does simple, fat-forming greed qualify as a theme in view of the fact that All You Can Eat places have recently given way to All You Can Eat and More places, and Too Much Ain't Enough places?

Probably not, unless the menus and draperies are spun of cheese and chocolate. (The gingerbread house to which the witch lured Hansel and Gretel may have been the first theme restaurant, at least for the proprietor.)

But even when Americans aren't eating in theme restaurants, or in great French restaurants, they're still eating out. If we're not putting on the dog, we're packing away the hot dogs. And sometimes we're doing it very, very fast. ("Let me show you how to cut your eating time in half, and triple your consumption in five days," wrote Marshall Efron and Alfa-Betty Olsen, fooling around in a humor book.)

America's speed eating: it's the rock on which Ray Kroc founded his empire.

PUTTING IT ON:
We're fat because of french fries and Fribbles.

7 Fast Foods: From Oeufs à la Neige to Egg McMuffin

She helped him to lean, and she helped him to fat,
And it look'd like hare—but it might have been cat.
—REV. RICHARD HARRIS BARHAM

ALMOST NO ONE breathes who hasn't at one time wondered just exactly what the hell—galoshes? pulverized shells? porcupine meat?—was in the hamburger he'd just bitten down on, but Ray Kroc's burgers aren't hare or cat or shredded Band-Aids, either; according to him, they're 100 percent beef.

Kroc sold more than twenty-five billion hamburgers in less than twenty-five years, and shared with the world his life story in a book he wrote with Robert Anderson called *Grinding It Out: The Making of McDonald's*. ("Work," he wrote on page 15, "is the meat in the hamburger of life.")

A feisty kid who disliked school, except for debating—"I would not have hesitated to bite a debate opponent if it would have advanced my argument"—Kroc was feisty but fifty before he struck it rich. He'd been a traveling salesman, hawking, at different times, coffee beans, paper cups, and Multimixers (machines that agitated six milk shakes at once).

In 1954, he came to San Bernardino, California, where he encountered two brothers, Maurice and Richard McDonald, who owned a drive-in restaurant.

"It was a restaurant stripped down to the minimum in service and menu, the prototype for legions of fast-food units that would later spread across the land," Kroc informs us. "Hamburgers, fries, and beverages were prepared on an assembly-line basis, and to the amazement of everyone, Mac and Dick included, the thing worked!"

(The McDonald brothers hadn't invented the fast-food business, they'd simply tapped into a strain that ran deep through the American character. "In stagecoach days," wrote Gerald Carson in *Cornflake Crusade*, "when the tavern keeper rang the dinner bell, the customers rushed from the washing pump to long tables, just as they later learned to slide on and off the stool of a railroad café in fifteen minutes . . . The pattern was 'gobble, gulp, and go.' The American gentleman, whom Mrs. Trollope characterized as 'George Washington Spitchew,' ate with blinding speed, shoveled his victuals in with his knife and swore while he did it. Afterwards and briefly, he cleaned his teeth with a pocket knife.")

In addition to their San Bernardino place, Mac and Dick McDonald had licensed ten other drive-ins, but Ray Kroc was scornful of such limited vision. Why not a hundred McDonald'ses? Why not a thousand?

No thanks, said the brothers, they didn't want to work that hard. If Kroc would like to push ahead, they'd sign a contract permitting him to use the McDonald's name, idea, everything. The deal was simple. Kroc would find suitable locations and landlords willing to build restaurants to his specifications, and then he would issue twenty-year licenses to franchisees. The franchisees would pay 1.9 percent of their gross profits to Kroc, who in turn would give the McDonald brothers .5 percent of his take.

"It requires a certain kind of mind to see beauty in a hamburger bun," says Kroc in his book, but he saves his real eloquence for the McDonald's hamburger patty, "a piece of meat with character. The first thing that distinguishes it from the patties that many other places pass off as hamburgers is that it is all beef. There are no hearts or other alien goodies ground into our patties. The fat content of our patty is a prescribed nineteen percent and it is rigidly controlled."

A glib talker (his tongue as fast as his food) and a ferocious adversary ("More than once at two o'clock in the morning I have sorted through a competitor's garbage to see how many boxes of meat he'd used the day before, how many packages of buns"), Kroc built a sultanate, and somewhere along the way he fell in love with a blonde named Joni, which falling caused him to dump his wife of thirty-eight years. "She wound up getting everything I had except my McDonald's stock. She got the house, the car, all the insurance, and $30,000 a year for life. I was happy to pay the alimony. I respected Ethel . . . she was a lovely person and a wonderful homemaker . . ."

As it developed, the McDonald's stock in which he so fervently trusted ("I believe in God, family, and McDonald's—and in the office, that order is reversed") would keep the wolf from Kroc's door, although Joni, his adored one, disappointed him by deciding not to leave her husband and child. Old Ray kept on trucking. "Hamburger University" was started in the basement of a McDonald's store outside Chicago, and there students came to learn how to be more perfect McDonald's employees. ("We award them a Bachelor of Hamburgerology degree with a minor in French fries.")

Kroc married a second time, built a dream house, took McDonald's stock public, became a millionaire, and in 1966 began experimenting with inside seating for those customers who had grown tired of eating in their cars.

In 1969, Joni finally elected to become Mrs. Kroc, to which end she divorced the mister. Now Ray had to deep-six Mrs. Kroc number two, who seems to have surrendered without a whimper. "Jane still lives in our Beverly Hills home," wrote Kroc in his book, "and I continue to see some of her relatives who are long-time McDonald's operators."

So it shouldn't be a total loss.

Kroc kept pushing into places where other entrepreneurs might have feared to go, partly because a Kroc cohort, Luigi Salvaneschi, had evolved a theory called "the monotony index."

"Luigi's idea was that the higher the level of monotony in a town, the better McDonald's' chances of doing business there," Kroc recalls. "'In big cities with all kinds of shops and restaurants, you are only one of thousands of choices,' Luigi said. 'But when you go into areas where there is nothing to do on Sunday afternoon, and people do not know how to spend their free time, your rate of frequency will go up dramatically. And there are literally thousands of areas where the monotony index is very high. These are people forgotten by industry and bypassed by superhighways and shopping centers, yet they are important to us. The heart of America is still in the boonies.'"

The behind of America, too. Good thinking, Luigi. Makes you realize how much business McDonald's could have done if the company had been able to break into Sing Sing or any other slammer where the monotony index is mandated by the State.

Over the years, McDonald's added to its menu. Some of the additions, like Filet-O-Fish, Big Mac ("two all-beef patties, special sauce, lettuce, cheese, pickles, onions on a sesame seed bun"), Hot Apple Pie, and Egg McMuffin (which opened up a breakfast trade for the chain) were winners. Others, like the Hulaburger, which combined pineapple and cheese, and was invented by Kroc himself, flopped.

An occasional fiasco didn't mean that Kroc needed to worry. He owned seven million shares of McDonald's stock, a condominium in Chicago, a ranch in California, and the San Diego Padres baseball team. He turned the running of the Padres over to his stepson-in-law after the commissioner of baseball, Bowie Kuhn, fined him $100,000 for daring to say he'd be interested in buying certain baseball stars for his team if said stars became free agents. After his dustup with the commissioner, Kroc was—briefly—downcast. "The fun is all gone for me," he said. "Baseball has brought me nothing but aggravation."

(For starters, he'd suffered aggravation when the Padres were training in Yuma, Arizona. Before heading out to the ballfield on a sunny afternoon, Kroc had decided to check out a McDonald's franchise and, to his distress, was recognized by the man behind the counter. "I don't understand it," he complained to Buzzie Bavasi who was managing the Padres at the time. "I just walked in and ordered a hamburger like anybody." Bavasi, according to columnist Red Smith, said sure. "In Yuma, Arizona, Ray, a guy pulls up behind a chauffeur in a white Rolls-Royce and orders a hamburger every day.")

Shortly before Christmas of 1979, Ray Kroc suffered a stroke, was taken to a hospital in La Jolla, California, and later moved to an alcoholic treatment center because "I am required to take medication which is incompatible with the use of alcohol." He was seventy-six years old, and his luck seemed to be fading, but nobody looking over the tip sheet that dealt with his past performance would bet against him.

At the time Kroc's book came out, in 1977, McDonald's had just opened its four thousandth restaurant. Kroc dreamed of five thousand.

"I've been dreaming all my life, and I'm sure as hell not going to stop now." By summer of 1979, McDonald's boasted more than 5,200 units in the United States alone.

Six years earlier, impressed by the success of Big Mac, *Time* had run a cover story entitled "The Burger That Conquered the Country." Inside the magazine, tastemakers (aesthetic as well as culinary) testified for and against McDonald's. Craig Claiborne and Julia Child were high on the French fries, Gael Greene loved the Big Mac ("an incredibly decadent eating experience"), Jim Beard admired the packaging and the help and said the food might be "more honest than some things you get at higher prices."

On the other hand, writer Vance Packard charged that McDonald's embodied what was worst about America, "blandness and standardization," writer Vance Bourjaily took the chain's popularity as a sign that America was a "failing culture," and nutritionist Jean Mayer said we could all get scurvy from "a steady diet of burgers, French fries and synthetic milk shakes."

Scurvy and terminal bulge.

Because Bud Trillin's friend Fats Goldberg (now slender Larry Goldberg) was telling the truth, he didn't get plump from *coq au vin*. (See Chapter Four.) At one time, Goldberg weighed over 300 pounds, was a nonstop eater, and his specialty, Trillin has written, "was always junk food . . . candy bars. Lunch meat sandwiches on white bread. Sweet rolls. Hamburgers. Chili dogs. Coke. . . . When he talks about those days, a lot of his sentences begin with phrases like, 'Then, on the way to lunch, I'd stop off at the Tastee-Freez . . .'"

It was Larry Goldberg, by the way, who after listening to various suggestions about what to name 1979— The Year of the Lusty Woman (*Esquire* magazine), The Year the Giants Are Going to Have a Good Season (William Steig)—suggested The Year of the Fat Person.

He had his reasons. "I think inflation's going to hurt people and they're going to start to cut down and go to a lot of fast-food operations. A lot of burgers, fried fish, white bread." And, he added gloomily, "There are already 50 million overweight people in the United States." (This statistic varies with the speaker who utters it. Mike Wallace says 30 million, Larry Goldberg says 50 million, Joanna Wolper—a TV writer-producer—says 79 million.)

By the time The Year of the Fat Person rolled around, Ray Kroc's demesne had become so integral a part of the American scene that thinkers were moved to turn out serious disquisitions on McDonald's. A man named David Sampson, writing for the Op Ed page of the *New York Times,* appeared to favor the company because it catered to the poor (among whom he evidently did not need, thank God, to number himself). "I like McDonald's," he said. "I don't like the food. I don't like to eat there. I feel uncomfortable when I go in. But I like McDonald's because they seem to care a little."

Even with the poor *and* the rich approving of him, Ray Kroc wasn't able to rest. For ten years, Burger King (8 percent of the fast-food market) and Wendy's International (2 percent) had been chipping away at McDonald's 20 percent. In an ad campaign costing $50 million, Burger King pushed its Whopper as "the best darn burger in the whole wide world," while Wendy's "hot and juicy" slogan helped Wendy's grow from a single store in Columbus, Ohio, to fifteen hundred stores across the country. (Wendy's, by the way, is the only big chain that doesn't use frozen meat.)

With the 80s looming, fear, for the first time, struck the hearts of fast-food tycoons, fear that the boom of the previous decade might be over. The cost of beef was accelerating to the point where it could turn off the consumer. Prices had risen 30 percent in 1978, and another 50 percent increase was being predicted for 1979. "There's a big washout coming," said Wendy's executive R. David Thomas.

Gas shortages were blamed for some of the chains' anxieties. People weren't so ready to hop in the car and drive out for a bite. Also, the rise in the minimum wage meant the chains had to pay their employees better, and therefore had to charge more for their food.

Fast food accounted for 22 percent of total restaurant sales in 1971, and for 35 percent in 1978, but in 1979 (the Goldberg theory of inflation-luring-ever-greater-crowds-to-fast-food-joints notwithstanding) there was suddenly talk of market saturation and diminishing returns.

Howard Johnson, president of the company his father started (by cranking out homemade ice cream in his Quincy, Massachusetts, basement), confirmed that his restaurants had been hurt by the gas crisis in the spring of '79. The following summer, profits had dipped for the first time since Johnson could remember. Describing himself as a man who didn't like surprises—"not bad ones"—Johnson said his company might have to alter its ways. "If we're going to be affected this seriously by long-distance travel, we have to shift to local dining, higher average menu checks, and locations closer to airports." (September of

1979 saw Johnson performing an even more startling shift. Imperial Group, Ltd., Britain's sixth-largest corporation, offered him $630 million in cash for his orange-roofed realm, and he took it.)

Whether or not Americans' travel habits would change radically, the fast-food outfits faced modifications in their operations. Profits were down, prices were up, and customers were bitching. In a *New York Times* piece headlined "The Fast-Food Chains Get Indigestion," Edwin McDowell spoke of resistance to "menu prices that have been raised as many as six times this year."

If it came to the point where a hamburger was no longer a bargain, would customers say nay to it? Ray Kroc looked at the situation and took action. In the summer of '79, he bought TV time and made personal appearances to announce that McDonald's was going to help fight inflation at all company-owned stores by reducing the price of hamburgers and cheeseburgers a straight 10 percent.

The Marriott Corporation, daddy of Roy Rogers fast-food outlets, cried, "Us too," and knocked a few cents off Roy's hamburgers and cheeseburgers. Talk of a "burger war" ensued, but it was just talk. The rest of the fast-food chains stood pat. Or patty. "At this time we do not have any plans to respond in like manner," said a Burger King spokesman. Right on, cried executives of Wendy's and Ralston-Purina, which owns Jack-in-the-Box.

Nonetheless, all the chains were reviewing the sudden shift in their fortunes. Ralston-Purina considered closing a quarter of its Jack-in-the-Box units (the ones in the East and the Midwest); Sambo's, losing money, fired its president; Pizza Hut (owned by Pepsico) saw its profits fall off twelve million dollars in a single year, despite its introduction of a hot new item, the Taco Pizza; Denny's (based in California, with 760 fast-food units in the United States and Japan, not to mention 888 Winchell's Donut Houses) sank two million dollars into television advertising, hoping to fight a financial slump; and although Burger King still showed nice earnings, its parent company, Pillsbury, was "scaling back somewhat its expansion plans."

Chicken is cheaper than beef, yet the life of the Kentucky Fried Chicken company hadn't been all downy either. In 1964, Colonel Harlan Sanders sold out to a Louisville group, which in turn sold out to Heublein, Inc.—legs, wings, and secret recipe. The year was 1971, and the Colonel was expected to go on boosting the product, even though he no longer controlled it. In July of 1975, he gave a newspaper interview in Bowling Green, Kentucky, during the course of which he said the new extra-crispy Kentucky Fried was "a damn fried doughball stuck on some chicken," and pronounced the Kentucky Fried gravy "pure wallpaper paste."

A while later, the Colonel came to New York, and he and Mimi Sheraton went around to visit some Kentucky Fried stores to see how the product was holding up. The result was an exposé in the *New York Times*. "Finger Lickin' Bad" was Mimi's appraisal. The Colonel's response was equally devastating. He took a single bite and announced soberly, "This is the worst fried chicken I've ever seen."

Pity the poor account executives. Heads are said to have rolled at Heublein—they were paying the Colonel $250,000 a year to be a "goodwill ambassador" but they couldn't come right out and ask him to lie a little—and the story goes that the company had to set up a school to retrain its chicken cookers.

In 1979, the Colonel was still bemoaning the gravy. "It's hard to get the fellas I sold the outfit to to go back makin' the roux and stirrin' the gravy the way they ought to," he told reporter Ira Simmons. "They've had fourteen years doin' it the wrong way."

He wasn't thrilled, either, with a PR brochure entitled *The Colonel's Other Recipes* that included a recipe for barbecued chicken. "That barbecued chicken," said the Colonel to Ira Simmons, "that's a bunch of shit." The old gentleman, who died in December of 1980, continued to speak his mind, but toward the end, he seemed to have come to terms with the extra-crispy stuff—"There's a place for it," he said grudgingly. So the Kentucky Fried brass might have breathed easy again, convinced they were succeeding in their efforts to keep the nation fowl-mouthed, had they not found themselves being battered by other chicken outfits like Church's Fried Chicken, Popeye's Famous Fried Chicken, Tom Sawyer's Old-Fashioned Krispy Chicken, Inc., and Ron's Krispy Fried Chicken, all fighting for a share of the shrinking Yankee dollar.

Were fast-food chains in trouble? Apparently. Would they survive? You bet. "I'm rather bullish on the industry," said analyst William Hale, an employee of a research firm in Massachusetts. "Because if consumers have the dollars, they'll continue to opt to have someone else buy the food, prepare it, serve it, and then clean up."

Little chains might fold, but the big boys would prevail (dozens of frozen yogurt stores came and went; Tom Carvel and his ice-cream empire endured).

During the course of a speech at a nutrition conference in May of 1979, Columbia Professor Joan Gussow told her listeners that a poll had shown eating out to be America's favorite recreation. "It may say something about our tolerance for any kind of extended activity," commented the professor, "that several of my students did observations of people eating at fast-food restaurants and found that however many bites, chews, mouth wipes, or sips they took, they spent only seven minutes on the average polishing off a standard sandwich and a soft drink."

(The prof's point may be well taken, but I say a pox on those students. Isn't it bad enough we bolt our food, without having to be studied like caged apes while we do it?)

The fact is that, even in France, hamburgers and chili and fried chicken have become popular. A Parisian explained to Mimi Sheraton why she liked the casual American-style restaurants that had sprung up around Paris. If she had dinner in one of them, there was still "enough time to see a movie. When we go to a French restaurant, it takes the whole evening."

Keep moving, that's the ticket.

The American family on the move—before and between gas crunches—provided *Time* essayist Paul Gray with material for an entertaining piece on fast food. Printed in the summer of 1977, here in part is what it said:

"Tires hum along the interstate while an afternoon sun reddens behind exhaust fumes. The natives in the back seat are restless . . . The day's second rendition of '99 Bottles of Beer on the Wall' has petered out at bottle No. 37. Now sullen silence prevails, punctuated only by stage whispers to the effect that *some* parents *feed* their kids, for cryinoutloud. Egg McMuffined for breakfast, Burger Kinged at lunch, and Stuckeyed in between, the little ones are hungry again. For that matter, Mom and Dad deserve another break today. A pit stop is called for. Time to eat and run.

"No leisurely backyard picnic for this hypothetical family—or for the millions of real ones who will take to the nation's highways this summer. They want food fast, and fast food they get . . .

"The terms vary: fast food, road food, convenience food, service food or (to the distaste of its producers and the grim delight of its detractors) junk food. Whatever it is called, America's infatuation with such fare is nothing new."

Reasons for the infatuation are obvious. Compared to other restaurant food, fast food is inexpensive. Fast food is of a reasonably dependable quality—if you like a Big Mac in Hoboken, you'll like a Big Mac in San Antone. There are no headwaiters to snub you at a fast-food place, and nobody cares how you dress. There is tremendous—and growing—diversity in fast food, not only burgers and chicken and fish are available, but also Mexican food and Italian food and Greek food and Chinese food. (Remember Archie Bunker's plan to invest in a string of "Chink-aterias"?)

Fast food has become part of the street life of big cities. An article in *New York* magazine noted that, on the sidewalks around Grand Army Plaza at the southeast corner of Central Park, vendors displayed not only the usual hot dogs, but a dazzling variety of refreshments. The pushcarts of summer creaked under loads of nuts, dried fruits, tacos, quiche, cookies, chow mein, pâté, Brie, crepes stuffed with blueberries, iced soups, French sandwiches made of fresh-baked rolls and *saucisson*, pita bread filled with falafel, burritos, skewered chunks of lamb, onions, and tomatoes, hot buttered popcorn, cucumber and yogurt salad, bagels spread with peanut butter and jelly, and even five-ounce shell steaks on club rolls.

One of the Grand Army Plaza drummers, a chap named Tom Green who called himself Tomasino Verdi, hawked his wares like a costermonger out of Dickens or Fielding. "If you're on a diet, you don't wanna try it," cried he of his sausage and meatball heros.

"To Americans over 30," observes Paul Gray, "the glut, the avalanche of fast food may seem the miraculous fulfillment of childhood fantasy. They were raised when Popeye was touting spinach, and it was everyone's duty to finish his vegetables . . . and Mom's idea of dessert was a banana. . . . How did the adults that these children eventually became respond when the forbidden fruits of their youth began dropping down like hot dogs from heaven? . . . millions . . . took on a secret vice, and happily said, 'Pass the mustard.'"

Not all food arbiters consider the love of fast food a vice, but then, at this point in its evolution, the term fast food is an umbrella sheltering everything from spartan, salt-free, sugar-free, fat-free "health" offerings of grasses and grains to delicious greasy stuff that clogs the arteries and sweets that satisfy the soul while they rot the teeth. Talking to a graduating class of the Culinary Institute of America, at Hyde Park, New York, William Rice, executive food editor for the *Washington Post*, told students that fast-food operations had "exposed Americans to foods that once were considered repellant or dismissed as too exotic. Fish sales are booming in Middle America. Szechuan is becoming a household word. Real oregano continues to outsell pot."

We have, said Rice, "crossed a Rubicon in this country. We are now a nation that eats out; it's part of our way of life. In my middle-class boyhood . . . eating out was an occasion caused by a birthday or a visiting relative. Now we Americans eat all manner of foods in all manner of ways away from home. Only hopeless snobs, longing for a yesterday that was for an elite few can—and do—deny the excitement of it."

In February of 1979 (attempting to fight off the sneers of the elite few and the hopeless snobs), representatives of McDonald's, Kentucky Fried Chicken, and Pizza Hut went to Washington to appear before the Nutrition Subcommittee of the Senate Commission on Agriculture, Nutrition, and Forestry. (Want a connection I bet the senators never thought of between nutrition and forestry? Some bakers and food processors are feeding us wood pulp and saying it's roughage, and it's good for us. The "roughage" part is true, the "good for us" has yet to be proved.) Anyway, the fast-food folks wanted to tell the Feds that their provender was chock full of health.

If Mom's chicken dinner was wholesome, why was the Colonel's chicken dinner derided as fast food? demanded an indignant John Mann, vice-president of Kentucky Fried Chicken. The very term fast food, said Mr. Mann, "has become a quick and easy slogan that implies inferiority."

Some heavy hitters outside the fast-food industry supported Mr. Mann's position. "Just because you can get it in a hurry doesn't mean it's junk," said publisher Malcolm Forbes, and nutritionist Dr. Al Roberts of the University of Texas advised us—on television—not to throw all fast foods into the same vat, figuratively speaking, because some fast food was actually *good* nutritionally. "Pizza," he said. "Or a hamburger with lettuce and cheese on a bun." What was not so good were greasy fries and often milkless milk shakes, frappes, fribbles. No matter what you called these drinks, they were, said Dr. Roberts, "sugared oil and straight fat calories."

Consumer Reports, a magazine dedicated to raising the rabble's consciousness about being ripped off, tended to side with Mr. Forbes and Dr. Roberts. "Fast foods are not junk foods," announced *Consumer*

Reports, under the blurb "There's more than empty calories in the fast foods we tested."

The magazine had dispatched "sensory consultants" to check various outlets of Kentucky Fried Chicken, Pizza Hut, Long John Silver's, Arthur Treacher's, Arby's, Wendy's, Burger King, McDonald's, Roy Rogers, Hardee's, and Jack-in-the-Box. Results: The roast beef sandwiches tested ranged from "slightly tough" to "limp or soggy," the fish fillets were too sweet or too dry, the chicken wasn't hot enough, the pizza was skimpy in the tomato and cheese department, all hamburgers tested had "steamed flavor and/or aroma" (some burgers were also "gristly and/or greasy"), all fried potatoes had "slight cardboard flavor and/or aroma" (some fries were also "limp and/or raw tasting"), and most chocolate shakes had "a slight coating and/or gummy afterfeel."

Nonetheless, *Consumer Reports* came down—if not exactly squarely—on the side of fast foods. "Any of the fast food entrees plus French fries and a shake would provide about one-third of all the nutrients you should have in a day."

True, said the magazine, if you were on a sodium-restricted diet, you should watch out, if you were on a fat-restricted diet, you should watch out, if you were on a sugar-restricted diet, you should watch out. ("Our analyses for sugars showed about 40 to 70 grams—from 8 to 14 teaspoons—per shake.")

Still, even though fast foods were "high in calories, fat and sodium," they were "not entirely off-limits. They are acceptable when consumed judiciously, infrequently, and as part of a well-balanced diet."

Summing up, *Consumer Reports* issued a tip that echoed Dr. Roberts. "If you *do* eat fast foods often, you might think about skipping the fries and shakes."

Senator George McGovern, who had been acting as chairman of the Nutrition Subcommittee, was equally inclined to shake, waffle, and roll (and I'm not talking about eating and drinking). McGovern had studied fast foods and his studies had caused him to change his "previously negative opinion." He now believed that "on the whole, quick food establishments provide a nutritional addition to the balanced American diet."

Still, said the senator, almost as an afterthought, he did wonder what the fast-food people were doing to combat obesity and hypertension.

He'd been wondering for years. In 1968, the Senate Select Committee on Nutrition and Human Needs, with McGovern installed as its chairman, had been organized to look at "hunger in America." In 1976, it was still looking (not only at hunger but at obesity, while growing ever more fat and powerful itself) when a Senate study group recommended that it be disbanded and reorganized.

Fighting for its life, the Select Committee called a press conference and issued a publication called *Dietary Goals for the United States*. Congress was not moved, and the Select Committee died, or was at least transmuted into the aforementioned Nutrition Subcommittee with a smaller budget and a much reduced staff. But *Dietary Goals* made some headlines. Its seventy-nine pages contained testimony from experts who warned us that the composition of the average diet in the United States had changed radically since the early part of the century. Consumption of fruit, vegetables, and grains had declined, consumption of fat and sugar had risen. And because diets high in fat and sugar—diets to which low-income people were particularly prone—led to vitamin and mineral deficiencies, and therefore malnutrition, many Americans were starving even as they became ever more gross in appearance.

Twenty percent of the adults in the United States were "overweight to a degree that may interfere with optimal health and longevity," warned Dr. Theodore Cooper, assistant secretary for health, and Senator McGovern issued a statement contending that some leading causes of death—heart disease, cancer, obesity, stroke—were linked to the American diet.

Dr. Mark Hegsted of Harvard (who later became director of the Department of Agriculture's Human Nutrition Center) and Dr. Beverly Winikoff of the Rockefeller Foundation were among the scientists who agreed that America was eating itself into trouble. Dr. Hegsted suggested that we might be better able to tolerate our "increasingly rich" diet if we were more active, and Dr. Winikoff tendered an irony. "Nutrition and health education are offered at the same time as barrages of commercials for soft drinks, sugary snacks, high-fat foods, cigarettes, and alcohol. We put candy machines in our schools, serve high-fat lunches to our children—"

The mills of government grind slowly. It wasn't until the summer of 1979 that the Agriculture Department suggested schools ought not to be allowed to sell gum, sodas, or desserts unless these foods contained "5% of the basic nutrients in the Government's recommended daily dietary allowance."

Too little and too late, howled nutritionists. "Total cave-in to the snack food industry," accused Michael Jacobson, director of the Center for Science in the Public Interest. "They are banning nothing, not even jelly beans," said Columbia's Dr. Gussow, "when you consider how cheap and easy it is to fortify any food with a little vitamin C, and so qualify."

All fast food *isn't* junk food, but all junk food is certainly fast food, and the problem is, we *like* junk food. Kids like junk food and so do their parents. Read this testimonial to the Ohio State Fair, characterized as "the Cannes of junk food" by Michael Harden, an editor of *Ohio* magazine:

"Anything that is edible and can be impaled on a stick is sold at the Fair. There are hot dogs on sticks, roasting ears on sticks, Swiss cheese cubes on sticks, ice cream on sticks, bananas on sticks. There are bologna burgers, sandwiches made from pulverized chick peas, and enough Narragansett Bay fudge to repave the Ohio turnpike. There is a sandwich called the Schwarma made from highly seasoned meats and pita bread. It is delicious. But it leaves one with breath that could drop a chihuahua 15 yards away."

Many of the Fair's junk-food lovers "travel indiscriminately from stand to stand eating everything in sight," says Harden. Harden has a friend who insists junk food can't hurt you, but who adds a caveat. "Never eat anything you can't pronounce because that's always the first question they ask in the emergency room."

Even among the muscular and, one would expect, health-minded, a seeker after truth can uncover a longing for chili dogs. Take the case of Lynn Lemaire, a champion swimmer, marathon runner, bike racer, and avowed "junk-food fiend." Lynn (at 5′6″ and 148 pounds, she's no sylph) excuses herself on the flimsiest of pretexts. "It's hard to find bean sprouts on the road," she says.

One last observation: a hankering for junk food can lead to a double life, or we would never have had the wrenching confessions of Larry Groce, as served up in his immortal song hit, "Junk Food Junkie." Larry Groce, who sneaked home at night and unlocked his strong-box and took out "some Fritos corn chips, Dr Pepper, and an old Moon Pie," and then sat back waiting to be hit by "a genuine junk food high."

I'm a friend to old Euell Gibbons,
And I only eat home grown spice,
I got a John Keats autograph Grecian urn filled
up with my brown rice.

Oh, but lately I have been spotted with a Big Mac
on my breath
Stumblin' into a Colonel Sanders with a face as
white as death.
I'm afraid some day they'll find me just stretched
out on my bed
With a handful of Pringle's potato chips and a Ding-
Dong by my head.
In the daytime, I'm Mister Natural, just as healthy
as I can be
But at night I'm a Junk Food Junkie, Good Lord, have
pity on me.

Nobody could top that. A smart person wouldn't even try.

PUTTING IT ON:
We're fat because Sara Lee and Duncan Hines and Betty Crocker and Clarence Birdseye make it so easy for us.

8 Convenience Foods: Like Taking Candy From a Baby

I find no sweeter fat than sticks to my own bones.
—WALT WHITMAN

I REMEMBER arriving in Palm Beach once, coming in from the cold of New York. All over town, oranges were hanging from the trees, oranges lay fallen in the grass, and I went to a restaurant for breakfast and ordered orange juice. The juice the waitress brought me was frozen, or out of a carton, I can't remember which, I only remember my outrage.

For all the good it did me. Nobody in that restaurant was going to squeeze oranges; if God had meant us to squeeze oranges or shell peas or peel potatoes or bake bread or bone a halibut, He wouldn't have given us flavor enhancers and antioxidants and emulsifiers and thickeners and dough conditioners and Mrs. Paul's fish sticks.

And He certainly wouldn't have sent us the tin can. Actually, He didn't send it to us; He sent it to the English. A chap named Peter Durand conceived and patented the idea of using tin cans in the 1830s. (Even before this, in 1795, a Frenchman named Appert had worked out the *art de conserver les substances animales et végétales* by putting food into glass bottles and sealing and heating the bottles. This made the

French government very happy because it was trying to feed its army and navy, and the army and navy had their hands full fighting wars "with several hostile European nations," not to mention a revolution at home, and there was no time to go looking for Chinese restaurants.)

An Englishman may have started us down the road to tin cans, but it was Americans who became the biggest producers and consumers of canned foods in the world.

Joke from my childhood:

American to Englishman: "We eat what we can, and what we can't, we can."

Englishman to American: "Very amusing."

Same Englishman, an hour later, to another Englishman: "Americans are droll. They eat what they can, and what they can't, they tin."

We started tinning in 1839, and by the 1960s, we were packing 700 million cases a year with fruits and vegetables and milk and meat and fish and juices.

Trains were an integral part of the equation. From 1830 on (with a bit of slowing down for the Civil War), the country was connected by railroads carrying goods from one town to another. Local brands became national brands. Walter Baker could send his chocolate wherever he liked, Gail Borden could have his condensed milk—first marketed in 1856—transported, and the Kellogg brothers could cover the planet with cornflakes.

Looking at the history of dry breakfast cereals is as good a way as any to begin to understand the impact of convenience foods on American life. The first cold breakfast food, Granula—a mix of graham flour and water, twice baked, twice ground—was devised by a Dr. James Jackson in 1863. Dr. Jackson ran a sanatorium dedicated to water cures and vegetarianism; his patients munched graham crackers, talked about "swine poisoning," and threw away the medicines they had been given by more orthodox M.D.'s.

In 1878, Dr. John Harvey Kellogg began to manufacture a "health" cereal called Granola (he'd called it Granula till the Granula people sued) and in 1893, a fellow named Henry Persky invented shredded wheat. The people who first tried it said it was like "eating a whisk broom," but Persky hung in and improved his process. By 1898, C. W. Post had come out with Grape-Nuts, and Dr. Kellogg's company issued the first cornflakes. (There was pirating back and forth. C. W. Post got the idea for Postum from a coffee substitute he'd drunk while a patient at

Dr. Kellogg's Battle Creek Sanatarium, but Post never felt he was poaching. After all, Kellogg's cereal brew had tasted "horrible," whereas Postum was delicious. And if Post borrowed from Kellogg, hadn't Kellogg built on the work of Dr. Jackson?)

Americans were ready to reform their breakfast habits. Partly, they were worried about their children. (A. J. Bellows, in a book called *The Philosophy of Eating*, indicted Scotch and Irish immigrants for rejecting the oatmeal and barley cakes of their native lands, and falling into "our starch and grease eating habits," thereby causing their offspring to become "as pale, puny, and toothless as pure-blooded Yankees.") And partly, housewives welcomed their release from standing over hot stoves in the mornings.

Dry breakfast cereals became the rage. Wheat, corn, bran, anything that could be poured out of a box and into a bowl. Between 1902 and 1904, Battle Creek, Michigan, saw such a cereal and breakfast drink boom that people were comparing the fever to an oil or a gold rush. Forty-two food companies were founded in a city that had only thirty thousand inhabitants. In the year 1903, the Postum Cereal Company (which grew up to marry the Jell-O Company, and eventually became part of the General Foods Corporation) registered a net profit of $1,100,000.

With breakfast made easier, could lunch and dinner lag far behind? Particularly when there was so much money to be won, so much leisure to be gained, so much pleasure to be found in trying something new?

A General Mills salesman latched onto the idea of Bisquick after having a meal in a railroad dining car and discovering the chef kept a store of ready-mixed lard, flour, baking powder, and salt in an ice chest. This enabled the chef to produce biscuits in a matter of minutes, without bothering to sift or measure. General Mills substituted sesame oil for lard, but Bisquick isn't very different today than it was almost fifty years ago.

Another salesman thought up macaroni and cheese dinners ("How the deuce did you make this keen macaroni and cheese so fast? Why we just got home" says a 1937 ad) in order to help Kraft sell more of its American cheese. At ten cents a box, the dinner was a bargain, and the instructions on the blue carton that contained two ounces of cheese and six ounces of macaroni promised you could "make a meal for 4 in 9 minutes."

Glass jars, cans, and cartons are only part of the story. In the name of convenience, foods have been dried, desiccated, salted, pickled, frozen (Clarence Birdseye was doing experiments in 1917, but the first Birds Eye commercial pack didn't hit the market till 1929), and irradiated. Irradiation kills bacteria by subjecting it to ultraviolet rays. Irradiated ham and irradiated cheese went along on the Apollo mission in 1975, and in 1979, the Army said it had kept irradiated bacon for four years without refrigeration. The bacon was still "of acceptable quality." In 1979, the Army was also getting ready to try out repasts packaged in flexible pouches (which, again, had first been used by the astronauts). The pouch meals would include such fare as chicken à la king, and would be a nice change for soldiers on maneuvers, eliminating the need to carry heavy cans and to remember to pack can openers.

It was time noncoms got a break. In the Revolutionary War, soldiers had to steal to eat; in the War of 1812 and the Civil War, the men subsisted mostly on pork, flour, beans, and coffee, and during the Spanish-American belligerency, our War Department insisted it could feed a man on eighteen cents a day. What it fed him was meat, tired from standing on the docks in the sun. Antiseptics were sometimes added so the meat wouldn't kill the soldiers before the enemy could. The soldiers called this delicacy "embalmed beef."

Instant coffee appeared during World War I, Spam (canned lunch meat that could be eaten hot or cold) appeared during World War II. Technology achieved in the service of war was turned to peacetime use as soon as the fighting stopped, for which the housewives of many nations have ever since been grateful.

In the aftermath of World War II, we got instant puddings, instant coffee, instant tea. By the 50s, we had instant mashed potatoes, and Swanson TV dinners. Realizing the potential of quick-freezing, Carl Swanson, a Swedish immigrant, had gone into the food business in Omaha in the 1920s. He automated the plucking and gutting of the birds in his chicken factory, and he mass-produced powdered eggs. By 1951, his sons, Gilbert and Clarke, had introduced frozen chicken pot pie to the country, and by 1953, the first frozen turkey dinner had appeared, packed in the compartmentalized aluminum tray so many kids have grown up thinking of as the family china. (In 1955, the Swansons sold out to the Campbell Soup Company, but the Swanson name stayed on the dinners.)

In the 60s, our know-how had accelerated to the point where we could achieve totally fake foods. You've heard the maxim "Man proposes, God disposes"? Well, modern science turned that around. God proposed orange juice and cows (from which we got whipping cream), man disposed of all that natural jazz, and brought us Tang and Cool Whip.

You think you won't get fat if you eat faked whipped cream? Think again. "Packaged synthetic toppings," say Ruth Fremes and Dr. Zak Sabry, "are just as saturated as real whipped cream, and real milk or table cream has much less fat than whipped cream or the substitutes."

Fremes and Sabry (a Canadian team who worked together on a nutrition survey) charge that food labels seldom indicate the amounts of saturated fats used in processed foods, or even the kinds of fats. Powdered, frozen, or liquid coffee creamers use palm oil, coconut oil, and saturated fats interchangeably. And, demand Fremes and Sabry, "what of all the other products like chips, convenience spreads and cookies? What oil is in them? We don't know and won't know without some government regulations and industry cooperation. Until it becomes mandatory for manufacturers to declare the type of oil on the labels of food with vegetable oil listed, we would recommend that you stay away from all commercial snack foods, including potato chips, baked goods, crackers and all mixes."

Toward the end of 1979, the Food and Drug Administration and the Agriculture Department came together to announce that they were going to try to overhaul the food labeling laws, since more than half of all food being consumed by Americans was processed food.

The agencies' case was put by Carol Tucker Foreman, an assistant secretary of agriculture. "I don't think it should be necessary," she said, "for any consumer to go to the supermarket with a science background, a magnifying glass, or a Ouija board."

But on the basis of experience, getting a new labeling law through Congress would be easier talked about than done, and even if we finally achieve jars that tell us how many shrimp in a shrimp cocktail, there probably still will be some additives not listed on our labels.

I'm not talking about soybean substitutes, either.

In a piece he contributed to a book called *Junk Food,* Harry Crews writes of sitting in a motel dining room, watching an old lady finish off a bowl of soup and a little package of crackers. Once, he'd worked for the company that made the crackers. "My job at the cracker factory was to dump 100-pound bags of flour down a chute that led into a set of grinders resembling the gearbox of an automobile. The only trouble was that rats liked to tunnel into the flour bags stacked in the warehouse and live there. All day long I had to listen to the squealing of whole generations of rat families being shredded into cracker mix . . .

"I sat there watching that old lady eat and wondered whether or not Ralph Nader and his boys had succeeded in getting the rat hair and fecal matter out of those crackers yet."

Ugh, Harry. You and your pesky The truth shall set you free.

There *is* something called the "defect action level" that spells out the amount of foreign matter the United States government will tolerate in any given food. The FDA sets these levels for all foods—fresh, frozen, canned, dried—and if the levels are exceeded, the FDA can seize and destroy the offending foods. (For something like fresh shrimp, the "defect action level" tells how much decomposition is allowed.)

The amount of foreign matter acceptable to the FDA differs from product to product. A few examples:

Peanut butter. There can be "no more than thirty insect fragments per 100 grams," and only "one rodent hair per 100 grams."

Crushed pineapple (canned). The "microscopic mold count cannot exceed 30 percent," and if the crushed pineapple is found to have "slime mold," that "slime mold cannot exceed 20 percent" per 100 microscopic fields examined."

Canned mushrooms. The FDA allows "an average of twenty maggots of any size per 100 grams of canned mushrooms."

If that depresses you, be glad you didn't live in the 1800s. In *Food, Nutrition and You* (Prentice-Hall, 1977), Fergus Clydesdale and Frederick James Francis say we've come a long way down the road to safer foods. It wasn't until 1902 that "Dr. Harvey W. Wiley established what became known as 'Dr. Wiley's poison squad.'"

Back then, say Clydesdale and Francis, "there were no checks at all, people could add almost whatever they wanted to their foods, and as long as they didn't kill someone, these additives did not have to be tested or screened by any governmental agency. Volunteers for this 'poison squad' were recruited from among the employees of the Department of Agriculture. Dr. Wiley said, 'I wanted young, robust fellows with maximum resistance to deleterious effects of adulterated foods . . . If they should show signs of injury after they were fed such substances for a period of time, the deduction would naturally follow that children and older persons more susceptible than they would be greater sufferers from similar causes.'

"Twelve men volunteered. This squad was responsible for taking many dangerous food additives off the market . . ."

Even today, there are no federal standards of cleanliness for certain convenience foods. In a piece on pancake mixes, *Consumer Reports* found that most of the 222 samples of mixes and batters they tested contained insect fragments and whole insects. "Since the packages were tightly sealed, it's probable that the contamination occurred during processing," deduced the investigators. "The levels of contamination weren't what we'd consider a hazard, but they weren't what we'd consider appetizing, either."

A 1972 report from the U.S. Department of Agriculture said the American eater's shift from fresh produce to processed fruits and vegetables had resulted in a decline in "nutrients obtained from this food group," and mentioned in passing that potato chips and dehydrated potatoes ought not to be considered the nutritional equivalent of freshly baked spuds. Fried and dehydrated potatoes not only furnish less protein, but compared to the .1 percent fat in baked potatoes, potato chips contain 40 percent fat. (A baked potato, incidentally, has only 80 calories. It's the butter and sour cream we add that brings the calorie count up to 350.)

By 1980, the government was concerned not only with new labeling laws, but with the American diet in general. In February of 1980, HEW and the Agriculture Department jointly issued a series of dietary guidelines, and offered a 20-page booklet, *Nutrition and Your Health,* to any consumer who wrote and asked for it.

The booklet didn't contain really big news. "Scientists in the Government's food and health agencies" advised us to eat a variety of foods, to eat foods with adequate starch and fiber, to avoid too much fat, saturated fat and cholesterol, too much sugar, too much salt, and too much alcohol.

It was a call for moderation, not a prescription, said Agriculture Secretary Robert Bergland.

But quicker than you could say "Ah, the hell with it, pass the hot dogs," the recommendations (which weren't very different from the dietary goals issued in 1977 by the Senate Committee on Nutrition and Human Needs) came under attack.

"We feel that the Government should continue to openly acknowledge that the diet-disease issue is not resolved," said Merlyn Carlson, president of the National Cattlemen's Association. "By repeating statements about saturated fat and cholesterol, the Government is perpetuating a theory which is unproven."

Predictably, producers of eggs and dairy products weren't thrilled either, and even the American Medical Association had its doubts. Dr. Philip White, head of the AMA's Council on Food and Nutrition, said the government's guidelines seemed to "imply that all people now eat in the same way and would benefit from a reduction in fat or sugar or salt. The whole population should not be treated as if it were at risk or falling prey to diet-related diseases."

Carol Foreman, whose appointment to Agriculture three years earlier had not been uneventful ("Some of the farm and food industry was in total panic about a consumer advocate coming into the Department," she said, "but the roof is still on"), went serenely forward, talking about using leaner meat and less salt in school lunches, while controversy raged around her.

And still, some voices of sweet reason could be heard, calling for balance and moderation.

"Fortunately," wrote Mimi Sheraton in the *New York Times*, "good eating along traditional lines and sound nutrition espoused by the guidelines are not mutually exclusive."

As for Americans who had too high an intake of saturated fats, Mimi suggested those fats weren't coming from goose liver pâtés, "but from French fries, deep-fried chicken, and fried fish sandwiches sold in fast-food chains, or from processed foods that use coconut oil, lard, or solid vegetable shortenings, some for flavor, others for price or long shelf life."

Columbia University's Dr. Joan Gussow concurred. "Once in a while, if I feel like having a quiche, I do not want it to be made with artificial bits of bacon, and egg substitutes," she said. "And when I make mashed potatoes, they are full of real butter. I would rather have terrific mashed potatoes once a year than have them all the time if they taste like water."

Just so, said Mimi Sheraton. Have your hollandaise sauce, she told her readers, "and then don't eat any eggs or butter for the next couple of days. That is a far more satisfying solution than to prepare a mawkish imposter of a hollandaise sauce that combines safflower oil and artificial eggs."

Processed foods are not only heavy with oils, but they cost us more.

Again, a report from the Department of Agriculture, after a study comparing home-prepared foods with convenience foods: "The cost of home-prepared batter-dipped chicken was less than one third of the cost of the convenience product. Both chicken à la king frozen in a pouch and canned chicken salad spread were about 60 percent more expensive per serving . . . Consumers paid approximately 40 cents more per serving for frozen turkey dinner or tetrazzini than for the separate ingredients."

A lot of convenience foods, said Patricia Wells in the *New York Times*, weren't convenient. That is, they didn't save much time. "It is hard to imagine any kitchen preparation simpler and quicker than slicing mushrooms to sauté in butter, or blanching a stalk of fresh broccoli. But consumers pay dearly for the questionable convenience of an item such as frozen sautéed mushrooms selling for ninety-five cents per six-ounce package, or sixteen cents an ounce. Fresh mushrooms cost less than ten cents an ounce, while an ounce of real butter costs just two cents."

(For certain disconsolate gourmets, even fresh fruits and vegetables have lost their savor. Since produce can be shipped green—thanks to planes and to refrigerated trucks, trains, and ships—instead of being left to ripen on the vine or the tree or the bush, you have the paradox of strawberries appearing amidst January snows, and strawberry fanciers crying that they're tasteless.

The cry is worldwide. A British writer says brussels sprouts "are no good until they get the frost on them, the same applies to celery. It never used to be possible to get either before the first frosts, now they are forced and marketed all the year round.")

In her newspaper column, Miss Wells suggested alternatives to convenience foods—eggs ("they can quickly be turned into omelets and soufflés better than anything the frozen food case has to offer") or pasta, cheap and delicious, tossed with "a bit of garlic, oil, and fresh basil."

But she knew she was whistling down the wind. "We are a nation utterly addicted to convenience foods," she lamented.

Not just at home, either. Essayist Enid Nemy found herself amused by trekkers headed for Europe laden down with Hellmann's Mayonnaise, and Oreos, and Aunt Jemima Pancake Mix, and Mrs. Butterworth's Syrup, and Nathan's frankfurters. "The cans, bottles and boxes carried by traveling Americans to friends abroad (both American and foreign friends) defy reason," Nemy observed.

But a passion for Sara Lee has little to do with reason. People argue for and against convenience foods with so much brio that it takes only a few seconds to whip up a first-class fight.

Consider epidemiologist Elizabeth Whelan, a research associate at Harvard who also runs a radio show about health and writes books and articles on diet. Despite the fact that there are more than thirteen hundred food additives currently approved by the Food and Drug Administration for use as colors, flavors, preservatives, etc., Dr. Whelan says there is no processed food she's afraid to eat because it might make her sick. (There *are* foods she's afraid to eat because they'll make her fat. She once bought a jar of wheat germ, but read the label, found a tablespoon was 36 calories, and jettisoned the substance.)

Whelan is against smoking, against the careless dumping of chemicals, and against the "misuse of scientific data." We can, she says, "have good health *and* the benefits of technology."

The benefits of technology get a boost from the *Encyclopaedia Britannica* too. Its contributing editors appear to think more highly of meals prepared in factories than of meals prepared at home. "It is clear," says the *Britannica*, "that the modern food processor, with his scientific control, large-scale operation, and use of raw materials in their prime, has many advantages over the cook or housewife."

Clear to whom? ask the anticonvenience factions. The *Washington Post* reported that inmates of a Maryland jail, fed TV dinners, hurled their trays against the walls, but after a switch to fresh foods prepared by an inmate chef, complaints petered out. The *Washington Star* ran an editorial along the same lines, dealing with children rather than convicts, and praising the work of a public health nutritionist, Mary Godwin. "The pleasures of seeing, smelling and tasting food that looks, smells, and tastes good," asserted the *Star*, "nourish the personality with sensuous experience even as the vitamins and minerals are making their contribution to the growth of bone and muscle. An awareness of real people preparing and serving the food helps too.

"Which is to say that if you eat enough precooked, frozen, reheated foil and plastic packed lunches out of machines, part of you will starve to death. On site food preparation—most important of all—is, in her [Mary Godwin's] words 'a way of keeping children in contact with the real world rather than a highly mechanized, impersonal one.'"

So there. For the mommy who has everything, something extra. Along with Special K, special guilt. One reason convenience foods permeate American life is that women feel they need them. Women are working, women are tired at night, they don't want to cook from scratch, they don't want to come home and start scraping carrots and grinding spices and beating drops of oil into egg yolks to make mayonnaise, and as long as they have those darling plastic bags packed with broccoli and cheese sauce, they don't have to.

The food companies are responding to a real demand. But lots of women are having trouble letting themselves off the hook.

One of the bits of fallout from this residual female guilt can be noted in the weekend orgy. (Interesting sociological change: People used to go to restaurants for treat meals, and stay home for ham and eggs. These days, fast-food joints get much of the family's nightly dinner trade, and the big fancy spread is prepared, in conjunction with Julia Child, at home, on the weekend.) It's as though the genetic impulses are too strong to be tamped down. Talk to a woman who doesn't cook during the week—whether she's not cooking because she's out at Burger King, or not cooking because even though she's at home, Swanson's and Birds Eye and Duncan Hines and Betty Crocker and Kraft and Stouffer's have done it for her—and you may find an uneasy woman. If she then decides to invite guests for dinner on Saturday night, she's apt to spend hours fussing in the kitchen, rather than laying on something casual.

(Women who work at home are even more addicted to convenience foods than women who work in offices, according to a study conducted by the *Ladies' Home Journal*. The *Journal*'s interviewers found that 62 percent of the housewives they telephoned had used convenience foods in preparing the previous night's dinner, whereas only about 50 percent of the women who worked away from home had done the same. So we can assume that housewives must feel just as guilty as professional women about having bought themselves a couple of cans' worth of leisure.)

The English have noted the same phenomenon. Women suffering feelings of inadequacy because they use "prepared packets and tins." To compensate, says author Philippa Pullar, "they are cramming their husband and children with too much food." Pullar, who talks about a revised Darwinian theory—"The Survival of the Fattest"—views with regret and a certain amount of savagery the effects convenience foods have had on her country.

She goes back to 1874, and the arrival of canned meat from Australia, "coarse-grained . . . surrounded by an unpleasant-looking lump of fat. It was known to the navy, who had the doubtful benefit of being served up with it in their messes, where it was called Sweet Fanny Adams, after an unfortunate lady of that name who, in 1867, was murdered and hacked into steaks by her lover."

From there on, says Philippa, it was straight downhill. After fifteen years of food rationing, England awoke to the 50s and an age of conformity and blandness. "Science had . . . made off with the seasons. The shops were filled, no matter whether it was spring, summer, autumn, or winter, with the same millions of canned, frozen, and dehydrated vegetables, soups, meats, and ice creams."

The 60s were worse still. Although everyone, rich and poor, city folk or country, ate the same things, "an awkward fact was observed. There was malnutrition in the country, malnutrition and disease. But these were due to no shortage, or failure of harvest. Obversely, this was malnutrition owed to surfeit. A new disease had entered the affluent society: obesity. One in two people was eating more food than he required."

Same on this side of The Pond. And convenience foods do make us fatter. They make us fatter because they contain large amounts of sucrose (ordinary sugar), salt, corn syrup, and dextrose. (Saccharin, heavily used in diet products, came under fire in 1977 when the FDA proposed banning it by way of the 1958 Delaney Clause prohibiting the use of any food additives found to cause cancer in men or animals. Later, Congress acted to exempt saccharin from the law, and early in 1980, two new studies—one published by Harvard's School of Public Health, the other by the American Health Foundation—agreed that the exemption seemed justified. Reviews of the diet histories of thousands of cancer patients had turned up no hard evidence of saccharin's having played a "significant" role in cancer of the bladder, the kind of cancer that rats had developed when fed huge quantities of the synthetic sweetener. The National Cancer Institute had already—late in 1979—published a study offering the same conclusion. None of the scientists involved in the studies was willing to say saccharin was perfectly safe (all believed its excessive use should be discouraged), but nobody thought it was bad enough to make a law about it. Dr. Samuel Epstein, author of *The Politics of Cancer*, might not concur. Dr. Epstein thinks saccharin triggers the appetite and doesn't do a thing for the obese subjects it's supposed to help. He says animal studies showed that rats who were fed saccharin ate more than other rats, and got even fatter.

Packagers aren't putting sugars into their products just to be mean, they're doing it to make the stuff taste better to sweet-toothed customers. And Americans do have sweet teeth. In 1822, our average per capita consumption of processed sugar was 8.9 pounds a year; by 1971, it was 118.6 pounds a year.

For a while, baby food companies were accused of sugaring the mush destined to be shoveled down the maws of infants in order to please the palates of the mothers who tested it. But the idea that a preference for sweets is "learned" was recently questioned by a biopsychologist named Gary Beauchamp whose studies, he feels, show that a food can't be too sweet to please a newborn baby. The more cloying the taste, the better little Wuzzums likes it. Dr. Beauchamp credits evolution for our leanings toward the syrupy, suggesting that the sweetness of nutritious fruits and vegetables may have served as a lure to our ancestors, guiding them to foods that were good for them. (In the same way, they were warned away from poisonous plants by bitter tastes.) Now, says Dr. Beauchamp, we've "separated the goodness from the sweetness," and we may be in trouble.

Science strikes again.

We've been going along for years, eating this, eating that, and suddenly a bunch of experts blow the whistle and say quit. You're ingesting too much sugar. Who would have thought it? It's like aerosol cans. We believed they were fabulous. Then someone said, look, we've made a big mistake, we can mess up the ozone layer and give ourselves rare diseases. And even though we didn't know what the ozone layer was, only a few diehards with beehive hairdos hung onto their lacquer.

It's the same with sugar. Patterns change, and change again. Traditionally, we ate what we could get, and after we weren't starving anymore, we began to eat what we liked, and when, for the first time in history, the great mass of Americans could *afford* what they liked, more and more of the things they liked turned out to be bad for them.

It's easy for people who just wanted to eat salads all along. But the rest of us are like smokers. They always knew smoking wasn't the best possible hobby, but they were willing to flirt with danger. Then the Surgeon General appeared and said it isn't just chancy to smoke—smoking can give you lung cancer and will probably kill you.

That made it a whole new ball game, but it didn't make it easier for addicts to stop smoking.

Something similar is being repeated with sugar eaters. The impulse to diet used to be for the sake of beauty; now people are trying to moderate their behavior for reasons of health. And like a smoker who continues to smoke, a sugar lover may still be dumping four teaspoons of sugar into his coffee, but he doesn't feel so good about doing it anymore.

Already, nutritionists are having an effect on food processors. Companies are taking the sugar *and* the salt *and* the coloring out of some baby foods. And gradually, consumers are being educated to understand more about what we're eating. Research chemist Betty Li, working for the Agriculture Department, analyzed the sugars (not only table sugar, but glucose and fructose, which appear naturally in fruits and grains) contained in more than fifty breakfast cereals. Miss Li "declined to make any value judgments on the products tested," but the facts were laid out for all to see. A box of Kellogg's Sugar Smacks contained 56 percent sugar, Kellogg's Apple Jacks had 54.6 percent sugar, and only three of the cereals tested—Nabisco's Shredded Wheat, and Quaker Oats's Puffed Wheat and Puffed Rice—contained less than 1 percent sugar.

The battle over sugar in cereal goes back, appropriately enough, to Battle Creek, and the Kellogg brothers. It wasn't until Dr. John went abroad for a few weeks that his brother, W.K., dared to add malt flavoring and sugar to Kellogg's Corn Flakes because it made them taste better. ("The Doctor came back from Europe and had a fit," reported one of the Kellogg nephews later.)

Dr. Kellogg believed in a spartan diet—he suggested his patients go without tea, coffee, meats, strong spices, and alcohol—and he invented many "health" foods, including peanut butter mashed from steamed peanuts. Again, his brother waited for him to leave town before ordering the goobers roasted to improve their flavor.

Commerce versus unadulteration; it's not new.

In today's supermarket, there are said to be 10,000 items to choose from (fifty years ago, there were maybe 800) and nutritionists holler about lots of them. "It is now possible," says Dr. Joan Gussow, "to buy chocolate-chip-cookie-shaped breakfast cereal, fruit juiceless breakfast drink mixes, synthetic whipped cream, and hamburger sauce to make your homemade burger taste commercial. . . . A consumer selecting randomly . . . would very likely end up with an assortment of overprocessed, high-fat, high-sugar, high-salt food items of a kind widely recognized to be components of an unhealthy diet."

People choose what looks good, and what seems easiest to them, and we tend not to trust the FDA or government experts who tell us they've got our best interests at heart any more than we trust the food industry.

But even the most slothful among us—those who were comforted by pictures of the fearless Dr. Elizabeth Whelan defiantly feeding her two-year-old a birthday cake made from a mix, and crowned with canned topping—are beginning to exhibit signs of anxiety. Because we've been privy to news about PCBs in our eggs, pesticides in our carrots, rats starving to death on a diet of white bread, and murders blamed on the killer's fondness for chocolate bars. (When Dan White shot the mayor of San Francisco and one of the city's supervisors, his lawyers came up with what the press called the "Twinkie defense," after a psychiatrist assured the jury that White's compulsive consumption of cake and Cokes and candy was not only evidence of a deep depression, but "a source of excessive sugar that had aggravated a chemical imbalance in his brain.")

Maybe taking candy from a baby will turn out to be the only prudent course of action. Still, most Americans are middle-of-the-roaders, and even though we wish to be healthy, we won't quit eating everything we like. A few years back, when beef prices rose astronomically, and cholesterol was beginning to be a big story, General Mills made some low-fat meat substitutes out of textured vegetable protein.

Nobody wanted them.

And probably nobody will want to eat grasshoppers or worms, though every so often an explorer in the field of survival suggests these creatures as high-protein snacks for the adventurous. Or the really, really hungry.

It's only consumer resistance that is holding back more fabricated foods, according to Patricia Wells. "As soon as consumers learn to live with and like scrambled egg substitutes and dehydrated champagne, these foods will proliferate," she says. "Many foods, such as pizza, will look much the same as they do today, but the ingredients will change drastically. Instead of a spicy all-beef pepperoni and whole milk mozzarella topping, the pizza of the future might include a sausage look-alike made of textured soy protein and a mozzarella fabricated essentially from vegetable fat."

O brave new world that has such pizza in it!

Already, scientists have developed "a polyunsaturated cow" (Bossy is fed soybean meal mixed with corn and safflower oil, so her meat is lower in saturated fat) and a featherless chicken. But doctors at the U.S.D.A. poultry research lab in Maryland found the denuded chicken had so many "emotional and physical problems" that further work on producing bald birds was abandoned.

What about the emotional and physical problems among human beings who drink dehydrated martinis and eat prefabricated bacon strips? Some experts, says Patricia Wells, are alarmed that "scientists really do not know the bodily effects of a long-term diet of highly fabricated and processed foods." Other experts are more concerned with the effects on our heads. "If you take away from food the wholesomeness of growing it," says Wendell Berry, author of *The Unsettling of America*, "or take away the joy and conviviality of preparing it in your own home, then I believe you are talking about a whole new definition of a human being."

A piece appearing in the *New Yorker*'s Talk of the Town section (August 13, 1979) may have offered the last, best word on the foolish lengths to which we can travel in the direction of convenience foods. Discussing television commercials pushing Country Time, "a powdered lemonadelike product," the *New Yorker* writer said the idea behind the commercials was that "lemonade itself is *a thing of the past*. No one can *get* lemonade anymore. Only some rich people. Most people don't even remember lemonade anymore. *Only Grandpa*. Who has been bound and gagged and dishonored all these years out in the desert, like the decrepit warrior in *Star Wars*, only Grandpa even remembers *what it tastes like*.

"The rundown is like this: Lemonade died out when the Old Ones lost out to the Invaders. But some people with the knowledge of the Old Ones escaped to Mars, where they made a kind of synthetic lemonade, using materials available on Mars. It was a powder and became popular. In the meantime, life on Earth contracted. Now, in these recent days, adventurers from Mars, sensing our need, have travelled to earth with the powder. When the powder is given to certain of our remaining Old Ones, they are made happy and remember lemonade. The idea is persuasive. It causes you to forget that you can make lemonade *any time you want* by squeezing some lemons in some water and adding sugar. People don't know. They really don't know that you can make lemonade any time you want. That's right. Lemonade is still available. Right now. Lemons are everywhere. You can make lemonade right now if you want to. It's great. Lemonade is still totally within our capacities."

"There is a mean in all things," said Swift.

American women aren't ready to give up their cans of soup, their boxes of gingerbread mix, their bottles of spaghetti sauce, their jars of chunky peanut butter, their cartons of frozen Tender Tiny Peas, their shiny little envelopes filled with dried salad dressing mixes, or the freedom from kitchen labor these goods have brought them.

But some women are mixing it up more, at least part of the time. They're rediscovering fresh green leafy vegetables, they're baking potatoes, they're patronizing orange juice stands that squeeze actual fruit in front of their very eyes. Because few human beings, given the choice, would vote for a totally processed world, mechanized, packaged, without allowance for the individual quirkiness that produces not only a great French meal, but also somebody's grandmother's really terrible banana bread.

Technology is miraculous; we can take what we want from it, and leave the rest. Some of what we leave may be fat we didn't need anyway.

PUTTING IT ON:
We're fat because we buy the cookbooks and eat more than their words.

9 Cookbooks: Your Basic Joy of Cookerie and Like That

They lard their lean books with the fat of others' works.
—DEMOCRITUS TO THE READER

WE WENT from being an agricultural nation to being an industrial nation; we went from growing our food to buying it at the store.

"The *whole* process of readying food for the table was no longer carried out in the home," say Root and de Rochemont, writing of a time after the Civil War. "The first steps, often the easily abandoned ones of drudgery, were handled by some nameless enormous factory which delivered preserved, prepared or half-prepared foods to housewives who might have little more to do about them than to warm them up. The arts of cooking were communicated less and less from mother to daughter, but were learned from the directions on the label provided by the manufacturer, or, an intermediate step, from a cookbook."

The use of cookbooks may indeed have become more prevalent as nineteenth-century America became more urbanized, but the printing of recipe collections was nothing new.

In 1796, the very first American cookbook—that is, the very first

American cookbook not swiped from the British—had been published "According to Act of Congress." It was called *American Cookery, or The Art of Dressing Viands, Fish, Poultry, and Vegetables, and the Best Modes of Making Pastes, Puffs, Pies, Tarts, Puddings, Custards, and Preserves, and all Kinds of Cakes, From the Imperial Plumb to Plain Cake. Adapted to this Country, and All Grades of Life*. Its author was listed on the cover as "Amelia Simmons, an American Orphan."

In the preface to her 48-page masterpiece (the title is nearly as long as the book), Amelia avowed that an orphan must be pure in word and deed. "It must ever remain a check upon the poor solitary orphan," wrote she, "that while those females who have parents, or brothers, or riches, to defend their indiscretions, that the orphan must depend solely upon *character*." (Actually, what she said was, "the orphan muft depend folely upon," etc., but I can read that early American Kitchen Kaffir. Otherwise, Amelia would have run me crazy with her news about the "beft" beef having a "coarfe open grain, and oily fmoothnefs.")

Amelia was a fount of practical advice. She told how to choose a fresh fish—"deceits are used to give them a freshness of appearance, such as peppering the gills . . . or wetting with animal blood"—and gave her opinion of "Garlicks," which, "tho' used by the French, are better adapted to the uses of medicine than cookery," and she became Old Testament lyrical when addressing herself to the preservation of plums. "Take your plumbs before they have stones in them, which you may know by putting a pin through them, then codle them in many waters till they are as green as grass . . ."

If you were planning to make a syllabub, Amelia suggested you "milk your cow into your liquor," and her loaf cakes were richer than Jean Paul Getty. The recipe for Loaf Cake # 1 begins, "Rub 6 pounds of sugar, 2 pounds of lard, 3 pounds of butter into 12 pounds of flour, add 18 eggs—"

I have to tell you that Amelia was rather cross with "the person" she hired to help her put the book together, if the "advertisement" on the last page is to be credited.

The person, said Amelia, "did omit several articles very essential in some of the receipts, and placed others in their stead, which were highly injurious to them."

Then followed a list of errata.

On page 35, for example, a cake recipe had been wrongly presented. "For 9 pounds of flour, read 18 pounds," urged Amelia.

Eighteen pounds of flour in a nice plain cake. Prodigal were our forebears. (It's a kinder word than fat.)

Women's work was not dainty in post-Revolutionary days. Amelia tells us quite a bit about dressing animals—"put the guts into another vessel, open them with a small pen-knife end to end, wash them clean—"

Still, nothing in Amelia's commands to readers was so bloody as instructions found in earlier books from the mother country. *A Book of Cookrye*, by A.W., printed in 1591 "at London," suggested that the culinary artist "Take a red Cock that is not too olde, and beate him to death, and when he is dead, fley him and quarter him in small pieces." A few pages later came a directive that has the earmarks of an order to a Mafia enforcer. A quail should be roasted "with his legs broken and knit one within an other."

In 1596, exactly two hundred years before our American Orphan's recipes first saw print, another English cookbook, *The Good Huswife's Jewell* (by Thomas Dawson), told its readers, I regret to say, how to boil larks (some people just don't care about music), how to bake a gammon of bacon ("You must first boyle him a quarter of an hour before you stuff him"), and how "to boyle a carpe in green broth, with a pudding in his bellie."

A New Booke of Cookerie (J. Murrell, London, 1615) told how to prepare many dishes "on the French fashion," but Gervase Markham's *Countrey Contentments* (also 1615), despite its tendering of recipes for "*quelquechoses*," was rather hard on foreign influence, and said a huswife's diet ought to "proceede more from the provision of her own yarde, then the furniture of the markets, and let it be rather esteemed for the familiar acquaintance she hath with it than for the strangenesse and raritie it bringeth from other Countries."

You want to learn how to make "Sauce for a Pigge"? See Gervase Markham. You want to find cures for "the Hemeroides"? For "dimme eyes"? Gervase will share his secrets. For inflammation of the brain cells, he advised squirting beet juice up the patient's nostrils; for hairlessness, he liked to mix wood ashes and oil and anoint the bald spot ("It will breede hair exceedingly") and he also proffered hope to men who had suffered a falling of the fundament. (Never send to know for whom the fundament falls. Or what the fundament is, for that matter.) "If a man's fundament fall downe through some cold taken or other cause," Gervase says, "let it be fourthwith put up againe; Then take the powder of Towne cresses dried, and strow it gently upon the fundament—" Honey also enters into the prescription, along with powder of cumin and more strowing and anointing. "Ease will come thereby," Gervase promises.

What have fundaments, or Elizabethan cookbooks, for that matter, got to do with fat in America? you may be asking. Well, as to the first, I have no answer, but as to the second, sit tight. "Elizabethan cookbooks and culinary traditions were transmitted to the new world by early colonists," says Lorna Sass, author and connoisseur of Elizabethan feasts, so "patriots who consider themselves as American as apple pie" may be surprised to discover J. Murrell's "Pippin Pye."

Other days, other ways. When American women began turning out meals, they didn't have self-cleaning ovens, they didn't have any ovens at all. In the early part of the seventeenth century, food was cooked in kettles or frying pans over wood fires. There was no running water. Baking was done in a metal box that sat on the hearth and had one side open to the flames. (The iron cooking stove didn't materialize until the 1870s.)

In 1742, *The Compleat Housewife, or Accomplish't Gentlewoman's Companion*, by Eliza Smith (an English work), was pirated by a Virginia printer named William Parks. He helped himself to such recipes as he thought would be suitable to the tastes of the citizens of Williamsburg, and ignored those he felt would "swell out the Book and increase its Price." (*The Frugal Housewife*, by Susannah Carter, published in Boston, and *The New Art of Cookery*, by Richard Briggs, published in Philadelphia, were also reprints of English works.)

Then, in 1796, came poor parentless Amelia Simmons, who was adopted by the American public. Amelia's work went into four editions, and inspired Lucy Emerson of Montpelier, Vermont, to issue a book called *The New England Cookery*. Mrs. Emerson's was an easy book to write; she simply copied out Amelia's recipes and had them reprinted.

"A Society of Gentlemen of New York" produced the *Universal Receipt Book or Complete Family Director* in 1814, following the formula (already noted in Gervase Markham's work) of offering not only recipes but also medical help and general household hints. You could learn how to cure "boloney" on one page and jaundice on the next.

Published in 1824, *The Virginia Housewife*, by Mary Randolph, was, writes Evan Jones, "the first genuinely regional cookbook available to Americans . . . in Mrs. Randolph's pages there was a candid breaking away from the English past . . . she was loyal enough to her region to be the first to recommend fresh, young turnip tops 'boiled with bacon in the Virginia style.'"

To make gelatin for desserts in the days before Mr. Knox brought us his magic powder required dedication of a high order. If you were fresh out of isinglass (obtained from fish bladders or animals' hoofs), *The Virginia Housewife* explained that you could take a calf's stomach, hang it up to dry for a few days, turn it inside out, and slip off the curd "nicely with the hand."

Although more cookbooks bloomed in the North than in the South—the best southern cooks, having been slaves, were for the most part illiterate—other contributions from Dixie did follow: *The Carolina Housewife,* compiled by "a Lady of Charleston" (Sarah Rutledge) in 1847, for one, and thirty years later, in 1877, *Housekeeping in Old Virginia,* edited by Marion Cabell Tyree (granddaughter of Patrick Henry), for another.

Mrs. Tyree (the same lady referred to in Chapter One, who hoped to keep American husbands out of hotels and saloons) had gathered tips from "two hundred and fifty of Virginia's noted housewives," and her book was praised by "many distinguished American women." Said Mrs. President R. B. Hayes (from the Executive Mansion in Washington), "I am very much pleased with it."

The press also gave Mrs. Tyree credit. "If two hundred and fifty matrons of Virginia cannot teach their sisters in other states something these sisters don't know about housekeeping, then corn bread is a failure, and Lady Martha Washington a free and independent American myth," said the reviewer for the *Chicago Inter-Ocean.*

Listen, it was a terrific book. Mrs. Tyree alternately encouraged and whipped up her readers. "Resolve that you *will* have good bread," she says, "and never cease striving after this result till you have effected it. If persons without brains can accomplish this, why cannot you?"

She was a bit hard on the help ("After having tried many new and patent [ice-cream] freezers, some of the best housekeepers have come to the conclusion that the old-fashioned freezer is the best . . . especially as servants are so apt to get a patent freezer out of order") but extremely solicitous of the sick. "Avoid whispering," she tells us, "as this excites nervousness and apprehension on the part of the sick. Do not ask in a mournful tone of voice how the patient is. Indeed, it is best to ask the sick as few questions as possible."

One of Mrs. Tyree's contributors advised eating the roots of peonies as a cure for epilepsy, and another had a novel treatment for fresh cuts. "Varnish them with common furniture varnish." There was news of a way to destroy bedbugs, and a way to get rid of mice (or at least to make them sneeze). "If a mouse enters into any part of your dwelling, saturate a rag with cayenne in solution and stuff it into his hole."

A woman of definite opinions, Mrs. Tyree protested "against the unwholesome custom of frying steak in lard," and assured her readers that the portions of the cow most suitable for soup were "all the unsightly parts."

Her Brunswick Stew called for "a twenty-five cent shank of beef" and "a five-cent loaf of bread."

Food was cheap in the 1800s—cheap, copious, and varied—so the privileged class, which performed no manual labor, found itself piling on the pounds. *Housekeeping in Old Virginia* carried a page advertising Dr. Scott's Electric Corset (featuring steel "magnetods" that carried "magnetic power into constant contact with all the vital organs"). For three dollars, a lady suffering from "a tendency to extreme fatness" could buy Dr. Scott's corset, and be cured. Extreme fatness, the doctor informed readers, "is a disease."

A disease the cause of which was not hard to uncover.

Even a relatively spartan cook like Mrs. Horace Mann, who implored housewives to use less butter and oil and lard, and had high compliments for vegetables, featured in her 1861 cookbook *(Christianity in the Kitchen)* a cake that called for twenty eggs. The exercise required to make the thing was its most healthful aspect, since Mrs. Mann suggested the batter be "vigorously beaten" for three hours.

Because of the plenty that prevailed, Eliza Leslie of Philadelphia, a veritable queen of cookbook writers—her output included *Seventy-five Receipts* (1827), *Directions for Cookery* (1828), *Pastry, Cakes and Sweetmeats* (also 1828), and *Domestic French Cookery* (1832)—used raw materials lavishly. She would give a recipe for soup that included pounds of meat and vegetables, then tell the cook to strain these out, throw them away, and keep only the broth. She also advised lovers of "omelette soufflés" to avoid failure by hiring a French cook "to come to your kitchen with his own utensils and ingredients and make and bake it himself."

Miss Leslie offered dozens of recipes for venison, hare, pheasant, plover, salmon, and sturgeon. Catfish caught near the middle of the river were "much nicer than those that are taken near the shore where they have access to impure food," she said.

Mrs. J. Chadwick's *Home Cookery* (Boston, 1853) also reflected the prodigal gifts nature had squandered on America. She called for a hundred oysters in her gumbo, and ninety egg yolks in a wedding cake.

During the time that Mrs. Chadwick and Miss Leslie were flourishing, E. Hutchinson of New York came out with a *New Family Book, or Ladies' Indispensable Companion and Housekeepers' Guide; Addressed to Sister, Mother and Wife*. E. Hutchinson wasn't just a recipe pusher, either, E. Hutchinson was a humanitarian. "Never give medicine to a very young child," E. Hutchinson warned. "Many have thus lost darling children. It will, if not murdered, be permanently injured."

E. Hutchinson disapproved of picking one's teeth with a fork, and admonished ladies not to lace too tightly. A tight-laced woman was unfit "to be a wife and mother." Not to mention that a tight-laced woman might faint dead away after packing in the roast pig and the hot biscuits and the sweetmeats.

Cookbooks multiplied like wire coat hangers. Formulas for *bonnes bouches* poured from volumes by Mrs. Rorer, Miss Ann Chase, Miss Beecher. The names had a fine, prim ring, in contrast to the profligate richness of butter and cream and chocolate and sugar they espoused. And then, in 1896, Fannie Merritt Farmer published the *Boston Cooking School Cook Book* and became the Julia Child of her day, our first national (as opposed to regional) culinary star.

A picture of Fannie in her prime, black ribbon around the throat, hair skinned back into a topknot, glasses with a bridge high above the nose, is enough to scare you silly and make you mind your manners. She doesn't look as though she would brook impertinence.

Actually, Fannie was treading hot on the trail of Mary Johnson Lincoln, the first director of the Boston Cooking School. Fannie attended the school, was graduated in 1889, and began at once to teach, herself becoming director in 1891. *Mrs. Lincoln's Boston Cook Book* had come out in 1884; twelve years later, Fannie's book appeared, borrowing liberally from Mrs. Lincoln, and not troubling to give that lady credit. Mrs. Lincoln had been one of the first cooks to concern herself with accurate measurements (she translated "butter the size of an egg" to mean one quarter of a cup) and Fannie continued this trend, approaching the arts of the kitchen with less gusto and more science than had many of her predecessors. "Food is anything which nourishes the body," Fannie wrote solemnly, and recited the percentages of each element ("oxygen, 62½ percent") that entered "into the composition of the body."

John and Karen Hess call Fannie "the maiden aunt of home economics," and say that because she became "the patron saint of American housewives," her helping herself to other people's recipes "contributed to the moral climate of the cookbook world today, where plagiarism is the norm."

Some of Fannie's notions seem odd to us now. She suggested cooking string beans for three hours. Even so, across the years, she was responsible for the sale of more than three million books. (Smart little dickens that she was, she paid for the first printing out of her own pocket, so she got to keep all the profits.)

As time passed, Fannie's work was amended and added to—her heirs, wishing to be *au courant,* loaded the sixth edition with canned and frozen products, and what Craig Claiborne has described as "other horrors."

In 1979, Alfred Knopf brought out a brand-new edition of *The Fannie Farmer Cookbook,* after having hired Marion Cunningham, a renowned cook (from Los Angeles, not Boston) to eliminate the "horrors," restore some of the original recipes, and explain how modern tools such as food processors could be used to whip up previously time consuming dishes.

(Example of a horror removed: the recipe for guacamole in the eleventh edition. "They used onion, tomato ketchup, and chili powder, which are certainly foreign to the original," Mrs. Cunningham told Craig Claiborne. "I went back to the more traditional chopped onion, green chilies, garlic and lemon juice.")

Mrs. Cunningham, whom James Beard had suggested for the job of fiddling with Fannie, was at first "scared to death." Four years, and 1,839 recipes later, she and her associate, Jeri Laber, had finished their task.

The new edition's editor, Judith Jones, who has worked with James Beard, M. F. K. Fisher, and Marcella Hazan, and who is credited with discovering Julia, says there are two kinds of people who buy cookbooks. "People who want to be fooled, who'll buy the books promising easier methods, cheaper foods, something with a gimmick. And then there are those who really care about cooking."

All in all, Jones told *Publishers Weekly*, Americans had come a long way. "Once you've developed a taste for what's good, it's hard to go back."

In our time, cookbooks are big business. To give you an idea of their growth during a ten-year period, compare these figures. In 1969, 229 new or revised cookbooks were published. In 1978, 403 cookbooks appeared.

To be sure, there have always been the standard reference works, guides to boiling-water-and-baking-ham that every new bride bought, or had bought for her. Not only Fannie Farmer, but the *Joy of Cooking*, by Irma Rombauer (published in 1931, it sold six million copies in the next thirty years), *The Better Homes and Gardens Cookbook, The James Beard Cookbook* (written in 1959, it became a best seller, and by 1966, had sold 500,000 copies in paperback), all offered basic information needed by a man or woman unfamiliar with the kitchen.

But once the phenomenon of food consciousness, the interest in cooking of all kinds, broadened, the market for cookbooks became so vast that specialization was possible. *Julia Child and Company* (to pick a recent winner), first published in 1978, sold 100,000 copies in hardcover at $15.95, and another 350,000 in paperback at $9.95.

And the same way people buy Julia for French cooking, they buy Marcella Hazan for Italian cooking and Paula Wolfert for Moroccan cooking, and Diana Kennedy for Mexican cooking. These women are great classic cooks; clearly, good cookbooks sell. But so do bad cookbooks and indifferent cookbooks.

Chinese cookbooks sell, so do cookbooks about Creole and Cajun cooking, and books by people who first took lessons from Alice B. Toklas, and books that use yogurt as the basis for every dish, and books that feature bananas from first course to last, and books restricted to recipes with carrots.

Do you own a pressure cooker? There are pressure cooker cookbooks. And there are microwave cookbooks, and there are vegetarian cookbooks, and cookbooks of nothing but desserts. And there are cookbooks about how to fill the stomach for pennies (these are in the honorable tradition of Mrs. Lydia Child who in 1835 produced *The American Frugal Housewife, Dedicated to Those Who Are Not Ashamed of Economy*). There are "natural" food cookbooks and cooking-with-wine cookbooks and cookbooks with edible chocolate covers and a cookbook called *Cooking With God*. Shirley King has written a cookbook called

Dining With Marcel Proust, which re-creates the roast goose, the chocolate cream, the skate with black butter of Proust's memories, and Israel Shenker has written a cookbook called *Noshing Is Sacred: The Joys and Oys of Jewish Food*. (Shenker asked Isaac Bashevis Singer why all Jewish mothers were reputed to be great cooks. Because, said Singer, "their sons were big liars.") There is even a cookbook entitled the *I Didn't Know What the Hell to Call It Cookbook,* which its author offered to mail to anyone who sent him $16.50.

And since technology marches inexorably forward, there is now on the market a machine that looks like a baby television set, and that will project pages from your favorite cookbook onto its small screen. The whole *New York Times Cook Book,* for instance, has been captured in eight—that's right, eight—microfilmed cards; one small box can hold cards on which dozens of books have been reproduced. If you have $325, the CuisineVu can be yours.

Any day now, Craig Claiborne says, he expects publishers to run out of subjects for cookbooks. Satirizing the volumes that cross his desk each year—"They have titles like the *How Not to Dirty a Dish Cookbook,* or the *How to Feed a Family Without Cooking Cookbook*"—Claiborne declares they aren't "worth the printer's ink it took to produce them." Though Claiborne and John Hess are not obvious soulmates, here Claiborne would seem to agree with Hess's stern judgment that most cookbooks "aren't worth feeding to your furnace."

James Beard states the case more mildly. "I think some cookbooks are put together like paper dolls, there's no feeling of humanness in them. I write about things I like, done the way I like to do them. I think your cookbook should reflect *you,* and what you do. That's what I've tried to achieve."

Although health problems have caused Beard to alter his own habits—he can't eat salt or sugar—he has little use for diet cookbooks. "Most of the ones I've read are very bad. I don't think they take into consideration flavor or taste. They're being oh so honest, they don't give a damn whether you like the stuff or not. There's this school that makes an ersatz ice cream and an ersatz sauce and an ersatz something else. Who the hell wants it?"

Does Beard (whose cookbook sales burgeoned, along with those of lesser writers) think the food explosion after World War II led to fatter people?

"I know it did in France," he says. "People had been so severely deprived that when it was over they all started eating their heads off. I was astounded. Prisoners of war who came home died, they really burst from excess."

But that was a response to starvation, rather than a discovery of truffles. What about America? Aren't the restless trendies moving into another phase, all jogging, and anxious about cholesterol? Will people continue to buy Jim Beard's books and Julia Child's books?

"It's going to be half and half," says Jim Beard. "You're going to have half the people who are fast-food addicts and diet addicts and nutrition addicts. And then you're going to have another half who are still going to want to live pleasantly. And they're going to do it until they get knocked down by the doctor."

Barbara Kafka, a food authority who was associated with Beard on a giant book called *The Cooks' Catalogue* (see Chapter 11), is one of the few who thinks the food boom is about to bust. "The idea that all cookbooks sell is erroneous," she says. "It used to be that any cookbook published could sell three to five thousand copies. Even today that's true, but now more books need to be sold in order to make money. Three to five thousand copies isn't enough to make anybody rich and famous.

"A Julia Child phenomenon has to do with television. I don't mean she isn't a superb cook and personality, but the exposure that she got through being that person on television made her sell the incredible number of books that she did.

"The Time-Life series of cookbooks was a function of Time-Life and direct mail; it was not a function related to normal publishing.

"A James Beard is a phenomenon some forty years in the making. You must remember, too, when you talk about the increase in this kind of material, that the women's magazines have been turning out food articles for fifty, sixty years. It isn't new. I think it's interesting that people have got more involved in food in the last ten years, but if I were writing this book, I would be concerned with the coming end of this fad, not the beginning."

Kafka (who edits for Cuisinart the monthly *Cooking*, which George Lang, another wizard in the food field, has called "the only magazine for us professionals") became an authority on food and wine and restaurants in the 50s. Fresh from college, with a degree in English and "lofty ideals," she ended up at *Mademoiselle*, doing copy editing. Leo Lerman, whose copy she handled, knew she wanted to write and offered to introduce her to Allene Talmey at *Vogue*.

"I was very innocent, and all set to go off, when he said, 'What are you going to tell her you write about?' 'Don't be silly,' I said, 'I'll write about whatever she wants me to write about. I'm a writer.' And he said, 'Oh, no, dear, you have to write about *something*.' Most of my friends were painters, so I said, 'All right, I'll write about art.' 'No,' Leo said, 'you can't write about art for *Vogue* because Allene Talmey writes about art for *Vogue*, and she's not going to let you do it. You cook divinely, why don't you write about food?' And that's how it started."

Can Kafka document her hypothesis that the American infatuation with food is dying down? She can, and she will. "We are a media-conscious society," she says. "Involved in many stimuli. And we have fads. In the 60s, it was fashion. You couldn't pick up a paper without reading about designers and clothes, without knowing who was who's hairdresser, and who was invited to what party. They were all fashion people.

"In the 70s, the fad was food. True, food is a more primitive craving, and I don't think the people who learned to cook will stop. It won't all go away, there will be a residue, but it won't have that fashion impetus it had all through the 70s. I think one can begin to hear people say, 'Oh, I can't cook anymore, I just don't have the time.' They're the same people who ten years ago were telling you how they were learning to make their own bread."

Like Barbara Kafka, Nika Hazelton recognizes that there are "fashions" in eating. But unlike most famous food writers (in thirty-two years, she's turned out twenty cookbooks, among them books on the cuisines of Italy, Switzerland, Germany, Belgium, and Denmark) she is baffled by the very explosion to which she's so richly contributed. "The contemporary preoccupation with food is something that I just can't understand," she told Harry Zehner, who interviewed her in March of 1979 for the *New York Daily News*. "And the gourmet cooking craze also seems a very odd phenomenon to me. Maybe it's a hobby, like polo used to be."

Her own philosophy is simple. "Food should taste good. Plain or fancy, it should be prepared to the best of one's ability and with the best ingredients one can afford. Because I don't have the patience, I myself don't make complicated dishes."

To Hazelton, the idea of wasting precious time making your own pasta is ludicrous. "The pasta machine as a status symbol just beats me; it's a fad, like painting flowers on porcelain."

Occasionally, to be sure, a difficult recipe is included in one of her books. "What I tried to do in those national cuisine books was to provide the most representative foods in their cultural contexts. I selected the recipes that pleased me most, simple or complicated, high or low caloric."

High caloric. What visions of pastry shells stuffed with sweetness and custard and heavy cream those dear words conjure up!

But we don't get fat eating words, we get fat eating cannoli, so maybe in the end we shouldn't blame our fat on cookbooks. Particularly since, for certain cookbook collectors, cooking never ensues. Cookbooks are a hobby. We croon over the pictures until, mad with hunger, we lurch into the kitchen and discover there's nothing but week-old bread and a quarter of an inch of dried-up peanut butter in a jar that somebody left the top off of.

Still, cookbooks continue to spawn, bringing us recipes from Pagopago, recipes from the Junior League of any city that numbers more than thirty-seven people, recipes from any magazine that has printed enough menus so the editors feel called upon to compile them into a volume readers can keep forever. Or until the binding breaks, whichever comes first.

Is anybody getting fat from cookbooks? The publishers, if they're lucky.

PUTTING IT ON:
We're fat because we go to school for it.

10 The Teaching Game: Quiche Me Quick, and Lead Me Down the Road to Salivation

Who's your fat friend?
—BEAU BRUMMELL, OF THE PRINCE OF WALES

OKAY, we've done cookbooks.

What do cookbooks lead to?

Fat, right? You thought I was going to say fat because fat is what I keep yammering about. You thought wrong. Cookbooks lead to—and from—cooking schools.

Despite Nika Hazelton's bewilderment over "the contemporary preoccupation with food," the beets go on, and so do the Turkey Orloffs. Or Turkeys Orloff, as the case may be. Almost anybody with a cleaver, a wristwatch and a charge account at Gristede's can set up shop in his or her apartment and give lessons.

Fortunately for insatiable New Yorkers, some of the best and brightest and beefiest cooks and cookbook writers also run cooking schools.

Some of the prettiest, too. Remember Annemarie Huste, who went to work for Mrs. Onassis? Annemarie was a peach, and like many a peach before her, she was canned.

Did she snivel and wither away in the blaze of Jackie's displeasure? Not a bit of it, she opened a cooking school, where she leads ten students a week through a demonstration course (the students don't get to touch a lettuce leaf) at a cost of $400 a head. Which makes Annemarie almost as rich as her former employer.

The superb Marcella Hazan, who was a biology teacher before she started cooking ("because I married a man who could cope with many bad things in life but not with a bad meal"), teaches in Bologna, Italy, from May to November, but after November, she sets up shop in Manhattan, charges $350 for five lessons in how to do pastas and other good Italian dishes. Diana Kennedy (Mexican cooking), Maurice Moore-Betty (Continental menus), Simone Beck (provincial French cuisine), Madhur Jaffrey (Indian dishes), and Perla Meyers (seasonal food) are some of the other big names offering courses in the city.

But it isn't only jaded New Yorkers who seek fresh thrills for their tired palates—jaded Californians are searching too. In the Napa Valley, the famous French chef Michel Guérard was imported for the laying on of hands and truffles, and each student lucky enough to put in a week of study with the master got to pay $1,700 for the privilege.

Jim Beard usually teaches in Oregon during the summer, thus giving the other coast a glimpse of the glories we effete Easterners have access to the rest of the year, while in Columbus, Ohio, the heart of the country, a lady named Betty Rosbottom runs a school called La Belle Pomme to which she has brought guest chefs such as Jacques Pepin (he flew over, cooked the kinds of things he used to cook for General de Gaulle, flew out again three days later). And how you gonna keep 'em down on the farm, after they've tasted Paree? Mrs. Rosbottom's school has been most enthusiastically greeted by those citizens of Columbus who used to claim there wasn't a single good restaurant in town. Some students admit they come more for the meals than for the learning.

When great chefs won't come to you, you're still free (maybe free isn't exactly the right word) to wing off to France, where you can pick up as many pointers as you've got francs for, in the same way that young ladies of quality have been doing for generations. But even in Paris, there can't be more passion for cooking than has recently flowered in New York. "Some classes are booked two to three years in advance," says Patricia Wells, in the *New York Times*. "Students compete for spots in the best schools the same way youngsters do for entry into prep schools. In some cases, it's who you know that gets you in."

Even knowing somebody, you'll probably have to wait to study with the masters. For Jim Beard, says the *Times,* "students line up around the block . . . classes are large and somewhat chaotic, and Mr. Beard is a bit impatient with those slow to follow instructions . . . Classes are taught in his spacious, though rather disorganized kitchen, and include careful and attentive instruction by Mr. Beard and his able assistant, Richard Nimmo. The recipes are honest and uncomplicated, the food and company worth the price of admission."

Sitting in the living room of his brownstone on East 12th Street, like a merry incarnation of Buddha, round and rosy among the Chinese statues and plates he collects, Jim Beard roars with laughter, and his reflection shivers in the smoky mirrors. "This place looks like something in an amusement park," he says.

Beard is a man of enormous good humor, but he is not amused by what he considers idiocy. People are fat? Let them diet, then. But he isn't going to teach diet food, he's going to go right on teaching "good" food, and if something calls for cream and butter, cream and butter will be used.

"Let's go back to that much overworked thing called *cuisine minceur,*" says Jim Beard. "Which after all was started for people who wanted to reduce their caloric intake, and to eat more simply. More simply! By the time they're through cutting out little pieces of vegetable to put around the plate, the food is so gussied up when you get it you want to throw up on it instead of eat it. That's the only way you can face what you see."

Beard teaches somewhat differently than he did twenty years ago. "I do much more improvisation. But I never follow one school of cookery. I'm not Julia, I'm not Madame Française."

All twelve to sixteen students in a Beard class participate. "I think one learns by getting one's hands and feet into it, and if something flops, it's not my fault." Again, the laughter wells up.

Is he never bored with class after class after class? He says no. "We're always doing something new, and we're always getting new people, which is fun."

Fun and profitable. Beard charges $75 a class.

All over town, if you've got the bread, you can learn to bake it. You can take lessons in Egyptian cooking, and discover how to stuff a squab with cracked wheat and pine nuts, you can learn plain French or fancy French, plain Italian or fancy Italian, heavy Italian or light Italian, you can study cake making and cake decorating, and how to put together a

Roman banquet, you can learn *nouvelle cuisine* and Tibetan cuisine and Japanese cuisine and Chinese cuisine.

New Yorkers love Chinese food, so New Yorkers take lessons from Madame Chu and Jean Chen and Millie Chan and Dee Wang and Anna Wong and Lilah Kan and Karen Lee and Eileen Lo.

I myself once took a Chinese cooking course. I didn't have to know anybody to get in, I just had to have $60 (it was the bargain of the decade), and I was so enraptured with the teacher's accent I kept forgetting to stir-fry. I once wrote about the teacher's accent, which so enraged the teacher that she threatened to sue. She said she didn't talk like that, she talked perfect. So far as I was concerned, she talked perfect; I loved every word of it. She called an old city an "ain-sint shitty," she fancied cartilage in meat ("If you cook long, the carteridge still chewy, carteridge is pro-ting, it's a good stuff"), and she confessed that she took a nip from time to time ("Most Chinese ladies don't drink. Habit or customer. I different. I drink").

My teacher was proud that Craig "Craiborne" had changed his mind about Chinese food. "Ten, fifteen years ago, Craig Craiborne, he don't like Chinese food, he dislike. Now after finally getting into it, he don't mind to adjust."

Sometimes, when my teacher went on demonstration tours, she would meet with a foolish audience, which irritated her. "I was in Indiana. There was two hunared ladies. So I say, 'Any queshings?' So one lady say, 'Yes, what kinda grasses you wear?' Ooh, I was so mad. I say, 'No queshings about dishes? Only my grasses?'"

She waves her collapsible spectacles, and tells us how to choose a sea bass—"When the eye is mean and stare at you, that's a fresh fish"—and that onions should be "nice and sweet without mushy" and that we should put a little pork "in the block-a-lee."

Some vegetables are not so easy to decode as "block-a-lee." The first time you hear "fresh binker," your mind doesn't leap to offer fresh bean curd, and "cucumbers are horrow" doesn't instantly conjure up the cavity that inhabits the cucumber.

On the other hand, "frank steak" sounded more decent, more honorable to me than flank, and when my teacher peeled the rind off animal or vegetable, it was for a good reason, namely that she had found "some un-dee-zyble sking."

Ask her a straight question, you got a straight answer. Did she prefer peanut oil or corn oil? "They both I like it." She also instructed us about birds' nest soup, made logically enough from birds' nests. But "Chinese people very par-tic-oo-lar," she said. "Got to take the dung and feathers out."

Forthrightness in a cooking teacher has always been valued. Consider Mrs. Rorer, of the *Philadelphia Cook Book*. In 1893, she opened the Philadelphia Cooking School. (The Boston Cooking School and the New York Cooking School flourished at the same time.)

In a biography called *Sarah Tyson Rorer, The Nation's Instructress in Dietetics and Cookery*, Emma Seifrit Weigley reveals that Mrs. Rorer never cooked until she was thirty years old, but once she got interested, the feathers flew.

Mrs. Rorer was a showwoman. Mrs. Rorer was smart. Mrs. Rorer had been pale, listless, and sickly until she discovered fresh air, exercise, and plain food, the news of which she elected to spread wherever she could. And Mrs. Rorer had a heart. She pioneered lessons in cooking for the sick, she taught working women and finishing-school girls alike, she suggested that domestics organize, thereby striking terror into the hearts of her upper-crust students, whom she'd already appalled by insisting that they learn how to clean up in the kitchen before presuming to direct servants in such matters.

All in all, Mrs. Rorer wrote some fifty-four cookbooks and booklets, and any number of magazine articles. She lectured across the country, gave exhibitions of her culinary art while gowned in pale colored silk upon which she never got a spot, and worked (when she had the time) at Philadelphia's Midnight Mission teaching "fallen women" cooking, in order that they might have a means of livelihood after their other charms had fled.

Believing that salads should be eaten 365 days a year, Mrs. Rorer was hell on fats ("Banish the frying pan and there will not be much sickness either in city or country") and sweets, although she was a wizard cook, and could show her pupils how to fetch up the very dishes she most disapproved of.

"Under protest," she would say, "I shall make for you some new desserts, which I hope none of you will think of imitating. Remember, desserts are both unhealthy and unnecessary."

Demonstrating how to prepare charlotte russe with chocolate sauce (and maybe a soupçon of schizophrenia), Mrs. Rorer would shake her head. "All these things look so good but they are so deadly." (Actually, Mrs. Rorer grew harder on sugar as she grew older. In 1891, she'd countenanced eighteen pounds of sugar a week for a family of ten, but by 1896, she was saying no adult who valued good health should consume "over two pounds of sugar a month."

Appalled by the use of vinegar and salt in salad dressing—if such a mixture could be used to clean brass and copper, what might it not do "to the delicate mucous lining" of the stomach?—she also went on record as saying that the "dirty Turk" was a more sensible eater than the average American. "Pork and mashed potatoes, white bread, stewed sugared fruits, hot sweetened liquids, layer cakes and stimulants kill the weak, ruin the middling, and help many thousands to hospitals for the insane." Besides leading to madness, the American diet, according to Mrs. Rorer, engendered crime, disease, and poor labor relations. "It is the ill-fed workingman who goes on strike, the well-fed workingman never."

Mrs. Rorer was sniffy about Boston, saying the Massachusetts city was "a great place for nervous prostration which is the result, not of brain exertion, as many Boston people claim, but of bean eating." Germany also drew her scorn. After a visit there, she declared she wasn't surprised by the high suicide rate in the country. "At four they take coffee and wafers, and then at seven in the evening bread, rye sandwiches with cheese, another glass of beer. Why would not one think death a joy after a month of such fare?"

Her economical ways with a meal brought Mrs. Rorer many converts. In 1894, she demonstrated how to produce a dinner for four—vegetable soup, sheep's liver with brown sauce, cole slaw, turnips, baked potato, bread, and tapioca—for forty cents. And it only took her forty-five minutes, start to finish.

Deploring waste, and the throwing out of leftovers, Mrs. Rorer explained that a clever housewife shouldn't even need a garbage pail. "We eat our garbage," she said. If there was any irreducible refuse in the Rorer kitchen, Mrs. R. put it in something called a "carbonizer," which fed into the stovepipe where the refuse was converted to fuel. The Arabs wouldn't have shaken Mrs. Rorer.

Some of the lady's tenets were unprovable—"Christianity and dyspepsia are never found in the same individual," she told a surprised Cleveland audience—but she was always interesting, whether she was running a session at the Philadelphia Food Exposition on the topic of "What I Have Learned from a Spanish Cook," or turning out articles about "What Nervous People Should Eat," and "The Best Diet for Bloodless Girls."

Mrs. Rorer exhorted her students and her readers to leave the table hungry, and she was wiser than the politicians about ways to feed the poor. "If the abundant and cheap vegetables and fruits of the summer had been canned," she wrote in her magazine, *Household News*, during the depression of 1893, "if wheat and corn at sixty and fifty cents per bushel respectively were used with judgment, and if the thousands of quarts of skimmed milk that are now daily emptied into our sewers (a wicked waste) were properly utilized, there would be but little room for complaint, even among the poor who are now but partially employed."

Years later, one of Mrs. Rorer's pupils recorded some memories of her training. "We learned the food values of proteins, carbohydrates, etc. We had ten lectures on chemistry and several on physiology and hygiene and we were taught that diabetic patients must avoid sugars and starches and nephritic patients must avoid proteins. We were taught to cook and to cook well. We had ten lessons on cooking for the sick, and emphasis was laid on attractiveness of trays and color schemes. Then we were examined and received our diplomas, and my classmates started out to lecture and to teach."

Although she herself was a fine robust figure of a woman, and no sylph, Mrs. Rorer was unsympathetic to overly fat folks who, she maintained, brought their misery on themselves. "If you suggest proper diet, they at once rebel and feel that it is all nonsense, that they probably inherit this fat . . ."

Mrs. Rorer was writing about obesity, says Emma Weigley, at a time when that topic "had received little attention."

"Reduce your flesh gradually before you get too fat," was Mrs. R.'s advice to American women. Obese women were worse off than obese men, she hypothesized in the *Ladies' Home Journal*. "The overfat woman . . . in thinking to hide a portion of this fat, draws in her clothing, pushing the fat from one place to another, pressing upon the heart, reducing the circulation until she really has more serious problems to contend with than obesity. Her face becomes purple, the end of her nose especially red, and she is really pitiful to behold. All this can be avoided if she has sufficient will power to now and then go hungry."

Cut down on sweets, starches, sugars, and of course, pork ("No product of the hog is fit to eat"), advised our heroine, and concentrate instead on fruit, green vegetables, a little lean meat. But how might a person know if she was overeating? "Fat," said Mrs. Rorer, "is the alarm bell."

The more things change, the more they stay the same. Roughly a hundred years later, nutritionists are still trying to get us to eat our lettuce and abandon our fats, while we lovers of pig cling, like Andrew Hedger in *Diana of the Crossways* ("'Hog's my feed,' said Andrew Hedger . . . 'Ah could eat hog a solid hower!'"), to our addiction.

Until the nineteenth century, society ladies hadn't often turned their feet toward the kitchen, so they hadn't required cooking instruction, but suddenly, toward the end of the 1800s, knowing how to cook had become fashionable. A New England man named Thomas Lawson went so far as to offer each of his four daughters $100,000 as soon as she had mastered the art of turning out a formal dinner. Mr. Lawson installed a cooking teacher in a cottage on his estate, so his darlings had no need to travel.

It was Pierre Blot, a visiting Frenchman, who started the New York Cooking Academy, which in turn became the New York Cooking School, run by Miss Juliet Corson. Miss Corson, says Evan Jones, foreshadowed "the health-food enthusiasm of the twentieth century" by lecturing about the "strength-sustaining values of lentils, fresh and dried peas, and beans."

Miss Corson taught elegant cookery to "ladies" (ten lessons, ten dollars) but, like Mrs. Rorer, she was also concerned about the disadvantaged. For fifty cents, said an article in *Harper's New Monthly*, "young housekeepers in moderate circumstances, domestics, and the wives and daughters of workingmen" were able to take a Plain Cooks' Class.

Helen Worth's first cooking students also paid fifty cents a lesson, which is even more amazing, because Mrs. Worth began teaching during World War II. The place was Cleveland, her hometown, and the purpose was to raise money for The Committee to Defend America by Aiding the Allies.

Eventually Mrs. Worth came to New York, where she started what the newspaper columnist Harriet Van Horne described as "the Radcliffe of cooking schools."

You don't go to Radcliffe for fifty cents. A two-and-a-half-hour private lesson with Helen Worth set you back $225.

She thought she was worth it, and none of her pupils, who have included Clare Boothe Luce and Betty Furness, disagreed. Mrs. Worth referred to herself as an "educator" (she offered concepts, not just recipes), and in the brownstone where she lived and taught, she discoursed on good kitchen equipment ("A carpenter can be no better than his tools") and the fact that she has had to watch her weight since she was twelve years old.

"In the long run, that's less painful than having to start being careful at forty."

I interviewed Mrs. Worth in the summer of 1979, shortly before she packed up and left New York to embark on a new marriage and a new life in Charlottesville, Virginia. She cited her habits. An "austere but nutritious" breakfast, and a lunch that might consist of "a sickle pear, one quarter slice of melba toast, and skim milk flavored with coffee ice cubes." This rigor is maintained so she can enjoy "whatever I like at dinner."

Americans are *not* getting fatter, said Helen Worth. "All you have to do is look at old photos. People are eating much more intelligently today."

Mrs. Worth said she did not believe in the pandemic obesity so many health counselors purported to see around them, and she wasn't repelled by the spectre of convenience foods, either. "When was the last time *you* milked a cow?" she demanded. (She herself used to hustle a sauce of soy and herbs and spices called Brown Quick, which she developed and in which she had so much faith that she continued to sell it though she figured she lost money on every bottle.)

Although as a child she was kept out of the kitchen—"I made the cook nervous"—the grown-up Helen Worth was not only at home on the range, but had so many irons in the fire that one of her listings in the Manhattan phone book read, Helen Worth Cooking School and Enterprises. She offered classes (called "Learn Your Lunch") for men only, she turned out cookbooks, among them the by now classic *Cooking Without Recipes* ("It took twenty years to get it published, it was that far ahead of its time, but since 1965, it hasn't been out of print"), she pioneered a course in "the practical and theoretical aspects of an appreciation of food and drink" at Columbia University, she was a wine taster, and she wrote poetry. "The kiss of satisfaction comes last. Love lying sweet along our mouths—"

But it isn't love, it's all that other stuff lying sweet along our mouths that makes us chubby.

And if you have doubts about engrossment with food piling on the pounds ("Another pound or two, what does it matter, Jim?" as Lillian Russell used to say to Diamond Jim Brady), come with me up the Hudson River to Hyde Park, where the Culinary Institute of America, also known as the "other" CIA, a cooking school housed in an old, pillared, stained-glass-windowed mansion that used to be a Jesuit monastery, turns out baby chefs.

Many of these white-toqued darlings, after two years of working with food, glorious food, are shaped like dumplings or, in the less charitable words of the school's chairman, expressed as he watched a group of 1978 graduates stepping up to get their diplomas, "A lot of these kids are overweight."

So, by the standards of puritanical, psalm-singing, calorie-counting, brown-rice-and-green-grass eaters, are a lot of the teachers. Observe Chef Wayne Almquist, noble chins resting one on another under his curled lip, as he scorns a student's hollandaise, and sends that student back to the whipping post to beat more lemon juice, or butter, or salt, into the offending sauce. Is Chef Almquist a man who cares about "cooking for fitness"? You can bet your béchamel he isn't. In fact, when the Dupont Company, hoping to demonstrate some no-stick pots, suggested such a seminar, nobody at the school dared to ask an Institute chef to run it. The long arm of the CIA had to reach out to La Costa, a diet spa in California, where a graduate student was "externing," and haul the extern back to cook a few dishes that might safely be indulged in by poor, health-crazed skinnies.

Chef Eric Saucy, another CIA teacher who has been described elsewhere in print as "pleasantly sturdy," says he thinks some of the *nouvelle cuisine* recipes are gimmicks. "If it's calories you're worried about," he told *Women's Wear Daily*'s Doris Tobias, "my feeling is that reducing a sauce by cooking it for ten hours will make it just as calorific as one that's cooked briefly with a little flour. As to all those purees and mousses, I'm against them. I like to bite into my carrots, not have them mashed up like baby food."

At the CIA, the chefs say they teach people how to cook. If

nutritionists get to them later, shaping them up—or down—that's not the chefs' business.

Even peripheral workers—meaning those who don't tend the stockpots—on the huge campus (which handles sixteen hundred students at a time) find themselves up to their ears in savoriness. Bill Primavera, the witty and energetic director of public and industry relations when I talked with him a year ago (he has since left to start his own PR firm), attested to that.

"I was a slim man when I came to this school," he said, "and my hobby was seventeenth-century wall stencils."

Eight years later, having sampled the wares of a thousand student cooks, Primavera declared his hobby had gone aglimmering, along with his waistline. No time for stencils now. "I jog," he said sadly. "I go to the gym."

And still the miracles of lunch in the Escoffier Room drew him—the chocolate torte, the trout fresh from the tank where it swam half an hour ago, the pasta, the wine.

The Escoffier Room is manned by students who are about to be graduated, and its patrons come from all over, having made reservations long in advance. The food is not cheap—one pays $21.50 for dinner (without wine) and $12 for lunch. The menu at lunch is basically the dinner menu, but without the cheese and fruit course.

"We used to have to drag people in there," said Primavera. "We couldn't advertise, because that would have been considered unfair competition by local restaurants. Now the word of mouth is so good the problem is to assuage the customers who can't get in for six months."

Males working at the Escoffier Room wear black trousers, white shirts, black bow ties; females wear black skirts and white shirts. All are eager to please, and most are a trifle nervous. A maître d' in training shyly murmurs that a suggestion has been made in class to chill the Beaujolais. A waitress, uncorking one bottle of wine, almost knocks over another, covers her mouth in horror, and looks up to see a confrere grinning encouragement from the doorway.

Each table is booked for one sitting only, and while critics have complained that the students aren't taught to cope with the real horrors and pressures of turnover as they exist in commercial restaurants, such captiousness didn't faze Bill Primavera. "They have enough to learn without that."

When Primavera came to the Institute, there were only three female students. "They had a very good time," he said drily. Today, the cast is 20 percent female, and they still have a good time. Once, nobody thought women could deal with the stresses of the profession. The life is hard, you lug heavy equipment, the kitchens are hot, the hours are long. On the other hand, the restaurant business promises great—and sometimes instant—upward mobility. You can be a dropout, a dreamer, and if you decide to knuckle down, and you have "some talent and sincerity" (Primavera's words), you can become wealthy and famous.

It costs as much to go to the CIA as to go to any good college—about $6,000 a year. When a student comes in, he or she is issued a briefcase containing a set of stainless steel knives and five pairs of whites. Then it's off to the classroom for lectures on hygiene and food costs (the CIA spent $1,700,000 on food in 1979, up 12 percent from the year before) and the uses of equipment. After the lectures comes the kitchen work—learning to fillet fish and knead dough and spin peacocks out of sugar and sculpt butter elephants.

Two semesters (thirty weeks) of baking, butchering, and ice-carving, to touch on just a few of the skills available to the dexterous, and the student is turned out to work as an extern in a restaurant kitchen for six hundred hours. His externship completed, the student comes back to school for two more semesters.

Sitting on a train that carries student hopefuls from the Poughkeepsie station into Manhattan, where they will be interviewed for jobs, an eavesdropper can tune in on the hopes and fears of the apprentice restaurateurs. "I've got an interview at 10:30 in the morning," one boy says to another. "They want a restaurant assistant to do all the slave work. I really hope I get it." His companion looks incredulous. "You *like* running all over like an asshole?" "I like serving," says the first. "I can't stand around like a captain."

Two other food enthusiasts are comparing notes ("Grand Marnier soufflé, I had that once, I have the recipe in my head. You take seven yolks and enough sugar to make a paste—") and across the aisle from them, a curly-haired kid in tattered pants and T-shirt is bending the ear of a patient old Oriental gentleman who is clearly one of the teachers from the Institute.

"Tomorrow," the kid explains, "I have to go to all my interviews for externship. The chef at Luchow's said he'd talk to me. He hasn't called me yet, but I might get a job with him. Plus I got an interview with

Restaurant Associates, and I'll check out the Rainbow Room and the Oyster Bar."

As the kid pauses for breath, the old man sighs. "Too many names. I forget," he says.

Not wanting to bore, the kid changes the subject. "When you make tempura, do you mix the flour and egg, or just beat it, you don't really mix it up?"

Again, the old man sighs. "Yeah, mix it up," he says.

Every three weeks, the CIA stages a nice noisy graduation ceremony in a hall hung with flags of wine-producing countries (a new class of sixty or seventy students starts every three weeks) and an Institute graduate is virtually assured of work in the food world. The average starting salary, Bill Primavera told me, is $13,500.

Each of the ninety-four chefs who teach at the school makes about $50,000 a year, because the Institute has to pay competitive salaries, or all the good chefs would go to work elsewhere. But there are advantages to teaching; few restaurant chefs can count on regular hours, and weekends off. Even Albert Kumin, the great Swiss-born *patissier* who baked at The Four Seasons, teaches at the school. Kumin had been working for the Carter White House until just before Christmas of 1979, when he suddenly quit. The Secret Service, the story went, was making it too tough for him to get fresh, unpasteurized cream. His "fragile meringues and delicate tortes could not survive a committee," wrote an editorialist in the *New York Times*, going on to confess that if given the choice of "what to O.D. on," he would choose "Mr. Kumin's chocolate velvet cake with whipped cream."

Once before, Kumin had been installed at the Culinary Institute, but that time, his old friend Joe Baum had pirated him back to perform miracles for the debut of Windows on the World.

"I could never get Joe Baum on the telephone," Bill Primavera said. "He was too busy. Then all of a sudden, he'd call. 'I think I'll drop up,' he'd say, and he'd arrive and go straight into the kitchens. It would be, 'Hello, how are you?' and next thing you know, everyone in the kitchen was gone, working for Joe."

Primavera's anger was fake. Joe Baum delighted him, and there are always plenty of good cooks willing to teach at the Institute, which has a growing reputation.

There are always plenty of would-be students on the waiting list too, Primavera said, among them a wide range of types including ex-Army officers, engineers, people who were beach bums until the spirit of Carême reared up and bit them.

Dione Lucas left the CIA her knives, Poppy Cannon left the CIA her books, many food and wine lovers support the school's annual fund through an organization called the Fellows of the Culinary Institute, but most important to the student is the fact that important restaurant men like Joe Baum and H. Jerome Berns, the god of "21", hire the school's graduates. (Berns, a colorful old-style entrepreneur, once awoke to discover that Mimi Sheraton had given "21"'s food a bad notice. "Everyone's entitled to his own opinion," Berns said philosophically. "I respect her. And I've instructed my people at the door to break her arm the next time she comes in.")

Before World War II, all great chefs were assumed to be foreign-born. Now such restaurants as Lutèce, La Caravelle, and Windows on the World welcome CIA-trained personnel, who arrive with "back of the house" and "front of the house" skills, and who seem to be totally dedicated to their chosen profession.

Even the cheers of the school's hockey team ring with culinary overtones ("*Mirepoix, mirepoix, roux! roux! roux!* Slice 'em up, dice 'em up, throw 'em in the stew!" cry rooters), and one student told a reporter he wanted to be a chef because it would help him "to please others in a more direct and rewarding manner than I can now as a tax accountant."

As though to prove that American cooks are the equal of cooks anywhere, 1977 graduates of the CIA took a bunch of gold medals at the World Culinary Competition in Switzerland, and the school has won verbal medals from many food authorities. "It's the best school of its kind in the country," says Craig Claiborne, while Julia Child observes that "We're very lucky to have it; there's so much demand for people with training."

To be sure, there are naysayers. Countess Marina de Brantes, who owns Le Coup de Fusil, an elegant restaurant on New York's East Side (and who runs a cooking school upstairs), says she wouldn't hire CIA graduates. "The training is good for the chain hotels, but not good for a fine restaurant."

Even among enthusiasts, an occasional reservation—no pun intended—is entertained. Roger Fessaguet of La Caravelle worries that the CIA degree "is now held in such esteem too many graduates come away with the feeling that they've learned all they need to know." Julia too says it takes more than a few semesters of training to make a great chef.

"You spend a few weeks in pastry . . . when what you need is ten years. You're really only an apprentice when you graduate."

A well-fed apprentice.

Chef and teacher par excellence, Wayne Almquist, described by one journalist as a man of "magnificent girth," says, "Food is my whole way of life." To see him is to believe him. Form, as the Bauhaus crowd used to insist, follows function.

As for the swelling student population, well, reports the *Christian Science Monitor*, "On the average a student gains twenty pounds at the CIA."

PUTTING IT ON:
We're fat because we have to amortize our toys.

11 Cooking Equipment: "Never Buy a Food Processor from a Thin Man"

When you have a mind to laugh, you shall see me, fat and sleek with good keeping, a hog of Epicurus' herd.
—HORACE

CARL SONTHEIMER, at Cuisinarts, has been doing a series of commercials for his company. He stands behind the Cuisinart food processor, offering various pieces of wisdom. One of these is, "Never buy a food processor from a thin man."

The Cuisinart food processor, a marvelous tool or a toy for grown-ups, depending on how you look at it, came here from France and found a good home. A million good homes. People own a Cuisinart who use it only to crush ice or to chop onions, though the thing can crumb and shred and slice and knead and grind and, for all I know, give you a haircut and paint your apartment.

Equipment to help us stay fat by helping us to eat more, and more easily, is everywhere—the merchandising fallout of the food boom.

In an essay written for the *American Heritage Cookbook*, Russell Lynes said the mechanical gadgets that filled our kitchens were "partly a result of the disappearance of domestic servants from so many households and partly a cause for their disappearance."

Enormous skill had once been necessary in order for an American woman to put a meal on the table, Lynes reminded his readers. "When one considers that in 1800 lavish two-course dinners were cooked on an open fire, that meats were roasted on spits or by metal heat reflectors, that pies and breads were baked in brick ovens preheated with hot coals or by burning twigs in them, it seems to us nearly incredible. 'It was a wonder,' wrote a household expert in 1900, 'that the women who ministered as cooks before those great altars were not devoured by the flames.'"

Although wood- and coal-burning stoves came in around 1840, gas stoves didn't appear for another fifty years, and electric ranges were scarce until the 1920s. For that matter, up until forty years ago, "the iceman cometh" was a simple statement of fact; electric refrigerators didn't hit the market until 1916, when they cost almost a thousand dollars apiece, and the prices stayed high until the 40s. "It was not until after the Second World War," says Russell Lynes, "that the home freezer had such an extensive influence on what got put on the American table, and delicacies that were once attainable only by the rich . . . became everybody's provender."

And utensils that would have been called "fancy" by Mrs. Rorer became everybody's playthings. To Mrs. Rorer, a well-furnished kitchen was more important than a well-furnished parlor—"Time, to the housewife, is money, consequently, purchase such machines as will save both"—but her taste in equipment was basic. Eggbeater, double boiler, meat chopper, and braising pan were Mrs. Rorer's indispensables, and she cautioned against the purchase of "all unnecessary and fancy utensils."

Paul Bocuse, the Frenchman many gourmets consider the best chef alive today, has a list that isn't much longer than Mrs. Rorer's. He requires "a good stove, a casserole, a cast-iron pot for stews, a frying pan, a whisk, a knife, a wooden spoon."

But Bocuse can fill in any gaps in his equipment with genius, whereas most of us hope that by buying this or that magical helper, we'll discover the secret of great cooking.

In 1977, *Time* magazine reported that a place in Hollywood would sell you a kitchen for $65,000, with "a Fasar range, which cooks by magnetic induction, a gas-fired wok, warming drawers, chopping-block islands with separate vegetable sinks, a rolltop condiment 'garage,' a fireplace, sofas, music, a soda fountain, and an indoor barbecue. . . .

But even outside Hollywood, *cuisiniers* pamper their kitchens with gadgets, widgets, and wonderizers that are worth more to them than yesteryear's family retainer."

One married couple told the *Time* reporter they could never contemplate divorce ("Who would get the Cuisinart, and who the Kitchen Aid mixer?"), and *Time* pronounced the sexual revolution dead. The Great American Love Affair, said the magazine, was "taking place in the kitchen."

It wasn't exactly hot news. Eleven years earlier, *Time*'s cover story on Julia Child had revealed that if Julia so much as mentioned vanilla wafers on a show, or used a fish poacher, the next day Julia fans went out and stripped the shops of vanilla wafers and fish poachers.

Practicing what Julia preached paid off, too. By the 1970s, a connoisseur like Chef Jacques Pepin was saying American cooks were the best in the world outside of France and China.

And we did it fast, coming from ham on rye, and Mom's apple pie with Velveeta, to a world we never knew, a world of truffles and *vol-au-vent* and rosemary and *roux*. The more adventurous among us evinced an interest in trying such delicacies as fried grasshoppers and rattlesnake meat. (Once, when I was planning a future in which I would be famous, I worked on preparing a few witty sayings so I wouldn't be caught short. One of my schemes would have been elaborate to set up, since it involved my being interviewed outside a gourmet store in the window of which tins of rattlesnake meat were featured. "You ever eat rattlesnake?" the interviewer would ask. "Yes," I would say. "How come?" he would say, and I would smile shyly. "It was him or me.")

Zabar's, a store on New York's West Side that has been in the same spot for thirty-five years, reflects the changes brought about by the American frenzy to make our taste buds bloom.

Zabar's used to be a delicatessen, featuring lox and chopped liver and rolls and salami. Fifteen years ago, when Murray Klein became a partner of the Zabar brothers, Stanley and Saul, the three men added housewares.

To a food and/or equipment freak, Zabar's is fairyland. Colanders, salad washers, strainers hang from the ceilings. There are garlic squeezers and egg slicers and olive pitters and every kind of device for making tea and coffee. Popcorn makers. Yogurt makers. Food factories—four buttons, three speeds. A French balance scale. A wine cooler that chills wine in sixty seconds.

In the front window, fresh cappelletti and tortellini. The narrow pathway between the counters is traversed by men pushing dollies, making deliveries, hauling boxes. Every Tuesday, the coffee comes in in 200-pound sacks. Zabar's buys only enough for one week's worth, so it's always fresh.

Chinese vegetables, kosher soups, calavo dip in a can, honey in the comb. Sesame oil, safflower oil, apricot kernel oil, walnut oil. Rice sticks from Hong Kong, whole roasted chestnuts from France. Panettone. Amaretti in tall skinny cans, and in short fat cans.

Salami crusted gray, looking as though it had been found in the ashes of Pompeii, and salami with a brown, pitted casing, and salami strange and misshapen, with knots like gnarled arthritic joints. German strudel, Greek baklava, Russian coffee cake.

There is butter from an Isigny cooperative, somewhere between Saint-Lô and Bayeux; there's a section for chocolates; there are cheeses from Italy, Switzerland, Holland, Norway, Denmark. The names (Saracino, Racletti, Burchcrois, Caccioreale, Le Vieux Pane) stir the imagination. There's a pale cream-colored cheese, its top studded with green and purple pistachio nuts; there's a tray of mini-cheeses, each one looking like a piece of a soap eraser, cheddar, double Gloucester, five for a dollar. A tiny round of French cheese that could pass for a wheel of stamps, and a horseshoe-shaped cheese from Grasse called Baraka, the same as LeRoi Jones.

A man lumbers out of the kitchen carrying a roasting pan heavy with brisket, still steaming, agleam with peppers and onions, on its way to the meat section, where a fellow named Harold is king. And king-size. You could safely buy a food processor from Harold; he is not a thin man. A boy brings him a vat of chopped liver. Harold tastes it. If he says no good, the whole vat is thrown away. "We can afford it," says Murray Klein. "We are not a little store that needs the $20."

The noise is loud in Zabar's, customers and clerks counterpoint. A lady looks at a smoked, fat-free duck, and speaks, somewhat mystifyingly, to her companion. "It's like a living thing."

Harold asks another woman what she wants. "Everything," she says. "That's the trouble."

A young couple stands in the middle of the floor, in danger of being run down, stepped on, elbowed, but they are rooted there, eyes wide. "My God," she says, "there's nothing in L.A. to equal this—"

Zabar's has cold rooms, storage rooms, rooms for unpacking. The kitchen is long and narrow, and the chef, an Oriental gentleman, has been at Zabar's for eight years. Under his guidance, salads are made, meats are cooked, trays for parties are assembled, a whole salmon sliced and put back together so realistically it might fool the salmon's mother.

At the cash register, a woman wants to know if she can phone to order twenty loaves of bread and twenty pounds of potato salad for a gala she's contemplating. "You don't have to order, just come around," says a counterman. "For twenty loaves?" she says. He sneers. "For a hundred loaves!"

Zabar's is expanding. The corner store (two doors away) has been taken over, made into a European-style espresso bar that also sells pastries from Délices La Côte Basque, a French bakery. The store between the original Zabar's and the coffee bar has recently been absorbed too. (Even the single-room-occupancy hotel that rises over the delicatessen, and in which Stanley Zabar holds "a substantial interest," is scheduled to become offices, kitchens, and storage space for Zabar's, once the tenants who live there are relocated. Some of these tenants, old people who had been paying low rents for forty years, picketed the store, carrying signs that said "Zabar's—Illegal, Immoral, Fattening" and chanting, "People Before Fish," although Stanley Zabar, who dislikes being thought of as the Lox That Ate Broadway promised the protesters nobody would be evicted before he or she had someplace to go.)

In the window of the espresso-and-pastry shop on the corner, a page from *New York* magazine is reproduced. It shows a picture of Murray Klein beaming, and it lists this new Zabar enterprise as one of its "Best Bets." Ungratefully, Zabar's has put a sign beneath the magazine's commendation. "These dummies went all over the world looking for the best espresso and cappuccino and then found it right here at Zabar's," the sign says.

Taking a ten-minute lunch break, Murray Klein is standing at his espresso bar, sipping a cappuccino spiked with cinnamon and Sweet 'n Low. He wears blue pants, gray sweater, no tie. His hair is white, his face is sweet, but he is never still. If the button on the phone across the room lights up, he is over there answering it, although there has been no sound, no ring, and you'd have sworn his back was turned to the instrument.

"By nature, I'm a proletarian, not a bourgeois," says Murray Klein, speaking English with a Yiddish accent. "I came over from Russia to the United States in 1950. My aunt brought me. I lived for a while in Italy first. It was after the war.

"I worked in a supermarket on Broadway. After that, I managed for Zabar's a supermarket. They had several supermarkets. Then I left, went in my own business, made money, sold my business. The Zabars gave up the supermarkets, just kept the one store, and they asked me to come back as a partner."

There are food experts in the city who say Murray Klein is totally responsible for making Zabar's into the most successful retailer of food and cooking equipment on a per-square-foot basis (which is the way department stores figure such things) in the entire United States. Murray Klein says the success part is true—"We do ten million dollars a year"—but he isn't the only mover and shaker; he and the Zabar brothers have worked together every step of the way.

Still, it was Klein's notion to stock household equipment. Why did the Zabars agree? Klein smiles. "They agreed because it was successful."

Klein chooses the equipment. "The best of everything. A lot of it is European. I don't say the United States doesn't make good machines, but they do it better in Europe. We stock the things department stores have, but we sell it 30 percent cheaper."

If he doesn't think it's good, Murray Klein won't handle it. "We don't sell percolators in Zabar's. They use 30 percent more coffee, and the coffee's bitter."

Even in the corner coffee shop, copper pots hang from the ceiling, amid signs advising the browser that he can obtain such copper pots two doors down the street.

When he first came to work for the Zabars, Klein says he didn't know about food. "We used to have meetings, and they would take me out to restaurants, so I would develop a taste for better food. I like simple food, schmaltz herring, a boiled potato and salt, like a peasant."

He savors his cappuccino. "When you go to Europe, you have a coffee, it tastes like this. This you drink slowly, you want to enjoy it because it's good. You go in a coffee shop over here, you taste the coffee, you want to get rid of it. They buy the cheapest coffee. Even if it's only five cents a pound cheaper, and it doesn't mean nothing to them. That goes for the coffee, that goes for the meat, the chocolate, whatever they buy. You go into Switzerland, and the smallest restaurant has pastry like in the best restaurant. Good. And it's going to come over here like that because people want better food now, they don't want just to fill their stomachs."

Zabar's, says Klein, doesn't cater to a luxury trade. "Zabar's is for anybody. They have Fauchon in Paris, Harrod's in London, those shops are for rich people, middle class wouldn't go in because everything looks so that you're afraid to touch it. Here it's made for everybody, sawdust on the floor. You can come and buy a roll for twenty cents, we treat you the same as if you buy a pound of caviar for $250. Europe has a history of food thousands of years, United States is a young country. Now that people have traveled to Europe, they come back, they don't want to eat so much hamburgers, they want to eat a piece of cheese and an apple, you can make a meal of it. Or cheese and wine. Or a good sausage. Smoked salmon used to be lox. Only for Jewish people. Now it's not true. You don't eat it with cream cheese, you eat it with butter. It's a delicacy." Murray Klein laughs. "Sah-moan foo-may," he says.

As an example of people's changing habits, Klein cites his croissant business. "We sell eight thousand croissants a week. And they're not cheap, they're fifty-five cents apiece. People who have four children come around and buy six croissants for breakfast, to enjoy it in the morning. They're not going to eat a doughnut like they used to, they want a good thing. I could buy croissants for half what I pay, but it's not going to be as good. So I pay more, I make a smaller profit, but people are gonna come from all over for the croissants."

The Zabar brothers and Klein do all their own buying. "Nobody buys for us," Klein says. "We sample green coffee, and if it's a good lot, we buy it, roast it ourselves. Saul Zabar buys the fish and Stanley Zabar buys the coffee."

There's another brother, Eli Zabar, who has gone into his own fancy food business, but Klein brushes away any suggestion that Eli might be competition. "We have no competition. There could come a store right here next door wouldn't be no competition.

"People come from all over the United States to us, people are searching, there's just nowhere they can get what we got. We mail to California, mail out the salamis from here because it's better. To Texas. To Chicago. They come here because they can't get it there. They say, 'Why don't you open a store there?' We can't. We'd lose control. I come in seven days a week here. Everything we make in the store, if it's not good, we throw it out, we don't cut corners.

"People trust us. They come around. 'What's a good pâté? What's a good coffeepot?' New people come to visit in the neighborhood, their host says, 'Come, I'll show you Zabar's.'"

Inflation, says Klein, hasn't caused people to spend less, but more. "They buy now. They're afraid it's going to be more expensive next week. There's more cooking at home because it's very expensive in the restaurants now. We got here people that know food, they would rather do their own."

Klein has been around long enough to have observed many fluctuations in the food habits of New Yorkers. He's seen the fever for "natural" foods flare up and die down again. "Good food is natural," he says. "The only thing is now we have the bacon without nitrites, the ham without nitrites. But you see changes every year. The people who come to Zabar's are mostly young, twenty-five to forty-five. The older people come in to buy some lox, some chopped liver, but they don't buy the household equipment, they don't buy the good cheeses—"

Mention Barbara Kafka's hypothesis that the food boom is over and Murray Klein looks disbelieving. "People are more cholesterol-conscious, but the food boom is just started," he says. "For the middle-class people in the United States, it's just started."

His own success surprises Murray Klein. "I never dreamt of it. I consider myself a rich man. But now I have the money I haven't got the time to go spend it, I haven't got the time to go on vacations. If I leave Zabar's to go home early, I feel guilty."

Would he want his fourteen-year-old son to go into the business? No way. "Too much pressure. I go in at six o'clock in the morning (we open at eight), I start selecting, I gotta order, I gotta buy—" Suddenly, Murray Klein grins. "I couldn't do without it."

He thinks again about what Barbara Kafka has said, and shakes his head. "Food is never over," he says.

Still, it isn't only the food—in a big city like New York, there are many stores that stock delicacies; Bloomingdale's advertises quail eggs and crusts of salt "formed by the East wind blowing over the top of the water in the salt basins of Brittany"—but the food equipment that put Zabar's so emphatically on the map.

It—the equipment business—is part of the overall big business in cookbooks, in cooking schools, in restaurants, in fast foods, in gourmet foods, that has come out of the food boom.

The equipment mania seems to date from the 60s, when there was great national prosperity, and people didn't worry about money as much as they do now. Anyone who wanted a $19.95 kitchen tool just went out and bought it. And in the early 60s, we were Francophiles. Mrs. Kennedy wore Paris clothes and had a French chef, ever-increasing numbers of people who traveled abroad came back proclaiming the wonders of French cuisine, and on television, there was Julia, presiding over this latest French revolution. She not only said let them eat cake, but told them how to whip up the batter.

People watched her cook, and decided they couldn't live without flambé pans and aspic molds and snail-serving equipment. Suddenly, they were buying tools like toast tongs, which had only one use—silly gadgets along with sensible ones.

Later, when the Chinese cooking craze struck, woks, spatulas, and cleavers sold wildly, though anyone could stir-fry in a conventional skillet if he wanted to. But the consumer wasn't buying a way to fry, he was buying a way to have a whole new eating experience.

Consider the success of *The Cooks' Catalogue*, published by Harper and Row in 1975. It contained beautiful photographs and drawings, anecdotes about food, recipes, excellent research, but essentially the book was a compendium of thousands of items of kitchen equipment, described and organized, with prices, evaluations, and lists of manufacturers and suppliers; it was, in short, an oversized hardcover guide to cooking utensils. And it sold over 200,000 copies, dumbfounding Burton Wolf, the man Jim Beard described in the book's introduction as its "principal architect."

"I thought if we sold 15,000 copies, we would be fantastic," says Wolf. "I had no idea there would be this enormous interest."

No idea? Maybe some small idea. Because Wolf and a group of investment bankers in Switzerland put up $800,000 (with the paperback publisher, Avon, contributing another $100,000) to bring the volume out in the first place.

Practically $1 million. Wouldn't it be almost impossible to earn your money back on such an investment?

"Well, yeah," says Wolf, "but the book has led to a hell of a lot of other things."

In truth, the book has generated an industry.

Three hundred stores across the United States are featuring Cooks' Catalogue corners where computerized television furnishes advice for equipment shoppers. If you want to know how to make quiche lorraine, you consult an index, press a "Search" button on the machine, and quiche lorraine pops up on a screen in front of you, its preparation being demonstrated by—you got it—Burt Wolf. Not because he's interested in selling cheese and ham, but because he's interested in selling the mixers, the pans, the measuring spoons, whatever tools it takes to put together a quiche.

Barbara Kafka, to whom Beard ascribes most of the credit for the excellence of *The Cooks' Catalogue* ("I didn't do anything on it except be a consultant," Beard says modestly. "Barbara wrote the whole thing."), believes Wolf's goal in doing the book was to become "a food personality. I think he perceives that television is the great road to success in this part of the world, and this is one way of being an actor, being on these machines. They're in the stores, they're a novelty, and what the financial arrangements are, I have no idea."

The financial arrangements, says Wolf, are complicated. "It's a big business to me, to the department stores, to the manufacturers. I wrote the scripts, I produced the tapes. The idea was developed to meet the needs of stores—I'm a consultant to seventeen major department stores—which have a problem demonstrating complex equipment. Sometimes there's a demonstrator who can do it, sometimes there isn't. So I said, 'Listen, we could try this and this and this,' and the stores said, 'Wonderful. Do it.'"

There is coolness between Kafka and Wolf because Kafka believes she was treated shabbily. "I had a letter of agreement whereby my name had to appear on the title page of *The Cooks' Catalogue*. When the book came out—Burton hadn't even sent me a copy—Jim Beard called me and said, 'You'd better come over here,' and I went to his house, and he had the book, and my name did not appear on the title page. I just broke into tears, which was not very dignified, but three years of my life had gone into the work."

Wolf says it was the publisher's decision to have the book's title page bare of anything but the title. "He didn't want *anyone* on the title page, me, Barbara, Jim, anyone. He had the right to do that. On the staff page, five important people were listed." (The "staff" page says "Edited by James Beard, Milton Glaser, Burton Wolf, Barbara Poses Kafka, Helen S. Witty, and Associates of the Good Cooking School".)

Jim Beard may claim he didn't do anything, says Wolf, "and in the day-to-day selection of pots and pans, this was true, but none of us would have known how to direct the book without his thinking. We'd go to him, and he would play Socrates, he would say, 'No, that is not a category,' or, 'That should be dealt with here,' and while these seem like little things to him, they gave form to the book."

Burton Wolf is forty-one years old, and grew up with the housewares business. "My grandmother owned a housewares store; it wasn't called a gourmet shop in those days. I played in the store, unpacked all the stuff, put the prices on it. It was during the Second World War, when you couldn't get a lot of toys, and my first conscious memory is of playing in a graniteware roaster, making believe it was a boat. I was always paddling down the Amazon in graniteware roasters. I didn't know where the Amazon was, but it sounded exotic to me.

"In the mid-sixties, I moved to Switzerland, hung around in great restaurants, learned to cook, learned to eat. I was an investment banker, and I specialized in investments that had to do with food and fine arts, so I knew a hell of a lot about what was going on in the food and cooking equipment business. In the early 70s, I bought the rights to cooking equipment developed by the three-star chefs of France, people like Bocuse, the Troisgros. Nobody knew who they were in the United States. I bought the rights to about 150 or 200 designs, but I couldn't tell which would be the most commercial for the United States market. Tools that were essential to the German or the Italian or the French or the English kitchen were esoteric for America, and I wanted to check in and get updated, so I came back home and asked Jim Beard, 'What do I do with all this stuff?'

"Jim and Milton Glaser and I went to lunch one day, and got to talking about equipment, and realized there was no definitive analysis of what was available. 'Listen,' I said, 'I'll get the money together from my investors, the banking group, and let's do a book.' Shortly thereafter, I moved back to the United States, because the book wasn't something I could do in Europe, and I assembled the group that put it all together."

Among those assembled was Barbara Kafka, described by Wolf as "difficult, complicated, but worth it, because she can do things that are just wonderful."

Barbara Kafka says that merchandising may have been in Wolf's head when he approached her to work on the book, but it wasn't in hers. "If *The Cooks' Catalogue* had just listed the manufacturer of something, and the price at that given moment, it would have died very quickly. I think it didn't die because the material had never been codified before. Here was all this material of the kitchen, and I tried to conceptualize it, put it in a logical sequence that hadn't existed before.

"Cooking equipment has a long history. The first tools of which we have any record are grinding stones, and things for killing animals. Man could find shelter in a cave, and he'd been an ape very few millennia ago, so clothing wasn't his first requirement, but feeding himself was. And as he changed and evolved, he prepared food. Man seems to be the only animal that makes tools, and if that's true, our start up the road from being great apes was as toolmakers of cooking equipment.

"How to go from a griddle stone and a fire tool to a pot was an idea that interested me. It interests me in equipment and it interests me in food. There's a Claude Lévi-Strauss book called *Le Cru et le cuit* ("The Raw and the Cooked") in which he proposes a theory that the way people prepare food is as good a means of defining a society as language. He's a structuralist, so it gets a little silly for me as an American at times, but the basic premise that a society is definable by its modes of eating and of cooking is important. Lévi-Strauss says there was the cooked, there was the raw, there was the rotted. People are always a little aghast when you say the rotted, but the yeasts that make bread are the product of a rotting procedure, wine is a rotted product, soy sauce is a rotted product, the garum, a sauce used in Roman times, was based on rotted fish."

Off and sparking, Kafka's mind leaps from idea to idea, leaving a listener gasping for breath. Among the modes of energy, we have to count human energy, she says. "The Japanese and Chinese cut food up in little pieces to cook it because, historically, they had very little fuel. Whereas a North American Indian could roast a whole beast and be profligate with fuel—

"Another obvious variable is the cost of the food itself. The more expensive the food ingredient, generally speaking, the less time and labor and fuel are used to consume it. So that caviar comes straight out of the fish and is washed off and is never cooked and requires no human energy to prepare it. Logical continuum."

The American bias *against* self-indulgence is one of the reasons, paradoxically, that fancy cooking equipment sells, according to Barbara Kafka. If a new dress would cost you two hundred dollars, and a food processor would cost you two hundred dollars, "then your value system is going to tell you to buy the kitchen gadget because, after all, you're not really doing that for yourself, you're doing it for someone else. We're a puritanical society."

Our puritanism helps make us fat, too, which sounds like another contradiction, but which Kafka renders logical. "I lose weight when I go to France," she says, "because the food is so satisfying I only eat a little bit of it. But the idea of leaving some of that very expensive food is alien to most of our culture." (One of the food establishment's claims to superiority over weaker mortals is the way they get skinny on great French food by pushing heavenly morsels to one side; we've heard this now from Gael Greene, and Karen Hess, as well as Barbara Kafka. What the experts don't seem to take into account is that they're offered more opportunities to pig out than the rest of us, and can therefore build up their stoicism. After the thirteenth time you're invited to lay lip to, say, "an incredible rich sauté of *foie gras* served with an exquisitely silken sauce made of a strong reduction of white wine—more than a bottle, shallots—two cups chopped, and heavy cream—three cups, to serve eight,"* you and the other seven guys are probably ready to say thanks a lot, but alien to my culture as rejecting this expensive goose's liver is, I think I'll just choke down a light green herb mousse and a couple of calf's brains in marinade. Plus a glass seltzer water.)

Mais oui. Brought up to clean our plates, we clean 'em if it kills us. And it sometimes does, but that's another chapter.

Barbara Kafka may believe that the cooking madness is tapering off, and that the 80s will bring some other enthusiasm, but Burton Wolf, like Murray Klein, is unconvinced. "It could be true for the fashionable world," he says, "for the wealthy, sophisticated people who bore easily and read *W*, and know what's in and say, 'I've done that,' and move on to something else. But do you know what a small fraction of the population those people are?"

The middle class is different, Wolf says, echoing Klein's idea that with dinner for four costing a hundred dollars at a mediocre restaurant, more middle-class women—and men—will be going back to entertaining at home. On good equipment. Because if a tool costs a lot today, it will cost even more tomorrow, and a good knife can last fifty years.

Top quality cookware sells, says Wolf, even in hard times. "I saw a new pot and pan line—it was Magnalite—introduced at Bloomingdale's Housewares Fair last January. It did two million dollars in about ninety days."

That costs keep rising, there's no gainsaying. I asked Murray Klein if, as a result of mass production and wider interest, the prices of some

*Description, courtesy Craig Claiborne, *New York Times*, October 24, 1979.

equipment sold at Zabar's hadn't come down. "Nothing," said Murray Klein, "comes down."

In *The Cooks' Catalogue*, now several years old, a beautiful spatula from France was listed as costing $5.50. In November of 1979, writing in the *New York Times*, Pierre Franey said he had walked the town searching out decent spatulas, and the best he had found—again, they were French—cost eleven and twelve dollars apiece.

Clearly, Wolf and Klein are right. Don't buy it now, and it will cost you more later. Wolf says he can advise his client stores six months in advance about what equipment is going to sell and what equipment is not going to sell. "Because I've been in the marketplace for ten years."

He writes a weekly piece for the *Washington Post*, he mails a monthly newsletter to a hundred private clients—"key people in the food equipment industry"—and in addition to his TV demonstration tapes for department stores, he's been making 90-second television spots, produced by *Newsweek*, and seen all over the country on such programs as the *Today Show* and *Good Morning, America*. The series of spots is called "What's Cooking with Burt Wolf."

"My audience," says Wolf, "is six million ladies who are looking at me across an ironing board, and they're saying, 'Oh, *that's* how you tell a good mushroom.' They're trying to learn to live better, to get good food for less money, to have their kids grow up without the chemical problems our generation seems to be having. My customers don't even read newspapers, okay? They watch me because I'm free. If you add up the circulation of *Gourmet* magazine, *Cooking* magazine, *Food and Wine* magazine, what have you got, two million people? I'm not talking to those people at all."

Wolf's ladies write him wanting to know if convection ovens are dangerous, and what he thinks about microwaves, and where they can buy electric teakettles. He'll tell them those things and more. How to measure sticky stuff, how to buy two spectacular gadgets that cost less than two dollars each, how to season a pot, which cooking equipment they really need. He doesn't talk to his ladies about gourmet cooking, but he does talk to them about health. He is a bit of a crusader.

"In my apartment, there is a giant sign on the refrigerator and it says *No Processed Foods, No Fats, No Sugars, No White Flours, or Removed Grains*. There's only whole wheat here, whole rice here. I did a show about candy bars. A candy bar contains the same amount of sugar as eight apples. How many people can sit down and eat eight apples? I walk out into the street and see a kid knocking off two Milky Ways. That's sixteen apples. The body was never made to handle that kind of volume of sugar. That's why people are sick. And that's why people are fat."

Right, Burt. And yet, and yet. In the mid-seventies, when *nouvelle cuisine* and *cuisine minceur* were being widely touted, some eaters turned the other way. "Without butter, cream and *foie gras*, what's left of French cooking?" demanded Jack Lirio, who ran a cooking school in San Francisco. And even Chef Michel Guérard who, after gaining twenty-six pounds, pioneered the butter-free, oil-free, cream-free, sugar-free diet, couldn't conceive of rejecting *grande cuisine* in perpetuity. "Dietetic food will never replace it," he said. "That would be awful."

In an attempt to forestall such awfulness, Americans buy crepe pans and escargot pans and soufflé dishes and porcelain mortars and pestles and take them home to play with.

To the tune of billions of dollars. We are obsessed with food and ways to fix it and what to fix it in. How could we not be fat?

PUTTING IT ON:
We're fat because we want to be (or some of us say we do).

12 The Other Side of Fatness: Big Is Beautiful

W'at good eesa wife eef she don'ta be fat?
—THOMAS AUGUSTINE DALY

IN MODERN GREECE, the majority of the populace thinks that jogging is something indulged in by lunatics, and that fat is grand. A 1979 survey conducted by the Greek government showed that Greek women and children were, on the average, between twelve and sixteen pounds heavier than other Europeans, which finding so upset the government that it decided to take action, and promptly produced a TV commercial showing a plump diner falling dead at the dinner table, and captioned, "Fatness shortens life."

The awful truth, as revealed to journalist Paul Anastasi, by Dr. Spyros Doxiades, the minister of social services, was that Greeks "have traditionally associated obesity with health."

For the ordinary Greek citizen whose family has suffered from generations of malnutrition (as recent an historical event as World War II brought famine and death to thousands of Greeks), "heavy eating and fat came to be associated with life."

The lord of a Greek village was always "the man with the enormous belly who had a lot to eat," said Dr. Doxiades. "Similarly, Greek mothers stuff their already overweight children and are proud of their kids' fatness and appetite . . ."

Excessive eating, added Helen Dimou (another Greek government functionary), had become a national sport.

Even in France, where eating (a religion) is at war with fashion (a different religion), round women have their admirers.

"They go out with the thin ones, they go home with the fat ones," says the actress, Régine, munching contentedly, in a Claude Berri movie.

And if a large French lady finds herself ignored at home, she can make her way to an Arab country.

Moviemaker Jean-Jacques Annaud told *Women's Wear Daily* reporter Christopher Sharp about a friend of his who produces TV films in France. "She is so heavy that by necessity she has to travel first-class—she could not fit into a second-class seat. Five years ago, we went on a trip to Arabia, and she received so many propositions she was beside herself. Even the Shah of Iran and King Hussein wanted her."

What, you may wonder, has this nattering on about Greece (and France and Arabia) got to do with a book examining fat in America? Just this. There is in our country a segment of population which is as protective of its amplitude as are the Greeks.

Throwbacks to Lillian Russell and Aunt Jemima (the woman named Anna Robinson who modeled for the picture on the box of pancake flour from 1933 until the early 60s weighed 350 pounds), they're fat and proud of it.

In fact, "Fat . . . And Proud of It" was the title of a *60 Minutes* segment broadcast by CBS in December of 1978.

A group of hefties—The National Association to Aid Fat Americans—was holding a convention in Washington, D.C., and Mike Wallace took a camera crew and went to look and listen. "It wasn't going to be a diet seminar," Wallace told his audience, "nothing like Overeaters Anonymous. Instead, it would be a weekend dedicated to fat pride, fat liberation."

Wallace found 150 fat people, most of them female, willing to discuss their having come out of the closet ("I'm finally admitting I am a fat person, and starting really to enjoy life at thirty," said one), and the prejudices of the straight (and narrow) world.

Unlike the Greeks, whom their government wants to educate away from a simple enjoyment of food and the flesh that follows, American fat folk have complex emotional responses to their largeness. Heavyweights who choose not to be cured of their fatness, like homosexuals who choose to remain outside the mainstream, say they are fighting a lonely battle against societal pressure.

Here is testimony collected from various speakers by *60 Minutes:*

"Most people . . . do not like me because I am fat."

"Within the past two months, I have been the unwilling participant of a verbal attack in public . . . with vicious language . . . about my size."

"I was in the supermarket . . . and a woman said to me, 'You have such a pretty face. Do you enjoy being fat?' I said, 'I work very hard at it. It took me a long time to get this way.'"

"I want to be acknowledged, and I want to be loved for who I am. And I don't want to walk down the street and have people turn around and make fun of my package."

Fat Americans, Mike Wallace was informed, couldn't get jobs as easily as thin Americans. "I went to a representative on the Hill," said a woman named Betty. "He had an opening as an aide . . . He called my boss. He said, 'Mr. Kelly, I really like Betty. She's got a wild sense of humor, she dresses well. But I don't put fat girls in my office.'"

Romance was more difficult for fat women too. "Men would like to be with fat women in the open," said one, "go to restaurants and everything else, but society has put so much pressure on them, telling them, 'Hey, you have to go out to a restaurant with a skinny woman—'"

True enough, said another. "Many men seem to have a fantasy of going to bed with a fat woman. They enjoy it. And once they get there, believe me, they enjoy it. But . . . some of them don't want to be seen in public with us."

A man whose taste did run to fleshy females said he found it hard "when people ridicule the type of woman that you like, and say they're ugly, and they laugh at you when you walk with them arm in arm down the street. Some people like to look at fat people. I love to look at a fat woman on the beach. If I saw Marilyn Monroe or Gina Lollobrigida on the beach, they turn me off. It's just like looking at a board."

The more Wallace probed, the sadder his subjects appeared to him. Fat people were supposed to be jolly, said Wallace, but in this meeting room, "I wondered if I didn't detect a real melancholy."

Occasionally, a success story surfaced, certifying the convention's fat-and-proud-of-it theme, as when a couple who'd been married for a year (thin man, fat woman) told Wallace they were very happy. "It doesn't matter whether I weigh 150 pounds or 350 pounds, I'm still me," said the bride.

The staggered Wallace took a breath. "You weigh 350?"

"Three seventy-five," bragged the lady's husband.

On balance, *60 Minutes* concluded, no matter how pleased with themselves they claimed they were, more agony than ecstasy prevailed among these defiant fat folks. "More dollars are spent on worthless cures for obesity than for all medical research combined," Wallace said, "and America grows fatter. The fact is science simply doesn't yet fully understand the psychology and physiology behind obesity. And behind their mask of pride or joy or liberation, America's fat people, especially America's fat women, suffer . . ."

But some conventioneers were determined to suffer no more. The woman who'd told Wallace she was beginning to enjoy life at thirty added that she was "learning to accept myself, and go out . . . to the beach in a bathing suit, if I want to. And if they don't like to look at me, they don't have to."

"If they don't like to look at me," Wallace repeated. "That's a sore point with many fat women who feel that even advertisers who are trying to woo them don't much like to look at them."

He probably wasn't aware of it, but even as he spoke, a couple in California were planning to do something about this last problem. Fade to Carol and Ray Shaw in Century City. Mrs. Shaw, forty-three years old, 200 pounds, and extremely handsome, had just come home from a shopping trip without having bought any clothes. Because what the stores showed for fat ladies were "tents, caftans, and acres of peach polyester."

Besides being frustrated, Mrs. Shaw found herself, she told Jill Gerston, a writer for the *Philadelphia Inquirer*, "mad. I said to Ray, 'You know what's needed in this world? A magazine for fat ladies.'"

Mr. Shaw is as fearless as his wife. The couple rented an office, hired a staff, and began putting out "the world's first fashion magazine for large-size women."

Don't feel bad that you didn't think of it. It wasn't one of those we-took-forty-nine-cents-and-parlayed-it-into-a-combine-that-bought-two-small-countries-and-a-tropical-island deals; the Shaws invested $250,000 in the venture, and if things had gone differently, they might have watched their savings float away on a tide of printer's ink.

As it turned out, the time for Mrs. Shaw's idea had come. *Big Beautiful Woman* was swamped with subscriptions. (The first issue, March–April of 1979, sold out its entire run of 75,000 copies, even though it was circulated only in the West. Of the second issue, 150,000 copies were printed and sold, the third issue went national, and the fourth—November–December—issue was bought by 250,000 customers at $2 a copy.)

As editor of *Big Beautiful Woman,* Carol Shaw is fiercely protective of her fat clientele ("Fat is not a dirty word," she says, "it's a description, like tall, short, old, young"), and any size 22 who picks up the magazine will not have her eyes assaulted by skinny models, or articles about diets, or exhortations to exercise.

"There are 25 million women in the United States who are size 16 and over who have been treated like second-class citizens by the fashion industry ever since the turn of the century when rounded shapes went out of style," says Carol Shaw. "They've been brought up to believe that fat is synonymous with ugly. Well, it's not . . . our magazine is . . . telling these women to stop apologizing . . . Everyone, no matter what size she wears, is entitled to the most up-to-the-minute, fashionable clothes available."

Because she didn't know any better, Mrs. Shaw went out and called on manufacturers and retailers ("No one had told me it's supposed to be impossible to get advertisers for a new magazine") and her efforts bore fruit. "The response was amazing, we had to bump articles to make room for ads in the first issue."

Suddenly, manufacturers are making better looking clothes in large sizes, a fat woman can buy designer jeans if she wants them (Lane Bryant, a New York store catering to large women, advertises that "for the first time, the genius of Adolfo has been translated into special sizes just for you"), and she can also buy shirts with horizontal stripes, and dresses in colors once considered too lively for the titanic torso. Up until now, the manufacturers' reasoning has seemed to be, elephants are gray, therefore anything outsize should be colored like an elephant.

Altruism isn't what turned the tycoons of the rag trade around, says Mrs. Shaw, it was money. "As soon as manufacturers heard there was lots of money available in our fat little fists to spend on fashionable clothes, they jumped on the bandwagon."

A company called Madame Pompadour was founded by a young woman named Patricia Leonard with the sole intention of making silk dresses in sizes 18 to 26; manufacturer Samuel Robert is making up size 20s in the Ultrasuedes and tweeds for which his company is famous; a shop called "12 Plus" in New York's Saks Fifth Avenue opened in the summer of 1979, and was an instant success; The Forgotten Woman, a boutique that sells only sizes 14 to 46, was such a hit on New York's Lexington Avenue that its owner started two more branches, with others planned in Florida and California. Even panty hose are being designed with full fashion treatment—flower and butterfly designs, pretty colors—for queen-size legs.

Clearly, Carol Shaw was on to something.

She had been, she explains, a fat child. "I died of humiliation every time they weighed us in school. When I heard the popular song, 'I Don't Want Her, You Can Have Her, She's Too Fat for Me,' I was convinced someone had seen me on the street and had written the song about me."

Humiliated or not, Carol Shaw (then Carol Bennett) was fair of face, and a good athlete (she's still a strong swimmer), and she didn't suffer any lack of attention from boys. Brought up in New York City, she studied music, became a singer, but quit her career when she married Shaw, himself an entertainer turned businessman.

In 1965, the Shaws and their two little girls moved to California, and Mrs. Shaw went into a decline. Literally. Looking without respite at suntanned starlets with Scarlett O'Hara waistlines drove her to diets. She tried every kind, from staples in her ears (an acupuncture device that is supposed to dissipate food cravings) to Weight Watchers, went down to a size 9, and into a deep depression. She didn't want to spend the rest of her life dieting, her husband liked her the old way, and finally, she decided to let nature takes its course. Especially the dessert course.

Mrs. Shaw is that happy heavyweight for whom Mike Wallace was searching. She's full, and fulfilled. "I've got a clean bill of health from my doctor, I feel wonderful, and I like the way I look. My grandmother was a size 44 and lived till ninety-five, and I have every intention of following in her footsteps."

Big footsteps. The models in Shaw's magazine are big ("skinny models in fat clothes look ridiculous"), the circulation of the magazine is getting bigger, and the Shaws' bank account is doubtless swelling along with everything else.

Besides photographs of king-size beauties in up-to-the-minute duds, *Big Beautiful Woman* features pieces on gourmet cooking (for the only audience in America that permits itself guiltless stuffing) and complaint coupons. The coupons come in pairs. The reader can send a coupon to any store that doesn't stock a variety of clothing choices for fat women, or to any store where the help has been rude. (Traditionally, fat people have been contemptuously treated by saleswomen in clothing departments.) The second—duplicate—coupon goes to *Big Beautiful Woman*, so the magazine can pressure the stores.

But it's the letters to the editor that thrill Mrs. Shaw. "Women write and tell me, 'I'm fat, I feel terrific . . . I have a wonderful job, my husband thinks I'm sexy, and my family loves me. I don't want to live my life on cottage cheese and lettuce, all I want are some beautiful, fashionable clothes.'"

Suzanne Jordan, who teaches English at North Carolina State University, doesn't even care about beautiful, fashionable clothes, she just wants thin people to get off fat people's backs.

Thin people, said Ms. Jordan, in a rollicking essay printed by the ordinarily sober *Newsweek* magazine, needed watching. "Caesar was right. I've been watching them for most of my adult life, and I don't like what I see. When these narrow fellows spring at me, I quiver to my toes . . . All of them are dangerous."

What were Ms. Jordan's complaints against skinnies? Their metabolisms, chiefly. "They say things like, 'There aren't enough hours in the day.' Fat people never say that. Fat people think the day is too damn long already."

Thin people jogged and fixed screen doors and searched out new problems. "I like to surround myself with sluggish, inert, easygoing fat people," wrote Jordan, "the kind who believe that if you clean it up today, it'll just get dirty again tomorrow."

Wizened, shriveled, surly, mean, hard at a young age—this was the Jordan assessment of thin people. "Because they never learn the value of a hot-fudge sundae for easing tension." Why didn't thin people like gooey soft things? "Because they themselves aren't gooey or soft," but "crunchy and dull, like carrots."

Thin people wanted to face the truth, believed in logic, math, morality, "and reasoned evaluation of the limitations of human beings."

Fat people, said Jordan, didn't. Furthermore, fat people knew that a program for happiness such as thin people work out is "never better than a whole cheesecake."

Fat people, said Jordan, "will like you even if you're irregular and have acne. They will come up with a good reason why you never wrote the Great American Novel. They will cry in your beer with you . . . they will let you off the hook . . . They are gluttonous and goodly and great . . . What you want when you're down is soft and jiggly, not muscled and stable. Fat people know this. Fat people have plenty of room. Fat people will take you in."

The Jordan treatise so moved *Newsweek* readers that it made even thin ones feel guilty, which was a nice switch. "I'd gladly trade my size-five jeans for a hot-fudge sundae anytime," wrote one poor miserable creature, but "my insatiable ego won't let me do it."

(A small amount of righteous indignation surfaced too. "Speaking as an ex-heavyweight," wrote a San Franciscan, "I am outraged by Ms. Jordan's defense of fat people. Obesity isn't funny. It is a pandemic and a leading contributor to illness and death in the U.S.")

A few months later, the *National Enquirer*, a newspaper known, if not for subtlety and taste, at least for liveliness, also came out for more and happier fat people. "Your Extra Pounds Are Good For You," headlined the *Enquirer*, and cited authorities to back up this amazing proposition. "Some experts," the paper crowed, "say it's o.k. to be 35 percent heavier!"

Which experts? A Dr. Andres, "clinical director of the prestigious National Institute on Aging," for one, and a Dr. Seltzer, "a Harvard University researcher," for another.

Dr. Andres was quoted as saying, "There's something about being moderately overweight that's good for you" (though he did warn that obesity could be "devastating" for people with diabetes, high blood pressure, and high cholesterol), while Dr. Seltzer took a shot at those "ideal" height-weight tables used by insurance companies, pronouncing them off-base.

The *Enquirer* also referred to The Framingham Heart Study sponsored by the National Heart, Lung and Blood Institute ("the lowest death rates were among men and women aged forty to fifty-nine whose average weight was 15 to 20 percent over their ideal weight shown on the Metropolitan Life Insurance Company's tables") and hauled in for review a fourteen-year study conducted by Northwestern University. "'In that project, researchers found people with the lowest mortality were 25 to 35 percent overweight,' said Dr. Alan R. Dyer, Ph.D., associate professor of Community Health and Preventive Medicine, who co-authored the study . . ."

Isn't it pretty to think so.

In the end, Robert Morley, that lovely campy actor (I know, he isn't American, he isn't even Greek, so don't bother to write and tell me), most cogently puts the case for fat people who intend to stay fat because he makes no excuses. Health is not on his mind, nor are fashionable clothes, as he limns what he refers to as "the joys of fathood."

"It's all quite simple, really," Morley told columnist Colin Dangaard. "I'm fat because I eat a lot. And I am not prepared to accept boredom as the price of self-denial. I don't see the point of it. Fat men get knocked over by buses no earlier, or later, than thin men. And I, for one, have buried most of my thin friends."

What was happiness for Robert Morley? Easy, he said. "When I'm at home by the fire, my feet up, the television on—and a couple of poached eggs in my lap."

PUTTING IT ON:
We're fat because we're human and we're lazy, and we don't read the labels or count the calories, and they've taken away our cyclamates, and health food is a scam, and we've got fat cells left over from when we were babies, and fat babies left over from feeding them too much, and we're victims of advertising, and if there's anything I forgot, you can fill it in yourself, and if there's anything I've repeated more than six times, sue me.

13 Fat and the Health Crusaders: Fear of Frying

The fat-headed majority, intoxicated by the fumes of excess . . .
–THE LIFE AND ADVENTURES OF SIR BATH LAPSKULL II

THIS IS A catchall chapter (bringing to a close the Putting It On half of the book) wherein several subjects—each worth a series of books of its own—will get a quick airing, the hope being that the reader whose interest is piqued may be inspired to go forth and search out more details.

There is no way to write about the American obsession with diet and ignore the business—it *is* a business—of so-called natural foods.

"With its heralded greening," Jean Strouse wrote in the *New York Times Magazine*, "America's consciousness turned toward health, fitness, nutrition, and the natural in everything from whole grains to childbirth. Since chemical technology was seen to be poisoning us with DDT, DES, red dye #2, and MSG, only nature's foods and remedies seemed safe. But the back-to-nature impulse was full of contradictions. You can't stop breathing polluted air by growing your own tomatoes.

And people who religiously avoid Cantonese restaurants, aspirin, maraschino cherries, and beef seem to think nothing of swallowing fistfuls of vitamin pills and dietary supplements marketed as 'natural.'"

Unfortunately, reported Jane E. Brody in the *New York Times,* natural "means whatever the manufacturer chooses it to mean."

Some "natural" products come right out of the chemist's lab, yet an FTC survey showed that 49 percent of the people interviewed would spend more for food and drink labeled "natural," while 42 percent "believed that products presented as natural had no harmful effects and were safer . . . than other products."

Jane Brody analyzed a few products labeled natural. Hawaiian Punch has "seven real fruit juices and other natural flavors." But the fruit juices amount to 10 percent of the drink, the other 90 percent is water, sugar, and corn syrup. Quaker's 100% Natural Cereal contains "brown sugar [no more natural than white sugar] . . . honey [processed by bees that don't discriminate between harmful and innocent chemicals they extract from pollen] . . . 35 percent fat, mostly coconut oil, which is the most saturated of edible fats." Colombo's All Natural Sundae-Style Peach Yogurt has, in addition to milk and peaches, "non-fat dry milk solids, sugar syrup, modified food starch, peach flavor and other natural flavors, and annatto extract for color."

"From the standpoint of consumer health," wrote Miss Brody, "nutritionists are concerned that indiscriminate use of the word 'natural' has drawn people to some foods that are not particularly nourishing, and distracted them from others that do in fact contain healthful ingredients." (Cheerios cereal, for instance, has less fat, fewer calories, and just as much protein as the "natural" granolas. It also has almost no sugar.)

It's our search for health that has encouraged the ballooning of the natural food business, and that, of course, is not a new search. All through our history, certain temperate souls have cried out for alterations in our eating habits. Remember Mrs. Horace Mann instructing her pupils to use less butter and oil? Mrs. Rorer fixing desserts "under protest"? John and Karen Hess urging us toward soups and stews and greens? Even Julia Child advising moderation and the ingestion of fewer processed foods?

But it's only lately that vast numbers of Americans have begun to worry that they might be consuming their futures, along with their meals. Solemnly, doctors contribute to that worry. "I have a feeling that most doctors scare people," says Jim Beard. "They're like judges sentencing you to penal servitude."

The very savants who'd been comforting us with apple pies were themselves stricken. Big robust feeders like Beard—"When I was first put on a salt-free diet, I thought, 'Well, this is the end of the world, I will just never be able to enjoy anything again'"—found themselves in no worse case than Craig Claiborne and other small-portion fanciers. Sometime in 1979, Claiborne was told he had hypertension, and would have to cut back on sugar, fat, and salt. A salt addict, Claiborne drank soy sauce with his morning lime juice, and even while he began to plan a new cookbook of salt-free diet dishes, he said defiantly that he was going to cheat. At least on Thanksgiving.

Beard too falls off the wagon ("Who doesn't?" he demands), and though he refuses to teach or write about diet foods, he sounds sane and resigned on the subject. "You can cook with lime, you can cook with lemon, you can learn the value of the native flavors of vegetables, you can bake potatoes longer at higher temperatures until you get a wonderful hard crust. You can use a little vinegar for a lift. And garlic. I've eaten ten times more garlic since I've been on a salt-free diet than I ate before, and I ate a great deal before."

What about salt substitutes? "Dreadful," he says. "They're not worth sweeping off the floor."

If the salt have lost its savour, wherewith shall it be salted? we ask one another. "Your honey or your life," cry foes of sweeties, and fear of frying spreads.

In a free enterprise system, there are plenty of entrepreneurs to build on that fear.

At a conference on Nutrition and Cancer in 1978, Dr. William Darby told his audience that the millions "who make the fad diet quacks rich and the health food store the most profitable of food businesses are those not physically ill, but only anxious and misled by false hopes of better health, of freedom from cancer, heart disease, etc., if they follow a given dietary fad or take great quantities of X elixir or megavitamin preparation."

Snake oil and faith healing—you can find a lot of both in the nutrition game.

"Although we learned long ago to abandon magical thinking in connection with weather, crops, the care of animals, and other natural phenomena," wrote Ruth Gay, in an article for *American Scholar*, "it still has us in its grip when we think of our diet. Our latest thinking about food, based on fear, is proportionately retrograde—willing to accept, indeed seeking out, the consolations of magic, the mute practices of peasants, and the quaint devises of folklore."

John Houseman talked about "the crisis in food" in a segment of *Here's to Your Health*, a series first shown over public television during the summer of 1979. "We need meat for protein," Houseman said, "but the fat in meat is causing heart disease. We can't afford expensive cuts, but hot dogs contain carcinogenic nitrites."

And our soil was depleted.

"In the meantime," said Houseman, "health food stores are one of the fastest growing, highest yielding businesses in America. The speed with which large corporations and financiers are joining this movement is astounding. Controversies over chemical additives and pesticides, artificial fertilizers and wonder foods, all seem to pale beside the tremendous profits to be made. Nowadays most supermarkets have part of their stores set aside for so-called health food, and, in some cases, they are selling the same products on different sides of the store at different prices.

"Food issues are anxiety producing, and they express a larger concern, according to some sociologists, and that is a longing for the return of a simpler life, a regret for the loss of trust, the loss of control over basic needs. It is that classic struggle of the little guy against the giant forces of big business and Uncle Sam. The irony, of course, being that the arm of resistance, the health food supplier, is now part of big business too."

On the same television show, Dr. Anne Race, of the University of Texas Health Science Center, asked Dr. George Cahill, a professor at Harvard Medical School, what he thought was happening in the field of nutrition. "The United States probably has more resources for good food than any other country in the world," suggested Dr. Race, "and yet, in many ways, we abuse our products, we eat junk food, we're always on some kind of diet, we're grossly obese. Really, how does all of this fit together?"

Dr. Cahill replied that he couldn't offer a one-sentence explanation, but he thought Americans were going through a "kind of phase of national hysteria relative to food, diet, poisons, toxins, radiation. Part of it is sponsored by the media, obviously. . . . Part of it is good, but part of it has raised the level of anxiety of some people so that it's sort of overshot the mark."

According to Dr. Cahill, health food supplements could be "fun," and they could taste good, but "I can categorically say that there's no evidence that we need them at all."

As for an organically grown diet, that was more nonsense. "What are the chemicals in fertilizers? Phosphates, nitrates, nitrites, urea. They're all natural products which I put out every day in my urine and that I have floating in my blood. And the fact that they came from a chemical company—well, where did the chemical company get them? By digging up phosphates, old coral reefs, so it's organic anyway. And the farmer throws it out to make his plants grow better . . . it's still organic."

Dr. Cahill might get an argument from Robert Rodale, who publishes *Organic Farming Magazine*, and who is trying to make the world a healthier place. "We've always had this organic mission," says Rodale. He believes a family can raise enough catfish and carp in a backyard pool to feed that family for a year. Rodale, who won't take coffee, cigarette, or laxative ads in his magazines, is planning to start commercial production of a grain called Amarinth, which is high in protein and can be grown anywhere.

If Amarinth winds up being sold in a health food store, Dr. Cahill will surely buy it, but only because he's curious. "I'm in the nutritional side of things, and interested. But I'm offended by people who declare that this [health food] is mandatory for their health, and double the price. To me, that's unethical."

For saying pretty much this same kind of thing, Dr. Elizabeth Whelan (mentioned earlier, in Chapter Eight) and Dr. Frederick Stare, a professor of nutrition at the Harvard School of Public Health, were jointly sued by something called the National Natural Foods Trade Association.

In her Broadway office on New York's West Side, Dr. Whelan, who's executive director of the American Council on Science and Health (a tax-exempt, nonprofit organization started with the aim of bringing "sense and scientific judgment back to policy decision-making related to chemicals, nutrition, and environmental health"), sits behind locked doors. So many cranks have threatened her that she is cautious even about answering the phone.

Dr. Whelan is swimming against the tide. She resents the disappearance of cyclamates from her diet sodas, and she didn't find the suit against her one bit funny.

The natural foods people—"They're a billion-dollar-a-year trade association of manufacturers of health foods, and all the health food stores pay dues"—have a trade journal. "And they've said in their journal that they've put aside money to silence me and Fred. They didn't sue an organization, they sued Fred Stare and Beth Whelan. And they asked for $1.3 million. They said we conspired to undermine their business and cause them to lose enormous amounts of money. Therefore, they were requesting retribution.

"We had to hire an attorney, it cost us over $14,000 in legal fees, our legal response took weeks, the court took all my papers as evidence. It's very effective. If you really want to screw someone up, sue them. Whether you win or not."

The National Natural Foods Trade Association didn't win. A judge threw their case out of court, but Dr. Whelan still calls the matter "shocking. It's a problem of civil rights. They sued me for saying what I think. I could sue them back for malicious harassment, but that means spending more money. It's as if General Foods sued someone for saying their Sugar Pops were a terrible product. Can you imagine such a thing?"

Whelan doesn't even contend that all health foods are terrible products. "We just say there's no advantage to health foods over regular foods. The only thing healthy about health foods is the markup on their prices. All foods are organic, or derived from organic sources. It's an absolutely ridiculous distinction. What they mean is the food was grown without benefit of pesticides or herbicides or artificial fertilizers, and again, it bears no impact in terms of the nutrient quality of the food. It just happens to be more expensive to do it. It has a snob appeal. If you have a few extra dollars, and want to humor yourself, you can patronize health food stores, but most of us simply cannot afford their prices."

That the health food movement should have appealed chiefly to the middle class was probably predictable. (The poor are still trying to figure out ways to put steak on the table.)

It appeals strongly to counterculture types too (one newsmagazine says a home-building school in Maine makes "the irrelevant boast that half their students are vegetarians, and 99 percent are against nuclear power"), so it swings from whole-earth orgies to high camp, as demonstrated in the 1979 Christmas catalogue from Sakowitz. The

Houston department store offered a swimming pool in the shape of Texas to be filled with over thirty thousand gallons of Perrier water, at a cost of about $127,000. Another of Sakowitz's "Ultimate Gifts of Health" was an offer to air-freight and hand-deliver to the object of your affections "one delicious red apple" every day of the coming year. The apple treat was available for $20,000, or less than $6 an apple.

But silliness and snobbery aside, doesn't Dr. Whelan fear the effects of pesticides in the food chain? Doesn't she think *Silent Spring* was a bench mark by which the wise were warned of disasters yet to come?

"I think when Rachel Carson wrote *Silent Spring*, it was a time when we weren't concerned about our environment," Whelan says. "We were dumping, not thinking about the implications of poisons on various species. That's one extreme. The other extreme is to go the way we're going now, say everything is poison, and let's ban everything at the drop of a rat. The whole purpose of pesticides is to kill things that we compete with for food, but there's now tremendous surveillance in terms of residues, and what's more, the trace amounts that you might get have no known impact on the body. They've done studies of people who work with pesticides, inhale them, splash with them, and over thirty or fifty years, they have no unusual cancer patterns.

"I keep hearing saccharin causes cancer. And nitrites, and red dye #2, and beer and Scotch. And the general population doesn't understand all this, so I've been trying to speak up, put these things in some kind of perspective. When the Naderites call a conference and say we should ban nitrites, I get on the phone with the press and say, wait a second, here's the evidence for and against nitrites.

"We're not an industry group, we don't take money from any of the petrochemical or food companies we investigate, but we spend a lot of time looking at the facts behind the scares on food additives.

"The food additives we have now in use make up less than 1 percent of the chemicals in our diet. Everything is a chemical. There are over 150 chemicals, including arsenic, in a potato.

"Look at saccharin. The FDA wants to ban it, and we're against the ban. In debate, the Naderites say, 'If there's even a hint of a problem with something like saccharin, we should ban it.' I say that's absurd, don't ban something unless there's reason to. In simple-minded terms, it boils down to a political argument. There are people who think government should take care of everyone, even if it means doing something that you as a citizen don't like, because the government knows more than you do. I'm at the other end of the spectrum; I think people should decide what they want to do with their lives, and make choices of their own.

"I'm a typical user of saccharin, but I think it's been oversold, and I don't think it really helps me lose weight. Because when I have a couple of diet soft drinks a day, in my head, I say, 'I have now earned at least 200 calories,' and that means a couple of glasses of wine, or a dessert. If I couldn't have the diet sodas, I'd drink water.

"One of the cruel things of life is that calories build up fast. I was in the ocean off the Jersey shore, and a woman next to me was jumping up and down, and she said, 'Oh, this is wonderful, it will take care of all the martinis I had last night.' She was really trying to convince herself.

"I swim every day. I cannot help but look at a lunch and decide how many laps it is.

"Fat is the basic problem. And heart disease.

"The bottom line is that people are worrying about all these additives causing cancer, and it's distracting them from their real problems, which are smoking—you couldn't possibly have more clear-cut evidence that it's a threat to human life—and drinking and overeating.

"The irony is there's been an explosion of interest in nutrition, and everyone thinks that's wonderful. I don't think it's wonderful because it's been an explosion of misinformation. The truth is there's only one major nutrition problem in this country, and that's eating too much. Fat. Everything else is nonsense. We don't need special kinds of food with lecithin. But it's easier to worry about vitamins and nitrites, and keep on eating. It's just human frailty."

Whelan's position on saccharin got a boost in March of 1980 when the results of several new studies showed the synthetic sweetener to be a very "weak" carcinogen. This seemed to insure that an FDA ban would not be ordered, at least, said one reporter, "until a truly safe sweetener comes along." The same thing happened five months later with nitrites. Maybe nitrites could combine with other chemicals (in cooking, or in the stomach) to form cancer-producing nitrosamines, but, the government admitted, there was not enough evidence to warrant banning sodium nitrite as a preservative.

Scientist Harold J. Morowitz, a professor of biophysics and biochemistry, appears, in a new book, *The Wine of Life and Other Essays on Societies, Energy and Living Things*, to agree with Whelan that there are more experts than there is information in the field of nutrition, and because he finds such information as we have "indeterminate," he is almost as salty as Whelan about rat tests. Rats, says Professor Morowitz, have a different life-style from humans, and cites studies to show that people who eat fried foods seem to live *longer*. As do people who are married. You want to make something of it?

Richard Cooper, general counsel for the FDA, does. Freedom to choose one's own poisons in food is a dangerous freedom, according to Mr. Cooper. In an impassioned speech to some food and drug officials, Cooper said he didn't want to tell people "where to live, where to work, whom to marry, whether to have children . . .

"Here, too, we as a society believe with Augustine that the value of free choice outweighs all the harms and unhappiness that may result from decisions that may prove to have been wrong . . .

"When we come to choices among foods, however, the claims of individual autonomy are very different . . . I enjoy consumption about as much as the next person, but I am quite content to leave it to the Government to decide on safety grounds what substances may not be added to food I eat, or what pollutants may not be added to the air I breathe (should there be freedom of choice in pollutants?), or what defective parts may not be included in the engines of airplanes I fly in. In general, I believe that when the Government bans an additive or a pollutant, or a defective part, it doesn't interfere with my ability to live in accordance with my personal beliefs and values.

"I say in general, because there are exceptions. There are some substances that are peculiarly important and that people feel strongly about. Such substances are, as a practical matter, unbannable. Examples are alcohol and tobacco. I suspect we are learning that saccharin . . . is a third. In this democracy, if a majority of the people . . . want to go on consuming these substances they should be able to.

"But the public demand for these substances that have special appeal does not justify any general argument that the centerpiece of food safety policy should be freedom of choice."

In the foreword to a book called *Eater's Digest* by Michael Jacobson, Dr. Jean Mayer (the Harvard professor who served as chairman of the First White House Conference on Food, Nutrition and Health) tried, from the eye of the storm, to balance opposing points of view, and talk sense. "Enemies of additives," he said, "give us a nightmarish vision of a food industry dominated by a few malevolent men of great wealth who in their craze for profit are indiscriminately spraying their products with poisonous chemicals. By contrast, the Bull Mooses of industry have perceived any criticism of additives as an attack on Science, Technology, the American Way of Life, and Western Civilization."

The fact was, said Dr. Mayer, that food technology had helped to reduce disease and make food taste better. Without additives, he said, time-saving convenience foods (see Chapter Eight) would not exist. "Their texture, color, taste, smell, shelf-life . . . would be impossible."

But, he added, many new foods were "excessively high in fat and salt, or in sugar," and there was the risk of introducing new and unfamiliar chemicals into our systems. Not that new food additives were necessarily more dangerous than "the thousands of normal constituents of established foods; cancer and other degenerative diseases existed ever since the human race started, millions of years before the first food additive was synthesized. But any added chemical of necessity increases the risk, albeit by a small amount."

Pity the poor consumer, trying to figure out truths that evade trained experts, and set them to bickering. Some of us simply close our ears, and go on eating what we like, some of us try every promised panacea. In succession.

"The American preoccupation with body weight, worry over the side effects of food additives, and a general supposition that anything labeled *natural* is good have combined to create a $1.5 billion a year demand for the herbs, roots, raw grains, and vitamin compounds broadly known as health foods," said a piece in the *Wall Street Journal* in September of 1979.

Journal reporter Terri Minsky told of a man named David Shakarian who owned 700 stores—General Nutrition Centers, he called them—that brought in revenues of $200 million a year.

But, said Minsky, a backlash was building against such big operators, with small health food store owners complaining that they were being driven out of business. "And the government is investigating allegations that the health food industry has fallen into price-fixing and deceptive labeling."

Since 1970, health food sales have risen 30 percent a year, and the Federal Trade Commission is thinking of banning the use of the word "health" on the packages, because "no food is inherently healthful."

Fred Stare (Beth Whelan's codefendant in the lawsuit brought by the

National Natural Foods Trade Association) says health-food snacks, sweetened with honey rather than sugar, are a rip-off too. "Just because a product is labeled *all-natural* doesn't mean it's good for you."

"Even health-food retailers call their snacks 'junk,'" writes Terri Minsky. "But, one says, 'Our customers have a sweet tooth, and you have to sell them what they want.'"

A sweet tooth leads to fat, even among the health-oriented, so here we are, back to square one again.

There are those Americans who would like the government to take on not only the health-food industry, but also the advertising industry, which—aided by our natural sloth—pushes the fruits of ever more processing at us.

In the *Los Angeles Times,* A. Kent MacDougall wrote that food manufacturers "eschew minimally processed staples that command relatively low profit margins to concentrate their new product development on convenience, gourmet, 'natural,' and 'light' foods that can be promoted as adding value.

"Predictably, convenience comes high. Every penny's worth of sugar sprayed onto presweetened corn flakes at the factory adds about two cents to the price the consumer pays for the convenience of not having to spoon on his own sugar at the breakfast table. The additional vitamins and minerals that General Mills, Inc., adds to Wheaties to turn it into Total cost an estimated two cents, yet add about thirty cents to the retail price of a 12-ounce box."

And you buy it. Ain't you 'shamed?

The more new products that come on the market, the more novelties that appear, the less the consumer gets for his money, MacDougall said. "Because the steep costs of developing, promoting, and distributing the four out of five new items that fail to catch on with the public are inevitably loaded onto the prices of existing brands."

Breakfast cereals, dog foods, fruit drinks, soups, all compete for the shopper's paycheck, beer companies battle it out for the domestic market (Anheuser-Busch claims Miller's puts additives in its beer, Miller fights back by saying Annheuser's vaunted "beechwood aging" consists of nothing but running beer through tanks filled with beechwood chips), and food advertising is even beamed to babies.

Bill Moyers went on educational television to deplore the seduction of innocents by commercials.

The Federal Trade Commission, said Moyers, was considering a ban on advertising directed to the kiddies, an idea so horrible to the big food companies that it caused a lawyer for Kellogg to say crossly that "the last thing we need in the next twenty years is a national nanny."

Moyers pronounced himself astonished "that high-powered people with enormous skills and resources should have unbridled access to the minds of young children . . . If the government wanted to shower 20,000 propaganda messages a year on our children, we would take to the barricades and throw the scoundrels out. Yet the words of an advertising executive are treated as constitutional writ when he tells the FTC: 'Children, like everyone else, must learn the marketplace.'

"In the end, this debate is between two views of human nature; one treats young children as feeling, wondering, and wondrous beings to be handled with care because they're fragile; the other treats them as members of a vast society to be hustled."

While the FTC was mulling over ways to protect tots from sugar surfeit, news arrived that our dogs were being oversugared too.

Ten years ago, only 28 percent of American dogs were fat; today, it's closer to 60 percent. "Overweight dogs," says animal behaviorist Bonnie Beaver, "tend to be owned by overweight people."

Just as they don't want to deprive themselves of anything, they don't want to deprive their pets of anything.

"A lot of people who have fat dogs don't like to be told they have fat dogs," says Dr. Harry Stoliker, a veterinarian who works with obese animals. These folks go on shoving treats at Fido, overloading his circuits, making his heart work too hard, and his arthritis worsen.

Unlike a cat, a dog will eat as much as you'll give him, so Manhattan's Animal Medical Center advises dog owners not to buy dog foods containing "sugar and other unnecessary additives," and says there are three words that have much to do with disease in dogs: "fats, calories, and obesity."

So often do the dread words fats and sugar surface when experts talk that a poem came to me in the dark of a particularly hungry night. With apologies to Robert Frost, it goes:

Some say the world will end in fudge,
some say in fat.
Of ways to put on terminal pudge,
the one I favor most is fudge.
But if someone would drop a hat

I'd switch my vote to marbled meat.
To go like that
might be a treat
right where I sat.

I know that stuffing ourselves with poisons isn't really funny, but sometimes a person's head gets tired. If you tell me I may be developing cancer today because of something I ate thirty years ago, I can only reply that I have a lot of trouble remembering what I had for dinner last night.

Sometimes it's easier to understand the results of tests made with foreigners. Japanese women used to have very little breast cancer. When they come to America, and begin to eat like us, which means more fat, their breast cancer rate goes up.

Rats get bowel tumors from high-fat diets, and obesity seems to contribute to cancers of the colon, the ovary, the prostate, and the endometrium, according to Dr. Arthur Upton of the National Cancer Institute.

As for self-satisfied health food converts who tell you they never touch butter, and wouldn't mess with the kinds of synthetic fats criticized by Fremes and Sabry (see Chapter Eight), but stick to unsaturated fats, they're in for a rude surprise too.

You know those ads that brag that Mazola is 100 percent corn oil, with "zero cholesterol," and high in polyunsaturates? Well, says Dr. Kenneth Carroll, a cancer researcher at the University of Ontario, unsaturated fats are more dangerous than butter. When he fed animals cottonseed, olive, sunflower (sunflowers are a hot new cash crop in America's Red River valley), soybean, and corn oil, they developed twice as many tumors as animals exclusively fed saturated fats such as butter and meat fat.

And if the animals ate unsaturated and saturated fats together, the results were more tumors than either kind of fat produced alone. Nathan Pritikin, whose diet program (about which more later) produced a best-selling book, agrees. "Human experiments show that when certain people drink either heavy cream (saturated fat) or safflower oil (unsaturated fat), their blood tends to sludge and undergo capillary blockage. Both kinds of fats raise the triglyceride levels in the blood, but with safflower oil, they stay higher much longer. Polyunsaturates also deplete the body's vitamin E, are implicated in gallstone formation, and may well stimulate tumor growth."

After that depressing information, here's a bit of good news. Americans have less stomach cancer than they used to. Also, vitamin C is believed to protect us to some extent against cancer-causing nitrosamines, and there are chemicals called indoles (found in cabbage, brussels sprouts, turnips, cauliflower, and broccoli) that seem to protect many people against colon cancers.

Furthermore, before you demand that the government throw out every possible variety of food additive, hear this: Dr. Lee Wattenberg, of the University of Minnesota, says BHT and BHA (additives used to keep foods from becoming rancid) appear to block cancer in certain animals.

Pectin, a fiber found in some fruits and vegetables, alfalfa, wheat sprouts, and selenium (cabbage, onions, peas, and green peppers are full of selenium) also seem to be able to counteract mutagenic chemicals thought to cause cancer.

So the prognosis for the future isn't all bad. Except if you want to keep eating chocolate bars and salted nuts and prime beef and bacon and whipping cream and butter.

Since 1900, the amount of fat in the American diet has gone up 25 percent. It isn't that fat *initiates* cancer, explains Dr. Ernest Wynder of the American Health Foundation, but that it probably causes metabolic changes in the enzymes and hormones protecting against cancer.

Dr. Wynder? These days, he eats red meat once a week, and ice cream only "on rare occasions."

It isn't just doctors who can change their spots. Frank Nicholas, a man who worked his way through college selling candy bars, in 1973 bought Beech-Nut from the Squibb Corporation, and by 1975 had removed all the salt from the Beech-Nut baby products. In 1979, the sugar followed the salt. "When my wife and I acquired Beech-Nut, we decided we'd develop our own market research department, so we had three babies," Nicholas told a reporter.

The Swiss-based Nestlé Corporation, which has a United States holding company, recently acquired Beech-Nut, and Mr. Nicholas went along with the package—"I've been given the assurance that we will be autonomous," he says—which puts him into bed with some questionable characters, according to many nutritionists. Because Nestlé's drive to sell infant formula to Third World countries has infuriated church groups, government groups, and Dr. Spock, causing a boycott of the giant company, and leading Senator Edward Kennedy to ask the United States Senate the following questions: "Can a product which requires clean water, good sanitation, adequate family income, and a literate parent to follow printed instructions be properly and safely used in areas where water is contaminated, sewage runs in the streets, poverty is severe, and illiteracy high? . . . When economic incentives are in conflict with public health requirements, how shall that conflict be resolved?"

It was like rediscovering the wheel, wrote Jane E. Brody in the *New York Times*. "Scientists studying the chemistry of breast milk are finding that it is uniquely constituted to foster the health and growth of the human infant." Because mother's milk "harbors an arsenal of immunological weapons believed to protect the baby against infections and allergies for months until the baby's own defenses are more fully developed."

Take that, Nestlé.

Babies having babies are said to have added to the country's nutritional problems too. A few years ago, in a book called *The Malnourished Mind*, Elie Shneour said doctors were seeing more infants suffering "because of their teenage mothers' diet of potato chips and cola drinks. Deficiency malnutrition among the affluent but nutritionally illiterate middle class is a major problem which deserves attention."

Attention is being paid, even as this is written, ours being a civilization that runs through alarms and enthusiasms so quickly that whatever you care about will come under public scrutiny—briefly, anyhow—if you just wait a minute.

The tide ebbs quickly, though. Suppose you were fixing to open a health food store just about the time the Food and Drug Administration started telling consumers a few home truths such as:

1. Natural vitamins are no better for you than synthetic vitamins.
2. Organic (fertilized) eggs are no more nutritious than infertile eggs.
3. Raw milk is no better for you than pasteurized milk.
4. Pangamic acid, sold as vitamin B15, is not a vitamin at all.
5. Potassium chloride, fed to a colicky baby in large amounts (as advised by the late Adelle Davis in a book called *Let's Have Healthy Children)*, may cure the colic but it can also kill the baby.

"Scientific rebuttal of food and nutrition myths published and perpetuated in faddist literature often is futile," says FDA nutritionist Marilyn Stephenson, adding, a trifle sadly, that Dr. Edward Rynearson, recently retired from the Mayo Clinic, was once moved to observe, "Americans love hogwash."

The buts and the rebuts go on. You can find a doctor to support almost any point of view, and you can then turn right around and find a different doctor to oppose the first guy's opinion.

Dr. Denis Burkitt, a British surgeon and researcher (his fame is so widespread he's had a disease, Burkitt's lymphoma, named after him), is interviewed for *Prevention* magazine and says he likes bran, and if people would just eat more high-fiber foods, there would be less appendicitis, varicose veins, diabetes and fat.

Dr. Harold Harper, at the University of California School of Medicine, interviewed for a magazine called *Let's LIVE*, says hold on there, high-fiber diets can cause diarrhea, increase colitis, and that the use of some synthetic fibers—sawdust, for instance—in commercially baked bread "borders on the fraudulent."

A few years back, high-protein, low-carbohydrate feeding was the rage, but now, says anthropologist Lionel Tiger, the "protein mystique" in our culture has brought us to disaster's brink, and high cholesterol diets are a factor in coronary heart disease.

Other scientists argue that the cholesterol case is far from closed. The Irish ate lots of dairy products, but were too poor to buy cars, so they bicycled everywhere, and heart disease wasn't a big problem. The Eskimos, the Masai tribe of Africa, the Bedouins of Saudi Arabia, ate lots of saturated fats, and didn't begin to develop heart trouble until they added white sugar and other refined carbohydrates to their diets. (If your body hasn't got enough cholesterol, your liver will produce some; it's a source of adrenal steroid hormones, which we need.)

Dr. Helen Linskwiller, at the University of Wisconsin, believes that a high protein intake reduces the body's calcium, and may thin out your bones (which are among the few things we don't want thinner).

On the other hand, Dr. Teh C. Huang, a Chicago researcher, believes cholesterol-rich foods like eggs and liver are not only the source of protective nutrients—lecithin, choline—but that high protein intake, with supplementary cholesterol therapy, might enable men to live as long as women do.

Dr. Basil Rifkind, chief of the metabolism branch of the National Heart, Lung and Blood Institute, doesn't argue against nutritionists who implicate high-fat diets in heart disease, but says, "What's missing is proof that you can *prevent* heart disease by reducing cholesterol."

In the spring of 1980, all hell broke loose after the Food and Nutrition Board of the National Academy of Sciences issued a 20-page report suggesting that healthy Americans stop worrying about cholesterol. "Good food," the report said in part, "should not be regarded as a poison, a medicine, or a talisman. It should be eaten and enjoyed."

The Food and Nutrition Board did *not* urge eaters to run hog-wild; it suggested that overweight people *should* cut down on dietary fat, exercise more, and avoid fat diets; it said people with family histories of heart disease and diabetes should have their fat and cholesterol levels tested, and that we all eat too much salt.

Even this seemingly moderate advice came under lupine attack by opponents, who said the report was "irresponsible," "slipshod," and had been composed by doctors who were creatures of the meat and dairy industry.

For weeks, scientists argued pro and con. Dr. Michael De Bakey, the Houston heart surgeon, said he didn't believe in the dangers of dietary cholesterol. "A good 60 percent of the people who have arteriosclerosis do not have elevated serum cholesterol levels," he said. The American Medical Association also found the report sound, but the American Heart Association was outraged.

So there. Cholesterol is bad for you, good for you, or somewhere in between.

"While the American Heart Association claims that eggs may be hazardous to health, eliminating eggs from the diet may be equally hazardous," says an article in *Let's LIVE*, and a magazine called *Better Nutrition* headlines one story, "Protein Eases That Craving for Sweets."

Sweets pushers find few friends at court. Like fats, sugar raises the serum level of triglyceride (sugar also raises the level of cholesterol, but not so much), and triglyceride may have more to do with heart disease than does cholesterol. Worse, refined sugar is straight calories—no vitamins, minerals, protein. No nutrients. None. Nada. Niente. In 1975, the Public Health Service printed a pamphlet saying that this century's increase in the U.S. per capita consumption of sugar was related to our ingestion of "soft drinks, cakes and other bakery products, candies, syrups, jams and jellies, and other sweet manufactured products which have a high sugar content."

Consumer Reports was right there hollering, Yea, government! and giving facts and figures such as: "Shake 'n Bake Barbecue Coating for chicken is 50.9 percent sugar—more than five times the percentage of sugar found in Coca-Cola."

The dentists of California warned health food freaks not to feel smug. The sugar content of honey is almost 73 percent and can put holes in your teeth as quick as any other sweet.

But people continued to put their money where their addiction was; by 1979, the soft-drink business was calculated to be an $11.5 billion a year industry and still growing. (The U.S. Department of Agriculture's "Sugar Report" gave the 1975 figure as $9.4 billion.)

To be sure, in February of 1980, the Coca-Cola company, which was already using fructose sweeteners in Fanta, Sprite and Mr. Pibb, announced that henceforth Coca-Cola would also be sweetened with fructose (55 percent fructose, the product scheduled to go into Coke, is equal to refined sugar in sweetness, and was first marketed in 1979; it is made from corn).

"So important are sweeteners to the soft-drink industry that some experts have estimated a $20 million impact on annual Coca-Cola products for every one percent change in sugar prices," said the *New York Times*. "Coca-Cola buys more than a million tons of sugar a year, taking nearly 10 percent of all the sugar consumed in the United States."

After Coke announced its switch to fructose, there was "a brief setback in the sugar market."

But plenty of soda pop companies still use sugar—about six teaspoons in an eight-ounce container—and often we drink our soda with cookies because we've become, says *Newsweek*, "a nation of cookie monsters. Cookie Coaches roam the streets of New York City. Boston's Chipyard sells more than 30,000 cookies a day. And at the Giants' games in San Francisco, vendors hawk cookies to crowds that once fed only on hot dogs and peanuts."

If diabetes comes, can hypoglycemia be far behind?

Says a coed at the University of California, attempting to explain the cookie boom: "After you've eaten a few cookies, you feel so gross about how much weight you've gained that all other problems fade away."

Just when you think there's no one with a good word for sugar, you stumble across Dr. Richard Rivlin, director of nutrition at Cornell

University Medical College, who says, "I don't know that the evidence is conclusive that a high sugar diet is harmful. The story is much clearer with respect to salt."

Put it all together, shake it up, and you come to the following conclusion: Salt *may* give you high blood pressure and heart disease and strokes, sugar *may* leave you toothless and hopped up and less able to combat bacterial infections, meat *may* set your heart to attacking you, and all of it *will* make you fat.

Fat. You heard me.

Nutrition is on everybody's tongue, but in few people's ecosystems. "In the last few years, it has been revealed that there's more nutrition in the plastic whistle in your cereal box than in the cereal," says Erma Bombeck to her television audience, and Carol Channing takes her own thermos bottles full of special foods to dinner parties.

Though Carol is in a distinct minority, the chic, in an effort not to be the kind of people who would have alarmed Dickens's Mr. Weller ("She's a swellin' wisibly before my wery eyes") and to have enough energy for work, gym, and disco roller skating, have started consulting nutritionists the way people with ingrown toenails consult chiropodists. Angelo Donghia, the interior designer, goes to his nutritionist twice a year, and starts off each day with fruit juice full of bran, lecithin, wheat germ, protein powder, and twenty-five vitamins including "kelp and E's and B complexes."

The chic and the vegetarians we have always with us, the vegetarians determined not to lay lip to anything that has to be killed first. The chic and the vegetarians are thin, and so beyond the compass of this book. And the compass of the rest of us who will eat anything that won't bite back.

A recent dispatch from Bombay by Michael Kaufman said the Indian diet was often a function of caste or religion. "There are vegetarians and non-vegetarians as well as vegetarians who will eat eggs and those who will not. There are traditional Brahmins who will only eat food prepared by other Brahmins. There are Hindus who will not eat beef and Moslems who will not eat pork."

For the most part, Americans aren't like that. Whatever foodstuffs a new group brings to the melting pot are thrown in, stewed up, and tried by other Americans.

Americans eat, and all the time we're eating, we're worrying about how fat we are, but we're too self-indulgent, too lazy, too bombarded by conflicting signals and information to do much about it. I look out of my window, observe the various shapes in warm-up suits and running shoes huffing past each other, and tell myself they're doing it so that people like me can be free. And I salute them, and I have another beer.

"The notion that the American family is caught up in a regimen of calorie counting, cholesterol watching, jogging through the park, and other healthful pursuits was largely debunked in a national study released here yesterday," wrote Georgia Dullea on April 26th, 1979, in the *New York Times*.

The national study she was referring to, a Yankelovich, Skelly and White survey based on two thousand interviews, said most of us were suffering from too much stress, only 26 percent of us were watching our caloric intake more carefully than we had a year ago, and 76 percent of us were confused about "all the government warnings."

Strong psychological resistance would have to be broken down, declared the survey, if people were going to be convinced "to exercise regularly and to stop overeating, smoking, and drinking too much." Because while obesity was thought of as a serious health menace, "every third family" had at least one overweight member, and two out of three adults didn't exercise much more than their right thumbs and forefingers on their television dials.

Six months after the Yankelovich study appeared, Dr. Mark Hegsted, of the Agriculture Department's Human Nutrition Center, delivered another body blow. He said we were eating less. That is, we were consuming fewer calories. And we were getting fatter anyway.

"We probably have to conclude," said Dr. Hegsted, "that there have been rather large decreases in physical activity—shifts to more sedentary work—that the national jogging kick has not balanced."

It all begins to sound circular, doesn't it?

Babes unborn are in trouble (a mommy who eats lots of sweets has lots of sugar in her amniotic fluid and produces an infant who craves the stuff), and so are young children who grow more wide than tall (tortured by their thinner brethren, called names, wrestling with problems of self-esteem, some play hooky from school and hang around the kitchen eating), and so are teen-agers, some of whom elect (consciously or unconsciously) to stay fat so they won't have to deal with the terrors of sex. "A layer of fat against the world" is the way one writer described it.

We eat too much because there's security in food. We eat too much because our parents were Depression victims, and an overstocked larder comforts us. We eat because it tastes good. We eat because we're happy and we're celebrating, or because we're sad and want to forget our sorrow. We eat because there is temptation all around us.

In a world where starving still occurs, America's chief nutritional complaint, as so many of the experts quoted in these pages testify, is obesity. "We are the only country where people die early because they eat," says Dr. Eli Ginzberg, director of conservation of human resources at Columbia University. "Everywhere else premature death is caused by shortage of food."

President Carter's Commission on World Hunger concurred with Dr. Ginzberg, announcing in December of 1979 that "Today, there are more hungry people than ever before, and at least one out of every eight people on earth is still affected by some form of malnutrition."

Sol Linowitz, chairman of the Commission, in a letter to President Carter, added a personal warning. "A hungry world is an unstable world."

America has the technology and the production facilities to nourish the poor in developing countries, and, says the Commission, we have "a moral obligation to do so."

But to feed the hungry may be easier than to stop overfeeding ourselves. Particularly since, according to Dr. Richard Spark of Harvard, it's only that fat is ugly rather than fear of impending medical misfortunes "that compels the American public to be 'diet conscious,' to spend vast sums of money on diet foods and diet doctors, and to periodically propel the latest diet book to the top of the best seller list."

Which brings us to Taking It Off.

II TAKING IT OFF

TAKING IT OFF:
We diet because the entire middle class wants to lose five pounds.

14 A View From the Fridge

You never know where bottom is until you plumb for it.
—FREDERICK LAING

SOME SAYINGS of the formerly fat, the fearful-of-fat, the fat-watchers, and the lawyer of one-accused-of-fatness:

Cheryl Tiegs, model, recalling the early days of her now defunct marriage, when she grew from 120 to 155 pounds. "I would look in the mirror, burst into tears, go on these diets for three days, then midnight-binge and eat everything in the refrigerator. I sat home doing nothing for a couple of years. I was bored. I had three double chins and was so heavy that when I lay down on the bed, I couldn't feel my hip bones."

Susan Cheever, novelist, admitting to an "awful" adolescence. "I weighed ten pounds for every year of my age."

Dolly Parton, country singer, confiding that she has to struggle constantly against overweight. "I'm on a seafood diet. When I see food, I want to eat it."

Wanda Bork, housewife (who couldn't walk, broke chairs when she sat in them, and wore a dress that measured 141 inches around), after she dieted herself into a lecture career. "Anybody can do anything they really want to if they want it bad enough."

Robert Strauss, lawyer, suing National Airlines on behalf of Ingrid Fee, fired for being too fat. "How can you say four pounds overweight makes a terrible stewardess?"

Barbra Streisand, movie star, explaining (back in 1968) how she handled the battle between her love of eating and her need to discipline herself as an artist. "How do I handle it? I'm eight pounds overweight, that's how I handle it. . . . I'm a complete hypocrite about food. What I do is have chocolate soufflé for dessert, and put Sucaryl in my tea."

Colette, 180-pound genius of French letters, writing in the guest book at La Pyramide. ". . . the duck is succulent . . . the pastry is heartbreaking . . . and me, who wants to get slimmer. No, no, I'm never coming back."

Régine, queen of nightclubs, eating grapefruit out of a Limoges candy dish and confessing glumly, "I am always on a diet."

Bill Blass, fashion designer, telling journalist Enid Nemy that he diets (hating every minute of it), but projecting a cheerier time to come. "People are going to eat fat foods and exercise will be out . . . They're bored with the whole *nouvelle cuisine* thing, and with jogging and tennis." As for fancy bottled waters, "We're going to drink only tap water. Or maybe gin."

Betty Ford, former First Lady, as a young, 145-pound mother of four, studying her reflection and making a vow. "There's no way I'm going to die looking like this."

Valerie Harper, actress, after falling in love with the exercise coach who helped her drop thirty pounds for a bathing suit scene in the movie *Chapter Two*. "He's changed my life . . . I have more energy, I'm in good shape, and I have a man I'm mad about."

Jack Kroll, movie critic, commenting on Valerie Harper's appearance in *Chapter Two*. "You find yourself counting her tendons instead of listening to her lines. Why would such a lovely woman and appealing performer want to look so painfully emaciated?"

Why indeed?

Why does any of us want to be thin?

Partly, it's hero worship. The most adored movie stars are thin, the beautiful people are thin, ballet dancers are thin, models on television and in magazines are thin, and on some childish level, we believe that if we looked like them, we too could achieve love, money, respect, power, recognition.

Partly, we're hoping to hold back the night. If we get close to our bones, we'll stay young, lithe, light on our feet, we'll have the wonderful stringy bodies of teen-agers, death will be fooled, and so will disease and pain and the thousand natural shocks that (too much) flesh is heir to.

And then there's medical science, offering threats from the actual horse's mouth, as opposed to our own subjective intimations of mortality. Cassandra in her darkest hour never prophesied so much doom as the doctors do. Fatties, forget about a future. If atherosclerosis don't get you, angina will. Or hypertension. Or an inflammation of your weight-bearing joints, which have got together and decided not to support all that tonnage anymore.

Anyone who elects to go on eating chocolate cake is no longer able to enjoy it in peace, because even before the plates are washed, the doctors have us listening for the sounds of our endocrine glands playing taps.

We've elevated food to status, food to entertainment. We've reached beyond food as sustenance to food as pleasure. Now we're afraid we're decadent, and we feel gross. We're told we could feed the rest of the world on our garbage, and we have anxieties a proudly fleshy person living in 1905 wouldn't have understood.

Fat is no longer socially acceptable. Fat is a health hazard. We've got to banish our fat. This may have something to do with modern man's feeling out of control in so many other areas. We're not able to govern much else in our lives, but our bodies are our own, and we think we should be able to master them.

I've mentioned elsewhere that the statistics on overweight vary, according to which expert you're consulting.

"At least 79 million Americans are significantly overweight," writes Edwin Bayrd in *The Thin Game*. "At any given time, 52 million of them are dieting or contemplating a diet. We are, in short, a nation of compulsive dieters, given to periodic bouts of systematic fasting and punishing self-denial aimed at achieving—and then maintaining—significant weight loss. That few of us succeed in doing so is a fact to which anyone who has ever attempted to lose weight can attest; that many of us try, despite past failures, is evidenced by the fact that the diet industry has become a multi-billion dollar business."

Different cultures do things different ways. You might assume that something so universal as dieting—you're fat, so you go on a diet—would work the same way in any country with a hefty middle class. It doesn't. In America, it's less private, our weight loss is "produced," taking off weight becomes a consumer product. This human desire—to drop a few pounds—begets commerce. Americans are incapable of saying, I'm just going to eat less and move my body more; instead we support companies that rise to fill our needs, and losing weight becomes a series of MGM spectaculars. As we generate industries to put it on, so we generate industries to take it off.

The ways in which we attempt to work ourselves out of our fat predicament are often counterproductive, sometimes silly, occasionally dangerous, and they almost always cost money. But none of this stops us.

Like Jay Gatsby, dieters believe in the orgiastic future that year by year recedes before them. "It eluded us then, but that's no matter—tomorrow we will run faster, stretch out our arms farther . . . And one fine morning—"

One fine morning, we'll have a 22-inch waistline.

To that end, we patronize diet doctors, buy diet books, sign up for exercise courses, bind our thighs in Saran Wrap, let acupuncturists put staples in our ears, and swallow amphetamines that will run us crazy, but that, we hope, will suppress our desire for a hot fudge fix.

Rich people get—and lose—their lumps in fancy diet spas, other people try groups like Overeaters Anonymous, Weight Watchers, TOPS. Somebody goes on every diet that's printed, even if it features opossum livers, or boiled scars from the ends of eggplants. In the very midst of trying, we are tempted and confused. "You open up these women's magazines," says Larry Goldberg (Calvin Trillin's buddy, the Pizza Baron), "and they have two diet articles, and forty-three recipes for lemon meringue pie. You don't know which way to run."

While you're trying to figure it out, some expert who doesn't admire the shape you're in calls you a moron. For instance, Hugh Drummond, M.D., in the February/March 1980 issue of *Mother Jones* magazine: "The microwave-heated, prepackaged, chemically treated fast-food industry has produced a generation of gustatory morons for whom any sensation other than hot-salty or cold-sweet is too subtle," writes Dr. D. And he isn't done yet. "The sterile rottenness of our food has not reduced the amount we consume, however, as the prevalence of obesity testifies," he goes on to say.

Dr. Albert Stunkard, an acknowledged pioneer in the field of weight control, is more forbearing in tone, but he too sounds somewhat despairing when confronted by the facts: millions of Americans diet, lose weight, then put the weight on again. Over and over and over. Nobody has come up with a way to reorder the country's eating habits, and science appears to be losing the war against fat, which is considered our primary health problem.

"Most obese persons will not remain in treatment," Dr. Stunkard says. "Of those who do remain in treatment, most will not lose much weight, and of those who do lose weight, most will regain it promptly."

Curtiss Anderson, once a wunderkind editor at the *Ladies' Home Journal,* attests to the truth of the doctor's thesis.

When Anderson came to the *Journal,* its editors were Bruce and Beatrice Gould. "There was a series of makeovers that Beatrice Gould started," Anderson remembers. "It was maybe thirty years ago. Mrs. Gould had the idea of taking women from around the country, women who'd been overweight, and dieted, and gone from 300 pounds to 120 pounds, and found husbands, and had children, and houses in the suburbs, and featuring them in the *Journal*.

"There was a whole department set up to locate these women. We'd fly them into our offices and photograph them in the *Journal*'s studios in this beautiful pink setting among bouquets of flowers.

"We were dependent on their sending in snapshots of their former fat selves, but occasionally it would happen that someone would write and say, 'I am going on a diet, would you like to do a story on me?' That, of couse, was a great opportunity. You could photograph them fat, then wait six months or whatever and photograph them thin.

"A long time later, I got the idea of doing a follow-up on some of the women. It was to be a kind of survey. Mrs. Gould liked the idea. She thought we would show the makeover subjects living happily ever after. We went back over a period of twenty years, and located them. Ninety-nine percent had blown right back up to their old weights. They'd lost their husbands, been divorced, they were angry again.

"I was the managing editor then, so I went to Mrs. Gould and said, 'This is an even better story than the one we'd planned. Because it demonstrates that there are factors in the weight problem deeper than any of us have realized. Psychological factors.'

"Mrs. Gould was appalled. She didn't want to hear about it. 'I don't believe it,' she said. 'I don't believe it's true.'

"She wanted the world to be like her fantasy. She'd throw out the world if it didn't work right.

"We never published that survey. Some of it was wonderful. It was a study in how meaningless our stories had been, how meaningless diet aids are, how meaningless diets per se are, how dangerous some of them are."

Meaningless and dangerous or not, Bill Blass's prognostications to the contrary, the American rage to diet shows few signs of simmering down.

TAKING IT OFF:
Some children diet from infancy;
some children diet to death.

15 Born to Lose

The baby figure of the giant mass of things to come
—WILLIAM SHAKESPEARE

IF YOU WANT to live long, pick the right ancestors, geneticists tell us smugly.

Same with beauty. The apple doesn't fall far from the tree, and Sophia Loren looks like Sophia Loren because her mother looked like Greta Garbo. Something like that.

So too is slenderness a legacy, since nature and nurture are both parts of the fat equation. It isn't just that Mom's apple pie goes straight to your hips, it's that fat parents make fat babies. The shape of your genes helps determine the shape of your jeans. (In *Fat and Thin,* Anne Scott Beller lucidly outlines the boundaries of our free will: "We are what we eat only insofar as our basic heredity permits us to assimilate our own food and maximize our own growth within certain limits laid down for each of us at the moment of conception by the random but irrevocable throw of the genetic dice.")

It doesn't matter that your daddy's rich and your ma is good lookin'. If one of them is fat, you have a 40 percent chance of being fat. And if both of them are fat, you have an 80 percent chance of thickening.

Some inherit fatness, some have fatness thrust upon them. An appalling amount of obesity is fostered at the family dining table. But whether it's eating habits or biology or a combination of both that makes us heavy, our misery is the same.

Once upon a time, survival of the fittest literally meant survival of the fattest. An Ice Age child heavily layered in flesh could better survive until its hunter daddy came home with eats. To say nothing of being better able to adapt to the cold.

But in an age and country of steam heat and supermarkets, a baby who eats an egregious amount is encouraging his fat cells to swell and plague him throughout his life.

The problem begins as soon as we're born. Here's Anne Scott Beller again: "There is some question as to whether we come into the world with our full complement of fat cells all finished and assembled at birth, or whether overfeeding in infancy may not actually stimulate the infant's body to produce not only more fat, but also more fat cells to store the additional fat in."

Adults who have been fat since childhood have a large number of fat cells. Adults who got fat after they grew up have fewer fat cells, but engorged ones. You never get rid of your fat cells; the most a diet can do is shrink them in size.

And we get fatter as we get older, with the possible exception of the Witoto, a tribe living in the Amazon River basin. According to Nicole Maxwell, in *Witch Doctor's Apprentice*, chubby Witoto babies are given the leaves of an arcane curative plant and, after judicious chewing of same, grow up thin. The ancient Cretans are also supposed to have had a drug that permitted them to stay skinny while gorging.

But the magic leaves and the miracle drug being unknown in these parts, American kiddies have a less idyllic time of it. Often lubberly hulks of both sexes find themselves spending their summer vacations at fat kids' camps.

The camps solicit inquiries all winter long. On any Sunday, look at the back of the magazine section of the *New York Times*. One January paper offered the following ads:

1. Weight Watchers Camps for Boys. (Illustrated by a photograph of

a helmeted fatty on a Moped, and a drawing of two other boys sighting down the barrels of guns.)

2. Weight Watchers Camps for Girls. (Picture of a teen-ager in open-mouthed ecstasy at the good news she is reading off a balance scale.)

3. Seascape on Cape Cod Bay. (Girls from nine to nineteen were invited to "have fun and benefit from a program proven effective for lasting weight control.")

4. Multi-Million Dollar College Campus. ("Teen Girls 13–17" and "Young Ladies 18–29" were promised they could lose twenty to forty-five pounds apiece.)

5. Camp Clover. (Overweight girls could "lose weight the fun way.")

6. Camp Stanley. (A body building camp for boys, and "no harsh regimes, just days of fun" for girls.)

Despite the facilities—swimming, tennis, golf, horseback riding, dancing, gymnastics—available in most of the camps, they can differ greatly, one from another, as I discovered a few years ago.

I'd been assigned to do a magazine piece about places where parents could dispatch their overweight kids to be starved and reshaped, and I visited three camps, one co-ed, one for girls only, and one just for boys.

The co-ed camp was run by a cheerful lady who'd been a fat kid herself ("I know how they feel") and whose object was to make her charges cozy. She housed them in bungalows rather than barracks. ("We're depriving them of food, so I think we should at least give them a nice homey atmosphere.")

This lady had been told that fat boys and fat girls wouldn't like to go to camp together, which had turned out not to be the case. "Fat boys are better than no boys," one girl said practically, as she marched into the dining hall to wolf down a lunch of stringently measured macaroni, carrot sticks, and fresh fruit.

The camp director swore by a nutritionally balanced diet that had first been published by the Board of Health in 1952, though the camp substituted margarine for butter and eliminated rich desserts. (A sugar substitute was the only dietetic food used.)

The place reflected the easygoing nature of its director, who was willing to abandon exercise classes when the temperature rose—"On real hot days, we just go swimming"—and her compassion for "the girls with the skinny, gorgeous mothers. I can take the weight off a kid like that, but she won't keep it off. She can't compete with her mother."

(In *Eating Disorders,* Hilde Bruch also mentions the tension between skinny parents and fat children. "Whenever one hears a thin, even scrawny-looking mother speak with particular vehemence and disgust about the fatness of her child it is not a farfetched guess, and one easily confirmed, that this mother owes her fashionable figure to eternal vigilance and conscientious, semistarvation dieting . . . It is in families with this intense hostility about obesity that I have most often seen a malignant development of childhood obesity, with schizophrenia or anorexia nervosa as the final outcome.")

It's a no-win situation. Fat mother or skinny mother, the kid is in the soup.

The second camp I visited was very different from the first. To begin with, the owner-manager didn't believe in "homey" atmosphere. "Home is where the trouble starts," she said. "We want to *break* the pattern they have at home."

No doors in this camp, except on shower and toilet stalls—"You walk down a hall, hear whispering behind a closed door, and you wonder if they're talking about *you*"—and no boys, either. "A girl gets into a bathing suit, and she's got rolls of fat hanging out, she doesn't want a boy around."

There was a no-nonsense athletic schedule for the inmates, who were also tutored in "poise and posture." The camp owner demonstrated a "corrective exercise" that consisted of walking with a magazine held between her thighs, and explained how this particular course of instruction had evolved. "I consulted a model," she said. "She'd gone to Barbizon."

Lunch—some kind of turkey roll, beans, sauerkraut, and a sickly sweet red drink—depressed me.

The atmosphere at the third, all-boys, camp seemed less grim, despite the fact that the boys were kept on equally strict diets, and had to exercise for even more hours a day. They swam, wrestled, played tennis, ran around a track, and traversed an obstacle course covered with hurdles, rubber tires, and horizontal ladders. The obstacle course was referred to as "the circuit," and the head counselor was very proud of it. "It was constructed personally by this guy, I forgot his name already. He was a world-famous gymnast."

All the camp counselors were thin, which made it easier for them to perform the required acrobatics, but harder for them to wrestle 300-

pound kids. "Even if they don't know anything, you can't move 'em," the head counselor said.

Still, he told me, the summer before, 200 boys had lost 6,000 pounds. Three tons of flab. Left on the playing fields of non-eatin'.

What developed when the boys went home again wasn't the camp's business.

As it happens, most boys don't pile on—or suffer from—adolescent fat as much as girls do. You see chunky eleven- or twelve-year-old boys, but by the time they're teen-agers, they've lengthened out and thinned down. Girls have the exact opposite problem. They stop getting taller at the same time that their estrogens start developing, and estrogens, says Dr. Barbara Edelstein, "protect body fat. So dieting with females often becomes a game of how to outwit their hormones."

Dr. Edelstein, author of *The Woman Doctor's Diet for Teen-Aged Girls* (a follow-up volume to *The Woman Doctor's Diet for Women*), appeared on the TV show *Good Morning, America,* fielding questions from several fifteen-year-old females.

"How come some people can eat as much as they want and never get fat, while others struggle?" demanded one girl.

"Everybody is different," said Dr. Edelstein. "Some people lose weight on 1200 calories a day, some people maintain, and a few unfortunate souls actually gain. If you're at the wrong end of the scale, that's just the way it is. I think that's a big problem with teen-agers, the idea of dealing with it, that it's not going to change, and you've got to live your life around it."

Watchfulness was the keyword. "Teen-age girls think, oh, wow, they're going to lose weight and their problem will be over. Overweight is a chronic problem, it takes work, it takes determination, it takes nutritional knowledge."

A general diet for teen-age girls should be no different from "an intelligent diet for everyone," suggested Dr. Edelstein. "Three basic meals, maybe two snacks, avoidance of high-potency carbohydrates."

And lots of exercise. There was, the doctor said, no good diet pill. If there were, everyone would be thin. "What you're dealing with is mediocre pills that have moderate to high risks—of taking too many, or of drug dependency. Dieting is not a pill, dieting is relearning eating behavior, learning to control hunger by use of foods that won't make you fat. It's a way of living, and taking a pill doesn't help that way of living."

One of the teen-agers who had been listening intently raised her hand. "I can look at myself in the mirror and feel fat when others tell me I'm skinny," she said. "How do you know when enough's enough? When does dieting become anorexia?"

Anorexia, said Dr. Edelstein, had nothing to do with normal dieting. "Anorexia is an emotional disease that manifests itself by extreme weight loss. Part of the problem when dealing with obesity in teen-agers is body image, which forms early. You see yourself as heavy when you start to develop normally. You try to get back to that preteen skinniness that's impossible to achieve. You have developed body fat."

The girls giggled at this, but the doctor went on. "You've developed a bosom, you've developed a rear, and you've got to live within your physiology. It's a nice physiology. You don't have to look the way you looked when you were ten years old."

The segment with Dr. Edelstein and the girls having come to an end, *Good Morning, America*'s host, David Hartman, announced a commercial break. "We'll be back in just a couple of moments," he said, "after these words from Mrs. Smith's Pies."

It was a lovely example of schizophrenia, American style.

Children of the Great Depression, children of poor immigrants, were fed till they all but burst by mothers who would have sneered at the idea that a fat baby was anything but a lucky baby. My sister-in-law knows a woman who still urges her grown son to stuff himself at her table. "Eat, eat," she says. "For your father. Me you killed long ago."

The craziness of the mothers is visited upon the children. In regard to "the eating function," says Hilde Bruch, if a mother's reaction is "continuously inappropriate, be it neglectful, oversolicitous, inhibiting, or indiscriminately permissive, the outcome for the child will be a perplexing confusion. When he is older he will not be able to discriminate between being hungry or sated, or between nutritional needs and some other discomfort or tension. At the extremes of eating disorders, one finds the grotesquely obese person who is haunted by the fear of starvation, and the emaciated anorexic who is oblivious to the pains of hunger and other symptoms characteristic of chronic undernourishment."

Dr. Bruch, a psychiatrist who is probably the best known authority in the United States on the subject of anorexia, has treated hundreds of adolescents who eat too much or don't eat at all. "Food may symbolically stand for an insatiable desire for unobtainable love," she writes, "or as an expression of rage and hatred; it may substitute for sexual gratification or indicate ascetic denial . . . it may serve as a defense against adulthood and responsibility. Preoccupation with food may appear as helpless, dependent clinging to parents, or as hostile rejection of them."

Obese adolescents and anorexic adolescents share one problem: They don't feel in control of their own lives or bodies.

It was Sir William Gull, a nineteenth-century English physician, who coined the term anorexia nervosa. In 1874, he wrote that some young women between the ages of sixteen and twenty-three were "specially obnoxious to mental perversity," and he recommended treatment "fitted for persons of unsound mind. The patients should be fed at regular intervals, and surrounded by persons who have moral control over them; relations and friends being generally the worst attendants."

In her 1978 book, *The Golden Cage*, Hilde Bruch suggested that anorexia was really an inexact name for the illness because although the word *anorexia* means lack of appetite, the youngsters who suffer from it "are fanatically preoccupied with food and eating, but consider self-denial and discipline the highest virtue and condemn satisfying their needs and desires as shameful self-indulgence."

They are, those youngsters, mostly girls who have never made (previous) trouble at home or in school; they are also mostly bright, and mostly born to parents in comfortable circumstances. You don't find anorexia among the poor.

Some anorexic girls will shop for food, cook the food, serve the food, and force other members of their families to finish every morsel of it, while they themselves are starving and lying about it. "Of course I ate breakfast," one patient told Dr. Bruch. "I had my Cheerio."

Anorexic girls who go on food binges make themselves throw up afterward; they also take laxatives, and exercise until they are exhausted, driven by the terror of gaining even a few ounces. A 110-pound girl will go down to 70 pounds and still insist she's too heavy.

Dr. Bruch sees a connection between anorexia and the women's movement—"these girls want to show they're something special"—and a connection between the sickness and the modern conviction that fat is ugly. But the roots of the problem go deeper. Anorexics are desperately fighting against feeling enslaved and exploited, says Dr. Bruch. "In their blind search for a sense of identity and selfhood, anorexic youngsters will not accept anything that their parents, or the world around them, have to offer; they would rather starve than continue a life of accommodation."

They who have never misbehaved, never rebelled, suddenly call a halt; they stop seeing friends, stop playing team sports, stop having periods, stop recognizing the difference between fact and fantasy. Some of them look like victims of Buchenwald, but they go right on talking about how fat they are.

Although anorexia is seldom found in anyone over thirty, the German psychiatrist, Binswanger, wrote in *The Case of Ellen West* of a patient who, in the year 1900, had become sick at the age of twenty-one and who suffered for the next thirteen years. She kept a diary in which she recorded her pain. "I do not think that the fear of becoming fat is the real obsession, but the continuous desire for food . . . The fear of becoming fat acts like a brake. I see in this '*Fresslust*' the real obsession. It has fallen over me like a beast and I am helpless against it."

Psychoanalysis did not help Ellen West. She went on walking too much, eating too little, taking too many laxatives, dreaming of being a man and going to war "in the joyful expectation that I should die very soon. I look forward to it so that towards the end I can eat everything, even a big piece of mocha torte."

She fantasized a food "that would permit one to stay thin . . . All I want is to become thinner and thinner . . . I am really ruining myself in this endless struggle against my nature. Fate wanted me to be heavy and strong, but I want to be thin and delicate."

Eventually, she was hospitalized for depression, and after she was released from the hospital, she seemed more peaceful. On the third day after her homecoming, she ate full meals, including desserts, for the first time in thirteen years. That night, she took a fatal dose of poison.

In the 1920s and 30s, some doctors believed anorexia to be a disorder of the endocrine glands, but modern thinking is that the trouble is psychological. And, says Hilde Bruch, among high school and college girls, the incidence of anoexia may be as high as 1 in 200. (Bulimarexia, related to anorexia, is even more widespread, and almost as dangerous to mind and body. College health officials believe that up to 25 percent of freshmen women are putting themselves through this cycle of starving, going on binges, throwing up, and taking laxatives.)

Why? Dr. Bruch repeats what she's said before. "Our society places enormous and unrelenting emphasis on slimness."

Slimness and youth.

It's an indictment of our civilization that so many young girls don't want to grow into women, that some of them would rather starve themselves to death. And in any overview of our eating habits, behavior carried to its maddest limits—the spectre of dieting run amok—is instructive, and serves as a warning to parents.

Still, the fact is that most American teen-agers—girls and boys alike—are straight-out big mouths. The fronts of their faces are always open, whether to say "rilly" or "gross" or simply to stuff in the pizza. *New York Times* columnist John Leonard, referring to his own three teen-agers as the Gang of Three, called their behavior "revolting. It is one Long March to the icebox. It is a night of teeth."

His teen-agers talked to him, said Leonard, "through the fried thigh of a dismembered fowl, and then only to ask for money for popcorn."

They were eating the world. He feared for the cats.

But long before the cats are gone, and the world completely gobbled up, Leonard's children will probably turn into calorie-counting adults. For them, as for the majority, the struggle to lose weight won't be pathological. Only maddening.

TAKING IT OFF:
For the people who write the diet books, taking it off means raking it in.

16 Diet Books: Hoping for a Winner, Would-be Losers Buy 'Em All

If at first you don't succeed, try, try again. Then quit. There's no use being a damn fool about it.
—W. C. FIELDS

WHERE DIETING is concerned, Americans haven't paid much attention to the sage counsel of Mr. Fields. Leaping from diet book to diet book (the only exercise some of us get), we go on diets and fall off again, and with each new manual we believe we've been given a new chance to drop the same fifteen pounds.

Some figures born of analyzing tables from the National Center for Health Statistics:

1. 84.1 percent of all Americans seventeen years and over are either trying to lose weight or trying not to gain weight.
2. 78.1 percent of all U.S. males seventeen years and over are either trying to lose weight or trying not to gain weight, while 87.4 percent of all U.S. women seventeen years and over are either trying to lose weight or trying not to gain weight.
3. 13 percent of American men between the ages of twenty and seventy-four are classified as obese, while 22 percent of the women

between the ages of twenty and seventy-four are classified as obese. (An obese person, according to the FDA, is someone who is 20 percent above average body weight for his height and bone structure.)

Occasionally, a citizen bored with the subjects of food and fat takes pen in hand and tries to fight back. In November of 1978, one simply furious lady wrote to Ann Landers.

> What is happening in the world that is making everyone so diet-and-exercise conscious? The last time I looked at the *New York Times* best-seller list, three of the top ten books were on diet and running. (My doctor says they are a ripoff.) This morning when I asked the doorman to get me a taxi, he said, "You'd feel a lot better if you walked half way." I came close to clobbering him with my umbrella. About 3:30 this afternoon, I felt the need for some quick energy, so I went to the vending machine and got myself a candy bar. When I got back to my desk, a secretary I barely knew tapped me on the shoulder and said, "You don't need that." I looked at her in shocked disbelief. She then added, "An orange would be a lot better for you, and it's only one-third the calories." I told her they didn't sell oranges in the vending machine. She snapped, "Well, why don't you bring one from home?" I became irritated and announced that I wasn't interested in a lecture on nutrition. She replied, "The people who need it never are." Who started all this nonsense that "the thinner is the winner"? Why the sudden preoccupation with what we should eat? Frankly, I am
>
> BORED BY THE OVERKILL.

Ann Landers had her hands full that day, with a woman who hated cats (they jumped on her and ripped her panty hose) and a kid who was caught in a fight between his father and his aunt, but she took time out to address the weight question.

"Dear Bored," she wrote, "I agree that fad diets are for the birds—the cuckoos, that is—and there is entirely too much rubbish being published on how to lose thirty pounds in thirty days. Also, running is not for everybody. Today's joggers may be tomorrow's arthritics. We have learned a lot in recent years, however, about diet in relation to heart disease. We also know obesity is very unhealthy. I believe in daily calisthenics and walking whenever possible. But when it comes to denying oneself all the delicious things to eat in exchange for a figure like a broom handle, count me out."

Annie's just like the rest of us. Everybody wants to be healthy, nobody wants to deny himself "all the delicious things to eat."

What's more, we know the secret, unspoken even to ourselves: The only way you can lose weight is to shut your mouth. If you take in more calories than your body spends to keep itself going, you get fat. Still, we keep chasing the impossible dream, hopeful that the very next best seller will finally bring us a magic formula by means of which we'll be able to eat all we want, while flesh melts off our bones, and the few remaining pounds stay firm and silky.

The very first best-selling diet book—only a pamphlet, really—was called *A Letter on Corpulence, Addressed to the Public,* and was published in 1864. Its author, William Banting, a short (5′5″), plump (over 200 pounds) Englishman, was by trade a coffin-maker who had been heavy all his life. He had tried the cures of his day—leeches, purging, steam closets, everything, in fact, except cutting down on food and drink—to no avail. In 1862, suffering from an earache, he had gone to see Dr. William Harvey, who decided fat might be the reason for Banting's ear trouble, and put him on the first recorded high-protein, carbohydrate-free diet. Banting was permitted lean meat, vegetables, bran, fruit, unsweetened tea, and sherry. He was not permitted starch, sugar, beer, or ale, and he lost fifty pounds in one year.

In order to celebrate Dr. Harvey, and also to encourage others with weight problems, Banting published his *Letter* at his own expense. The booklet included his diet regimen and recounted humiliations to which he, as a fat person, had been subjected. "No man laboring under obesity can be quite insensitive to the sneers and remarks of the cruel and injudicious in public assemblies, public vehicles, or the ordinary street traffic," he wrote.

The first really popular American diet book was called *Diet and Health With Key to the Calories,* by Lulu Hunt Peters. It was a best seller from 1922 through 1926, and science writer Theodore Berland has a theory to account for this. "The 20's, the 60's and the 70's were narcissistic decades," he told the *New York Times*'s Ray Walters. "Dieters are predominantly women whose concern isn't their health, but a desire to appear 'sexy.'"

It makes sense that a diet book should have taken off in the 20s, when flappers, strapped, cropped, and straight as little boys, were turning upside down the previous notions of female allure. It also makes sense that the country enjoyed a respite from considerations of weight for the next three decades. During the Depression, much of the middle class had to worry about getting enough to eat, not about eating too much; after that came World War II, with rationing, and a certain amount of culinary deprivation. Then peace, escape from gray considerations of destruction and the woes of the planet, color, travel, exotic foods, hedonism, succulence.

"The whole cycle impenitently revolves," says the poet, "and all the past is future." We were headed for a new birth of narcissism.

Among the books that made publishing history in the 60s and 70s were *Calories Don't Count* (Herman Taller), *The Doctor's Quick Weight Loss Diet* (Irwin Maxwell Stillman and Samm Sinclair Baker), *The Last Chance Diet* (Dr. Robert Linn with Sandra Lee Stuart), and *Dr. Atkins' Diet Revolution* (Robert C. Atkins).

What constitutes a best seller? Take the Atkins book. It sold one million hardcover copies in its first seven months, and later, 5,117,000 paperback copies. That constitutes a best seller.

Throughout most of 1979 (for forty-four weeks), *The Complete Scarsdale Medical Diet* (Herman Tarnower, M.D., and Samm Sinclair Baker) was the number one hardcover nonfiction best seller on the *New York Times* list. The book went through twenty-three printings, sold 750,000 copies in hardcover, and by the time Dr. Tarnower died, in the second week of March 1980 (a few days short of his 70th birthday), more than two million paperback copies had been bought. (Tarnower, a man who preferred to be known as a good doctor, rather than a diet specialist, and who kept his personal life to himself, would surely have detested the furore that surrounded his passing. He was shot in the bedroom of his secluded house in Purchase, New York, by a longtime friend, Jean Harris, whose assistance in "research and writing" he had acknowledged in his diet book. Samm Sinclair Baker, Tarnower's coauthor, had asked Tarnower about the acknowledgment, only to have the doctor tell him it was a "private matter." With the killing, all private matters became public, tabloids screamed of a "love triangle," and the sales of *Scarsdale* soared.)

Even the tongue-in-cheek paperbacks of one time PR man Richard Smith did phenomenally well. *The Dieter's Guide to Weight Loss During*

Sex tickled enough people so they bought hundreds of thousands of copies, and Smith's subsequent *The Bronx Diet* sold well—though not *as* well.

Smith advises using food as a crutch—"a legitimate and happy substitute for misery, anxiety, bad sex, and a boring Monopoly game"; poses the question, "Why isn't a bowl of spinach as satisfying as a bowl of chocolate mousse?"; promises that a cheeseburger will clean and soothe "delicate esophageal membranes corroded by grapefruits and leeks"; and sets a few commonsense rules, among them "Avoid blue food" and "Eat only in one room. Moving about creates air currents that will blow away your spaghetti."

Some critics think you might as well listen to Smith as to the authors of straight, hard-core, best-selling diet books.

"We believe it would be desirable if, prior to acceptance for publication, books on diet or nutrition for the public were reviewed for scientific accuracy by several impartial and knowledgeable referees," wrote Dr. Jules Hirsch (of Rockefeller University) and Dr. Theodore Van Itallie (director of the Obesity Research Center at New York's St. Luke's Hospital) in *New York* magazine. "We think it unfortunate that the public believes that popular diet books contain important nutritional discoveries and that if they are condemned by the scientific establishment, it is out of prejudice and jealousy. In a free society like ours, the First Amendment rights of authors and publishers must be fully respected, even if nutritional nonsense in print is the outcome."

Theodore Berland, in a book called *Rating the Diets*, analyzed seventy-five different popular diets and concluded that most of them were "baloney," and a few were actually dangerous. The success rate of dieters in keeping off weight was put by Berland at 3 percent.

And still the books sell.

Looking back over some of the favorites of recent years—the Taller book, the first Atkins book, the first Stillman book—Edwin Bayrd makes the fascinating point that they are all "essentially the same book. Differing only in style, format, and particulars, they all offer versions of a high-protein, low-carbohydrate diet that first became popular [with Mr. Banting] more than a century ago."

So did the Mayo Diet (largely grapefruit and eggs), the Drinking Man's Diet, and the Air Force Diet (which had no more to do with the Air Force than the Mayo Diet had to do with the Mayo Clinic).

A high-protein, low-carbohydrate diet works, and works fast. Dr. Atkins (about whom more later) actually said you could eat as much as you wanted, as often as you wanted, because when you weren't taking in carbohydrates—the first fuel burned by the body—the body would be forced to burn up stored fat. In burning fat, you throw off ketones. Dr. Atkins's followers were supposed to check their urine with test sticks bought at a drugstore. If the stick turned purple, the dieter was in a state of ketosis.

Many nutritionists didn't think this was such a great state to be in. Without carbohydrates to burn, the body will attack its own lean muscle tissue, as well as its fat stores. Carbohydrates, says Hilde Bruch, "are needed in sufficient quantity to prevent ketosis and to minimize wastage of protein and electrolytes," and Edwin Bayrd explains that the human body needs carbohydrates "for two reasons—because our muscles work most efficiently while burning carbohydrates and because our brains burn nothing but carbohydrates in the form of glucose."

Take away our glucose, and the liver goes to work converting stored fat "to partially oxidized fatty acids known as ketone bodies, which the brain uses as a substitute source of energy in the absence of glucose."

Now do you understand ketosis? Me neither.

Ketosis does suppress the appetite. But it also puts strain on the heart and kidneys, and could cause a diabetic to go into ketotic crisis.

Furthermore, since carbohydrates retain fluids, a diet without carbohydrates causes quick water loss. The minute you go off the diet, the water—and the weight—comes back.

According to serious nutritionists, the only weight that stays off is weight that is lost gradually. And the only diets that should be contemplated are balanced diets including fruits and vegetables; milk, cheese, and yogurt; whole grains, enriched breads, and cereals; lean meat, fish, poultry, and eggs; and dried peas, beans, and water.

No quick-loss diet is balanced, and any diet that is out of balance, says Edwin Bayrd, "whether it favors protein, saturated fats, or carbohydrates, is inherently dangerous."

We are a country that diets dangerously.

Herman Taller took his readers off all carbohydrates and refined sugars, assured them that they could "live a full life and not gain weight," and set them to swallowing large quantities of unsaturated fats (eighty-four capsules of safflower oil every day).

"There is hardly a word of sense in the whole book," said Harvard's Dr. Frederick Stare. Even so, Taller might have gone on fooling some of the people most of the time if he hadn't run afoul of the FDA, which came to the conclusion that Dr. T. had written *Calories Don't Count* as a means of pushing the safflower oil capsules in which he had a financial interest.

There was a lawsuit, Dr. Taller and the manufacturer of the capsules were convicted of mail fraud, violation of federal drug regulations, and conspiracy.

Did Taller's followers lose weight? Indeed they did. Because they were ingesting fewer calories than they'd been accustomed to. It didn't matter that those calories were largely fat. Repeat: If you take in fewer calories than your body burns off, no matter what food group those calories come from, you'll get thinner. Your body can't tell 50 calories of fried pork rinds from 50 calories of sunflower seeds. (That you won't be healthy on a diet limited to pork rinds is a whole other matter.)

One of the lessons other doctors learned from Dr. Taller's case, says Edwin Bayrd, "was to market the idea but not the product, and subsequent promoters of Banting-type diets have been careful to avoid that legal pitfall."

The late Dr. Irwin Stillman (skinny, bald, crusty, amusing) was a winner on the *Tonight Show* and a winner in the bookstores. *The Doctor's Quick Weight Loss Diet* sold more than ten million copies; it prescribed lean meats, poultry, fish, eggs, cottage cheese, clear soups, coffee and tea (no cream, sugar, or milk), and a minimum of eight glasses of water a day.

Dr. Stillman "created" this diet when, at the age of forty, and greatly overweight, he suffered a massive heart attack. For him, high protein intake had worked wonders. In eleven weeks, he'd lost fifty-five pounds, and almost forty years later, he was still bouncing across the stages of America, charming audiences and influencing people.

In its heyday, Stillman's watery diet was the source of much merriment, because followers could never wander too far from a bathroom, and critics insisted that much of the weight loss the doctor achieved was the result of dehydration.

Since a dieter wasn't permitted a lettuce leaf or a green bean on Dr. Stillman's diet, there was nothing nutritionally balanced about it, and the director of the Department of Foods and Nutrition at the AMA was quick to point this out.

A Stillman acolyte with kidney trouble or gout or diabetes "would be a candidate for sensational trouble," admonished Dr. Philip White.

Dr. Stillman didn't give a fig for the balanced diet croakers. "Beware of those who advise you blandly, 'eat less,' 'eat half,'" he warned. "They are in large part responsible for so many people being overweight, for they indoctrinate the public with the warning that only higher calorie 'balanced eating' and 'balanced reducing' are correct—*even though that doesn't succeed for the vast majority of overweights!* Such 'experts' sustain their principles no matter what; the tragedy is yours as you grow fatter and unhealthier."

He was not, Dr. Stillman soon demonstrated, a man to sustain *his* principles "no matter what." Plagued by Quick Weight Loss dieters who whimpered that they were "bubbling over with water," or that they craved "a very dry martini," or were "dying for some vegetables," or "a little salad," or "a drop of milk," or "a little taste of cake," he turned around in *Dr. Stillman's 14-Day Shape-Up Program* and offered his new Protein-PLUS diet, on which you did *not* have to drink eight glasses of water a day, and you could have liquor, vegetables, salad, skim milk, and even "a square of Protein-PLUS Custard Cake."

(Stillman also produced *The Doctor's Quick Inches-Off Diet,* which was *not* high-protein, but low-protein—no meats, poultry, seafood, eggs, or cheese—and heavy on fruits and vegetables, and even featured a little spaghetti.)

"With consistency, a great soul has simply nothing to do." Emerson would have loved Dr. Stillman.

Dr. Robert Linn, however, had reservations. In *his* best seller, *The Last Chance Diet,* Linn wrote that "The Stillman diet [by which he meant the original Quick Weight Loss Diet] should be approached with utmost caution by anyone susceptible to high cholesterol levels. This is mainly a diet of animal protein and fat—which translates into lots of cholesterol."

What was Dr. Linn himself offering the American blimp?

A "protein-sparing" fast.

Not a total fast, but a fast accompanied by a "predigested liquid protein formula . . . with all the necessary amino acids, the components of protein."

On a total fast, said Dr. Linn (and regrettably, total fasts were becoming "a national fad"), only 50 percent of the weight loss was fat, "the rest is water and lean body tissue."

Terrible tales were told, said Dr. Linn, of total fasters. As in the case of a young Englishwoman who stopped eating for thirty weeks, lost a hundred pounds, and died nine days after she'd come off the fast. "An autopsy revealed that in those weeks of total fasting, she had used up more than half of her lean body mass—including part of her heart."

But with liquid protein "substituting for the sustenance you're used to," the doctor assured us, we could lose thirty pounds a month while staying in "nitrogen balance."

What was liquid protein made of? Sow underbelly. It would, Dr. Linn admitted, have tasted vile, if it hadn't been "heavily laced with natural fruit flavorings."

In *The Thin Game,* Edwin Bayrd took issue with Dr. Linn. When Dr. George Blackburn first developed the liquid protein diet, said Bayrd, it had been intended for "supplemental feeding of critically ill patients." Blackburn had not been thinking of it as a cure for obesity. Moreover, there was a danger on this diet of mineral loss (mainly potassium), which could lead to catastrophe.

Again, ketosis was indicated. "Because the liquid protein formula contains no carbohydrates whatsoever," wrote Bayrd, "the regimen is strongly ketogenic, producing . . . immediate water-weight loss and loss of lean body mass . . . And because it restricts the dieter to 300 calories per day, well below the 800–1,000 calorie per day minimum level recommended by most nutritionists, it quite naturally produces the adipose tissue loss associated with near-starvation diets. The worst, in short, of both worlds—and the deleterious side effects of both as well."

Dr. Linn had taken the precaution of telling his readers that nobody should use liquid protein without first consulting a doctor, but since the FDA had classified the stuff as a food, not a drug, it was sold over the counter, no questions asked, no prescriptions necessary. At one point, in 1977, it was estimated that two million dieters were swilling liquid protein. One woman I know said she had nothing against it except that it gave her bad breath. Dr. Linn's private patients were fed a liquid called Linn Modified Fasting Formula, but, mindful of the trouble earlier fellows like Taller had seen, he went to some pains to explain that he had "no direct or indirect financial interest in this product."

The tide of liquid protein—"It's not as thick as Jell-O, but it doesn't run like water," wrote Dr. Linn—turned once the FDA began investigating the deaths of some fifty-eight women who had been involved in protein-sparing regimens. Here, from the *FDA Consumer*, the results of this investigation:

"The Center for Disease Control found that in at least sixteen of the cases, the diet was highly suspect as a contributing factor in the deaths. In these cases, the victims were obese women between the ages of twenty-three and fifty-one who lost an average of eighty-three pounds after being on low-calorie protein diets for two to eight months. None had a history of heart disease. All died suddenly, without previous symptoms, of heart irregularities—either while on the diet or shortly after going off it."

After that, public enthusiasm for liquid protein abated.

Dr. Linn stonewalled, insisting that—under a doctor's supervision—his diet was safe, and that 80 percent of his patients had "kept all or almost all of the weight off." But, said Edwin Bayrd, Linn had "produced no figures to back up his claims. This had led at least one disgruntled colleague to observe that 'the key ingredient of Linn's diet is not protein but hype.'"

When Dr. Atkins came along with his diet revolution (which was not only high-protein and zero carbohydrate, but also high fat), certain cynics observed that the Atkins diet wasn't for welfare recipients. It was rich stuff for rich people. You could have spareribs and duckling and heavy cream, you could have mayonnaise, butter, shrimp, steak, lobster, or cheeseburgers (Atkins offered a recipe for quiche lorraine that included 1 pound of bacon, ⅓ cup of bacon fat, 2 cups of heavy cream, plus eggs and cheese), but you couldn't have sugar or starch.

"Some people actually don't like fat," said Dr. Atkins, "but I don't encourage a no-fat diet, ever. . . . I have seen women on diets so low in fat that they couldn't manufacture enough female hormones to have a regular menstrual cycle. Now, if your very function of being a woman can be impaired by going on a low-fat diet, low-fat diets are to be considered with extreme caution."

This kind of thing caused Dr. Stillman to become indignant. He said he'd had patients come to him who had *gained* weight by following Dr. Atkins's advice. Weight, and cholesterol. "The excuse that 'fat melts away fat' may appear valid on paper, but certainly not on the scale, or in your body where it counts," said Dr. Stillman. Furthermore, high-fat diets frequently produced nausea, and the American Medical Association had yet to track down Dr. Atkins's so-called fat mobilizing hormone.

The AMA did, in fact, declare the Atkins diet "grossly unbalanced," and in March of 1973, a lawsuit was brought against Atkins by an actor who said the doctor's diet had caused him to have a heart attack. The actor did not win his case.

Still, Dr. Atkins was wounded, if not in his purse, in his feelings. *Dr. Atkins' Super-Energy Diet* (written with Shirley M. Linde, the book came after *Dr. Atkins' Diet Revolution* and *Dr. Atkins' Diet Cookbook*) included a chapter headed "We Must Discuss the Controversial Aspects."

In this chapter, Atkins said his first book had become the fastest seller in the history of publishing. He said the publisher had needed five printers working full time to turn out 100,000 copies a week.

He said he'd always respected "my own organization, the American Medical Association," and had thought it would support him "if only as a way to solve the embarrassing problem of amphetamine-dispensing for weight reduction."

Had this happened? Not at all. The AMA had responded to his book with "a Pearl Harbor Sneak Attack," by issuing a 16-page press release calling the Atkins diet "unscientific and potentially dangerous to health."

His patients, said Atkins, were losing weight, feeling rejuvenated, and here was the AMA saying it couldn't be done.

As though that weren't bad enough, his own county medical society, the one representing New York City doctors, called a press conference and leveled "unsubstantiated charges upon my research."

Next came attacks from magazines, from writers who "had not even been curious enough to interview me or look at my files," but who were throwing around words like "quack, faddist, charlatan."

And then the lawsuits. Not just the actor, but other people. "In this country, anyone who wants to get some free publicity can sue a public figure," said Dr. Atkins, suggesting that the AMA or "the food industry" was really behind most of the nuisance suits with which he'd been confronted.

He had, said Atkins, appeared before the Senate Committee on Nutrition and Human Needs on April 12, 1973, to testify about amphetamines ("I had been working with a diet that had totally circumvented the need for them"), and had made a statement that included a "point-by-point rebuttal to the AMA critique on my diet."

Even so, said Dr. Atkins, he had run into a "brick wall of media resistance. My detractors were given free rein on the most important of network talk shows, but I was consistently shut out from the very shows that claim to thrive on controversy."

He had, admitted Dr. Atkins, done one exciting Merv Griffin show ("Merv knew the diet was great because he had gone on it") with Jean Nidetch, "the Weight Watcher lady, and the late Dr. Irwin Stillman and Adelle Davis. Ms. Davis, a grand and gracious lady I had never met before, gave me her enthusiastic support and told millions of viewers that she had used my diet successfully to lower her cholesterol and lose weight."

(Adelle Davis, herself a best-selling author—*Let's Cook It Right, Let's Have Healthy Children, Let's Get Well, Let's Eat Right to Keep Fit*—was also a biochemist and a much respected nutritionist. Back in the 50s, she was already railing against white "Styrofoam" bread, refined sugar, coffee, doughnuts, soft drinks, and synthetics, while praising wheat germ, fresh fruits, vegetables, and vitamins, but she did on occasion get carried away. Among her enthusiasms was raw milk; she said no one who drank a quart of raw milk a day would get cancer. Unfortunately for this theory, Adelle Davis herself died of cancer in 1974.)

Anyway, Dr. Atkins's books continued to sell and journalists continued to take potshots at him.

"If it works at all," wrote Toby Cohen in *New York* magazine (May 21, 1979), "the Atkins diet—despite what it promises—works by getting you to eat less. It is one of a number of diets like the Scarsdale diet and the rice diet (developed at Duke University) which, by excluding whole categories of food, cunningly manipulate your eating habits . . . For example, cutting out carbohydrates means passing up traditional dessert food, movie food, TV snacks, bread, potatoes, pasta, and *all the fats* we would have eaten by buttering, saucing, or smothering with sour cream the limited carbohydrates in bread, potatoes, or pasta. All these are eliminated without our having to worry about portion size, without having to be reminded every day that we are dieting."

While Dr. Atkins suggested that dieters could have all the bacon and eggs and butter they liked, Dr. Tarnower, sage of Scarsdale, took an entirely different tack, what might be called the Jack Sprat approach. The less butter, meat fat, shortening, milk, duck, eggs, and avocados, said he, the better. Dr. Atkins wouldn't let you munch a carrot stick? Dr. Tarnower wouldn't let you snack on anything else. (Carrot sticks and celery, to be precise.)

Dr. Tarnower, a cardiologist, internist, and founder of the Scarsdale,

New York, Medical Center, had, back in 1960, devised a weight control plan for his heart patients. This plan, known as the Scarsdale Medical Diet, had become immensely popular.

Scarsdale worked backwards. Long before the book appeared, the diet was famous. Mimeographed copies had spread from hand to hand, physical education teachers pushed it, joggers swore by it, restaurants featured its dishes on their menus. A vice-president of Bloomingdale's department store said he'd lost twenty pounds in fourteen days. Speaker of the House Tip O'Neill dropped forty pounds in two separate two-week cycles, and called the diet "a thing of beauty." Queen Elizabeth was rumored to be devoted to it. It was, wrote a *Time* reporter in the spring of 1979, "unquestionably the diet of the hour. Some socialites with no weight problems at all are following it simply because it is chic. 'Everyone's been on it,' declares a Chicago hostess, Donna (Sugar) Rautbord. 'I believe its appeal is its popularity.'"

Dr. Tarnower believed its appeal was that it was simple, "and time has proved it safe. People are willing to put up with the discipline and deprivation because they know it works."

The deprivation of Scarsdale wasn't simply in going fatless—a dieter was permitted no booze or sugar either.

The blessing of Scarsdale was that it took all decisions out of the hands of the dieter. For two weeks, you ate what Dr. Tarnower said you should eat, at every single meal.

With some patients, the establishment of a definite routine is most effective, says Hilde Bruch. "The monotony is an advantage, not so much because the patient will eat less because he gets tired of such a diet (this he does anyhow, with any type of diet) but because he does not need to think continuously of what he is going to eat next, and about how to improve the diet without cheating."

The Scarsdale breakfast was the same every day—half a grapefruit, a slice of dry protein toast, and coffee or tea. The Scarsdale lunches and dinners were high in protein (cold cuts, broiled fish, broiled steak, broiled lamb chops, broiled chicken, cheese), and everyone hated Thursday night. Thursday night's dinner featured "two eggs, cottage cheese, cooked cabbage, one piece protein toast, coffee or tea."

After a while, Dr. Tarnower gave up on eggs and cooked cabbage. By the time the book came out, in January of 1979, Thursday night's dinner called for all the chicken you wanted, "skin and visible fat removed before eating."

Scarsdale took off and sales of Thomas' Protegen Protein Bread doubled in many big cities, but soon it was Dr. Tarnower's turn to get knocked about by the experts. The point was made that besides the danger of ketosis (which we know by now is a product of *any* high-protein, low-carbohydrate diet) the Scarsdale diet didn't provide daily calcium and phosphorus.

The FDA, asked about Scarsdale, warned once again that high protein intake means high cholesterol, and that weight loss due to water loss would come right back as soon as carbohydrates were eaten again.

"Dr. Tarnower consciously encourages his readers to believe in chemical wizardry," complained Dr. George Blackburn of Harvard Medical School (he's the one who developed the liquid protein feeding for critically ill patients), "when he writes in *The Complete Scarsdale Medical Diet,* 'A carefully designed combination of foods can increase the fat-burning process in the human system, and this means weight loss.' There's no 'metabolic miracle' built into this diet, just tight control of what and when you eat."

Dr. Myron Winick, director of the Institute of Human Nutrition at Columbia University's College of Physicians and Surgeons, said the diet probably wouldn't cause "much trouble," since it was prescribed for no more than two weeks at a time. On the other hand, said Dr. Winick, "there is a tendency to lose water on these high-protein diets, giving you the false feeling of success."

Dr. Louise Light, of the Human Nutrition Center in Washington, D.C., said Scarsdale was "an effective short-term, quick weight loss diet, which is why it is so appealing to the public. But this is not a way of life nutritionally."

Ruby Good, a nutritionist with the New York Health Department, called Scarsdale incomplete. "You can lose weight on it, but it is low in calcium-rich milk and cheese, and the high amounts of protein would present problems if kept up for any long period."

Another Health Department nutritionist, Alice Heller, agreed. "No milk, so it is obviously inadequate in calcium. It is also low in carbohydrates, so it doesn't allow for complete metabolism of fats."

And from Vivian Schulte, a member of the New York Academy of Sciences, came a response to Scarsdale that was brief and uncompromising. "You give me a short-term diet and I give you a waste of time. You may lose weight, but it is a seesaw. You have to change your eating habits."

The seesaw of losing, gaining, losing, has been described by Jean Mayer as "the rhythm method of girth control." (The witty Mayer also wrote the immortal words, "If you *look* fat, you probably *are* fat.") Dr. Mayer opposes all crash diets. "They are nutritionally unbalanced, they make you weak, irritable, and dizzy. After the first thrilling plummet of the scales, the pointer inexorably creeps upward again."

But not everyone agrees (despite its promise of losses "up to twenty pounds in fourteen days") that Dr. Tarnower's is a crash, or fad, diet.

"The Scarsdale diet could be rechristened 'The Common Sense Book of Losing Weight,'" says Craig Claiborne. "Its principles are simple and sound. You avoid fats and sugars and high-calorie snacks, peanuts and other seemingly trivial between-meal foods."

Claiborne went to a dinner party given by Tarnower, and observed the doctor "helping himself to a sizable portion of rich-as-Croesus salmon mousse with lobster sauce," followed by chicken, baked zucchini in cream sauce, and "a fine apple dessert with a ring of sweetened whipped cream with chopped macadamia nuts." Craig was relieved to be told that the doctor considered the feast "one of his rare indulgences at table."

Ordinarily, said Tarnower, he existed on 1900 calories a day, but "as I said in my book, good food is one of life's great arts and great pleasures and should not be bypassed even by dieters."

Spread that on your carrot stick and chomp it.

In 1979, Dr. Tarnower's only real hardcover competition was *The Pritikin Program* (which won't be dealt with in this chapter, since it isn't really for people who want to lose weight, but for people who want to live longer, and who think Nathan Pritikin can prevent their having heart attacks).

But there's always a new diet book in town. Some people went for *Dr. Cooper's Fabulous Fructose Diet* because it was brilliantly promoted in ads that said the doctor, "himself a former 240-pound fatty, is a board-certified specialist in both family practice and bariatric (weight control) medicine."

What's fructose? Fruit sugar, found naturally in fruits and vegetables (and soon to be found unnaturally in Coca-Cola, as we've lately learned). Dr. Cooper says fructose is 50 percent sweeter than sucrose (table sugar) and he says it can help you to lose weight "without the torture of hunger and without the weakness and loss of energy that accompanies other, less natural diets."

You eat high-protein foods on Dr. Cooper's Fabulous Fructose Diet.

You eat fish, seafood, chicken, veal, beef, pork, and lamb. You also eat two large salads a day, "and regular small meals of sweet, delicious fructose."

If you eat foods with table sugar, the glucose in your blood rises swiftly, triggering insulin, which makes the glucose level drop just as fast as it rose. Fructose, on the other hand, says Dr. Cooper, "is absorbed into the bloodstream slowly and smoothly, without creating the roller-coaster blood sugar response. It eliminates both the hunger and the low-energy periods of conventional dieting. Some dieters report that they actually have to remind themselves to eat *because fructose turns off the hunger alarm in the brain*."

You can buy fructose in a health food store. You can buy Dr. Cooper's book at a bookstore. Or you can take the whole thing with a grain of salt, unless you're on a sodium-free diet.

Because in *National Health*, which calls itself The Consumer's Health Newspaper, a correspondent named Jane Glicksman published the results of her interviews with various doctors and nutritionists who gave their opinion of several diets, including the Fabulous Fructose.

"Americans love diets that hinge on a magic new ingredient or process for shedding pounds," wrote Miss Glicksman. "The more outlandish or contrived the method, the more appealing to an overweight public."

True, fructose was rapidly absorbed into the liver, true, diabetics might be better able to tolerate fructose than sucrose, but the fructose diet was really just one more low-carbohydrate (no alcohol, beans, bread, cereal, corn, milk, pasta, potatoes, or rice), high-protein regimen. With a gimmick.

In the absence of carbohydrates, David Salinger (consumer affairs officer for the FDA) told Miss Glicksman, the body was forced to break down fatty acids. "The ketones produced from this breakdown can also suppress the appetite." (I'm going to keep telling you this till you get it right.)

There was no scientific evidence, added Mr. Salinger, that fructose itself slaked the appetite.

The AMA's Dr. Philip White was skeptical too. "At nine to twelve dollars a pound for fructose, rewards go to the seller rather than to the dieter."

And to the writers of fructose diet books.

Edwin Bayrd, who hasn't a good word to say for most of the diet industry (unless you think the words "large scale consumer fraud" are friendly), told journalist Bonnie Lake about one of his public appearances to push *The Thin Game* in Minneapolis. "They put me on a talk show against the author of 'The 9-Day Wonder Diet,' which amounts to four days of fasting and then a terribly restricted diet. The man was telling the audience that his plan was a proven success.

"I said that I was sure people would lose, but the problem is keeping it off. Then I asked for a show of hands for those who had managed to lose fifteen pounds on the Stillman, Atkins, or Scarsdale diet. Maybe three fourths of the hands went up. Then I asked how many had kept the weight off. All but one hand went down."

You pays your money and you takes your choice. But for sure, you pays your money.

The probability is that you won't stay on any diet—even a best-selling one—long enough to really hurt yourself.

TAKING IT OFF:
Two who pass when the clams are fried.

17 Formerly Fat: Larry and Elaine, Among the 3% Who Have Really Done It

In which the heavy and the weary weight
Of all this unintelligible world,
Is lightened.
—WILLIAM WORDSWORTH

"I MET Kurt Vonnegut down at Trillin's house, and he said I should do a novel about losing weight, but I can't sit at a typewriter, I get twitchy," says Larry Goldberg, tucking into a pastrami omelet (well done), French fries, and a toasted buttered bagel, at the Gaiety Delicatessen.

Goldberg's adventures among the literati have not kindled in him an ambition to be an important author, though he has, despite his twitchiness, turned out not only a *Pizza Cookbook* but also *Goldberg's Diet Catalog*, which promised on its cover to deliver "everything you ever wanted to know about diet books, scales, over-the-counter diet medications, exercise equipment, diet spas, obesity programs, diet food, mind-control therapy, diet cookbooks, and diet groups." A new book, *Controlled Cheating: The Fats Goldberg Take It Off Keep It Off Diet Program,* is due this fall.

The *Catalog* offered hundreds of paragraphs with names, prices, phone numbers, and brief descriptions of the doctor, spa, or book in question.

But Larry Goldberg used none of the above. Larry Goldberg healed himself. He went from 320 pounds, in 1959, to the 160 pounds he weighs today, and he did it his way, which consists of fanatical diet days broken by judicious cheating days, a system he manages to make sound like the most ordinary common sense.

"I figured out," he says, "that a man can't look down the long road of life and never see a hot fudge sundae. So I developed this theory that worked for me. I think it would work for anybody because it gives you release. The reason dieters fail is the deprivation. It's like a tight band around my head when I'm not eating." He bites into his bagel. "I'm happier today than I was yesterday.

"People kid themselves," says Goldberg. "They know what's fattening, what they don't know are portion sizes. They don't know what four ounces of cottage cheese looks like as opposed to eight ounces, or what a ten-ounce steak looks like as opposed to a five-ounce steak."

Goldberg doesn't kid himself. Even if it's his birthday, and he's at a big fancy party, if it's a diet day, he'll avoid the pastries, and search the buffet until he finds something he can permit himself to eat. Last birthday, it was cold bass—"I ate 40 yards of it." As for exercise, he runs up the seven flights of stairs to his apartment in less time than it takes the elevator to get there, and his stationary bike is used so much he's had it fitted with a reading rack.

When he was little, Larry Goldberg lived over his father's store, Goldberg's Market, in Kansas City, Missouri, and he was the only fat one in the family. "My father weighed 150 pounds, my mother weighed 130, my sister weighed 120. My mother used to make six pork chops, three for me and one for each of them. My father never got hungry. He died at seventy-four, and he never got hungry. Used to force himself to eat, while I was inhaling everything I could get my hands on. My father always thought the A & P put him out of business, but it was me.

"I had a loving family, and anything I wanted was fine with them, but my mother said she had to stop breast-feeding me at an incredibly young age because she was getting fat keeping me in milk. I moved on to cereals right away.

"I weighed 105 pounds in third grade. In sixth grade, I had to sit in a chair at the side of the room because I was too fat to slide in behind a desk. By eighth grade, I weighed 240.

"If I hadn't played sports, I wouldn't be able to walk now. But my friends and I played hour after hour of basketball, football, baseball, and I became really well coordinated.

"As a little kid, I was always on diets. My mother would take me to the pediatrician, he'd say, 'Goldberg, you want to die in ten years? You're gonna die unless you lose weight,' and he'd give me a mimeographed sheet. You know the kind. One piece of whole wheat toast, skim milk, cottage cheese, tomato, all that crap I don't like. The first day, I'd diet through breakfast, then blow the whole deal at lunch.

"The doctor had me so scared I became a screaming hypochondriac. I wanted to join a TOPS group (that's run by the YMCA and the YWCA, it stands for Take Off Pounds Sensibly, it's way ahead of Weight Watchers); I'd read about it somewhere, and I thought in a group I wouldn't be so lonely, trying to take off the weight, but nobody in Kansas City knew what I was talking about.

"People in Kansas City wrote me off as a slob. I was always popular, because I developed a fast mouth, and I was funny. But I was afraid to go out with ladies, afraid of rejection, and fat gave me a wall all through puberty. I didn't have to date. I only had two dates in high school. Both were fixed up.

"I was known as Fats Goldberg, and in a way, I used being fat. It made me outstanding. I was protected, people felt sorry for me, I got a great deal of sympathy."

After he was graduated from college—he'd gone to the University of Missouri, in Columbia—Goldberg took his Army physical, "and it was the most embarrassing moment of my life. I was rejected because I was too fat. I went back to Kansas City, had four jobs in one year, and was written off by everybody.

"But I think being fat made me fight harder for what I've got. My theory is that the only people who count have been through a lot of crap in their lives, whether it's obesity or something else."

His serious dieting began for Larry Goldberg more than twenty years ago. He isn't quite sure why, at the age of twenty-five, he was able to start living another way, but there were many reasons that converged to spur him on. The fact that when he got to 320 pounds, he had to be weighed on a cattle scale, because most normal scales don't go above 300. The humiliation of the Army's rejection. "And I was sweating a lot, and I wanted to meet women, and the *Chicago Tribune* had given me an actual grown-up job selling space advertising, even though I only had one suit. And I didn't want to die."

Also, he'd read a book in college that said if you were going to lose weight and keep it off, you had to find out why you'd got fat in the first place.

"So I analyzed myself. I said, 'Well, why did you get fat, Goldberg?' Part of it was what I said before, fat made me outstanding, and I could hide behind it, hide my fears, my lack of self-confidence.

"But I realized I didn't want to be written off anymore. Instead of sitting in Kansas City getting fatter, and having some kind of crummy job, I wanted people to say, 'Look at Goldberg, he did something.'"

For a year, Goldberg stuck to a low-calorie balanced diet, no cheating, "and then I decided, I'm not going to be able to keep this up, and I began cheating on Sundays. I'd gain three or four pounds on Sunday, then go back on the diet. I got my weight down to 190 pounds.

"For the first ten years, I cheated one day a week. Then the *Chicago Tribune* transferred me to New York, and I went down to 180. Then I went into the pizza business, and I was standing in front of two 650-degree ovens all day long, and I went down to 160, and started cheating two days a week.

"When I go back to Kansas City to visit, I'll put back eighteen pounds in a week. I got nothing to do back there, and I horse around. They got some great barbecue, great doughnuts. Lamarr's doughnuts will drive you right up the wall. They're twisted, they're as long as a baseball bat, they weigh about twenty-six pounds apiece, deep-fried, heavy, crusted with cinnamon and sugar. And there's Zarda Dairy's banana split. They make it in a Sara Lee pound-cake container, with huge dips of ice cream. And there's hot fudge. They do something out there they don't do here. If you like chocolate, go into Baskin-Robbins and get a hot fudge shake—"

It is not the confession of a man who has grown indifferent to food. "It's always depressing," he says, "to come back to New York and go back on the diet, but I say, 'Goldberg, you can handle it now.' When I figured out I was thin enough so I could cheat every third day, I started counting my cheating days. I was forty-five years old. That meant thirty-three more days of happiness a year. What I plan to do is keep this up till I'm eighty, and then just forget about dieting, eat myself into oblivion. Somebody might have to mash up all the Big Macs and french fries and spoon-feed me, but I'm not going to fool around. After eighty, nothing's going to happen anyway."

The first Goldberg's Pizzeria (its sign now hangs in the Smithsonian Institution, along with Fonzie's leather jacket, a cultural artifact of our time) was opened in 1968 "because I thought New York had lousy pizzas, and I was bored out of my head with my job. I tried show business for a while, I was half of a comedy team, Berkowitz and Goldberg, but I wasn't funny enough to be a stand-up comic. I'm finally getting it into my head that I can't tell jokes.

"But Goldberg's Pizzeria is just an offshoot of show business. And so were Goldberg's Fortune Cookies. What I learned from the fortune cookie business is to stay in the pizza business. Everybody knows about Goldberg's Pizzeria. Even though I've franchised the two stores, I still go in all the time, mess around, say hello, because I like it."

Being fat, Goldberg says, was not all bad. "I don't regret it, there's a positive side to it." He says again that it gave him the impetus to try harder. "It made me write books, made me go in the pizza business, made me try the comedy act."

Also, he says, "It gave me an imagination. I'm a good voyeur. I can watch people eat a piece of apple pie on one of my diet days, and I can taste it, my fork is going through that crust, the butter, the apples, the juices, the cinnamon. I taste it, and I'm not eating anything."

Being thin, says Goldberg, is not all good. "Dieting is like getting up and going to work every day. You get up and you diet. It's as hard today as it was May 1st, 1959. Dieting is rotten. You have to understand that in my life, the three best things in the world are food, women, and air conditioning. Food is an obsession. I'm hungry all the time. I try to help other people who are dieting. I know what they're going through, the pain, the honest-to-God physical and mental pain of deprivation, the pain of being hungry.

"The cure rate for obesity is less than the cure rate for cancer. Only 3 percent take it off and keep it off. Dr. Hirsch, the adipose tissue guy at Rockefeller University, wanted to take some fat cells from my tush with a big league needle. I found out Rockefeller was interested in my body one Saturday night when I was schlepping pizzas—it was very busy in the place—and a guy comes in wearing a long, gorgeous cashmere coat, and says, 'Are you Larry Goldberg?' And when I said yes, he said he was from Rockefeller. 'Dr. Hirsch would like to talk to you.' Because in ten or twelve years of running an obesity clinic, they found out none of their patients had kept the weight off. Of course they had 500-pound people there. Friends would slip them chickens, sneak in sandwiches."

At the moment, Goldberg is classified as underweight. "On the chart, my doctor has written 'controlled malnutrition.' I think my system works, but you've got to keep it simple. Don't eat that bagel. Don't eat those French fries. Simple, but it's full-time work.

"People have the damndest notions about dieting. They think you do it for two weeks, and you stop, and you're okay forever. People still say, 'Goldberg, you don't have to diet anymore, do you?'

"I'm a rigid dieter. I won't change for anything. Yesterday, a diet day, I ate chicken salad and a bagel and a couple cups of coffee. And a grapefruit, an orange, a banana, and an apple. I eat straight through the day. Like I come here to the Gaiety for brunch every day, have a glass of milk, six tablespoons of raw bran. I drink ten to fifteen glasses of water a day. Water's the magic elixir.

"I won't change for anything. If it's a diet day, the angel of death could be sitting on my shoulder, a guy could have a gun at my head, but I won't eat. It bothers people. They say it doesn't, but it does. I don't drink, either. See, I never drank. I was too busy eating. I never smoked, I was too busy eating. I never even smoked grass. Food was the world to me.

"I've gotten smarter. Even when I cheat, I don't eat the real crap anymore. I save up for the good stuff. I'm saving up for Entenmann's chocolate doughnuts. I don't just go out and blow it on some Twinkie. I'm a class junk eater. I've changed."

Goldberg's favorite food when he isn't dieting is anything baked. Bread, cakes, pies. "And potatoes, corn. See, I think salads are for sissies. I don't like salads, and I don't like fruit. The only reason people eat salads is for the dressing. Nobody likes a dry salad, plastic tomatoes, and that bitter iceberg lettuce. Crunch, crunch, nothing's happening.

"I like bananas, but I would never touch an apple unless I had to, and forget the oranges. Anything healthful, I don't like. My mother and sister used to eat salads. Not me, man, I wanted the real stuff, I wanted grease running down both sides of my mouth.

"I like meat and potatoes. Nothing fancy, none of that French restaurant stuff. The Palm is my favorite restaurant in New York City—steak, potatoes, cheesecake, bread, and a lot of butter. No crapola. Mexican food is all right because it's fattening, all that fried stuff, and French is okay if you order right, but I ain't dancin' around with chocolate mousse and spending ninety-two dollars. Chocolate mousse is fine, but I'm not gonna spend a lot of money for it. I like Jell-O, tapioca, chocolate tapioca. The trouble is, what I figured out about eating is, it's just joy.

"I'm thin, but I'm still scared I could go back up. People say, 'Goldberg, you can cheat today, look how thin you are.' I say no, I can't cheat today. After twenty years, it's still the same. The problem with dieting having made me so rigid is that the rigidity enters other phases of your life. In the pizza business, I had to change, become flexible, but that was hard for me. People love to be rigid. They want specifics. They want to be told what to do. All the successful diet books are specific. *Scarsdale* is a brilliant piece of work, a low-calorie balanced diet, low in calcium, but people can't stay on it. And when they come off, they're not going to change their habits, so it's not going to work for them. It's the yo-yo syndrome."

Goldberg has little respect for most diet doctors ("I know more about dieting than they do"), but he praises Dr. Hirsch, and Dr. Morton Glenn, "a disciple of Dr. Norman Joliffe, who's dead, but who started it all. Dr. Joliffe wrote the New York City Health Department Diet, and ran an obesity clinic, which is what Weight Watchers came out of."

Having achieved his weight loss through his own efforts and determination, Goldberg also sneers at the science of behavior modification, even though he has certainly modified his own behavior. "I think life is simple, people mess it up. Behavior modification has you eat at a certain place every day, eat a certain amount, keep diaries. Weight Watchers is doing it, they're all doing it. My point is, if a person's that motivated, they don't need behavior modification. No one knows why people lose weight and keep it off. Food addiction is worse than drug addiction, worse than alcoholism, because you have to eat to live, and eating is fun. Sometimes food is better than sex."

"I've never been to therapy. I think it's bullshit. Thurber wrote a series of pieces in the 30s in the *New Yorker* called 'Leave Your Mind Alone.' I got so sick of taking out women in New York who'd say, 'Ah, Goldberg, you ought to go to therapy.'

"Okay, you find out you have a problem, you might have hated your mother when you were eleven years old. Then there's eighty-three more problems off that one. It's never-ending, the thing never stops. I just don't believe in therapy. Not for me. I just don't think it's good."

Goldberg considers what he's just said, and grins. "I am a little crazy. Being fat has residual results. I'm just a fat man disguised as a thin man. I've still got the same fears. I still want approval. And it's hard, because for so long, my whole life revolved around being fat. I would literally have killed for food. And your metabolism doesn't change. My appetite is just the same. I've finished this lunch, and I'm still hungry.

"When you lose all that weight—I lost a whole Goldberg—it's schizophrenic. You have to come to grips with that. You don't know what to do with your time anymore, because so much time was spent running around trying to get something to eat. You have to fill in with work, and women, with trying to get a lady.

"A fat man eats until it's all gone. I'll never leave anything on a plate. At Christmas, I was down at Trillin's. I carved the turkey, and I was out there eating it before anybody else got to it. I say, 'I'll cut the thing, I'm a natural-born waiter,' and I'm out there grabbing it with both hands, digging out the dressing, putting it in my mouth. And later I say, 'Well, I'll clean up now.' I want to clean up. I want to clean up the plates is what I want to do. I want to clean up everything. I'm gonna tell you this, I'm being very honest with you, when you took that French fry there, I got pissed for a minute. I said, 'She's taking my food.'

"See, at the University of Missouri, I would get pizzas and take 'em down in the toilet in the basement and close and lock the door and sit there and eat them. Nobody got any of my food.

"And when you hit those French fries—listen, my mother could be sitting there, and if she went for a French fry, I'd feel the same way. That's how a fat person thinks. No one messes with his food. You don't give bites, you don't share. Fat people get in there and pitch. They want all the stuff."

Larry Goldberg studies the empty plates on the table in front of him, and restates his thesis: "A fat man eats until it's all gone." Then he returns to the subject of dieting. "It's predominantly a twentieth-century phenomenon, because before that, people had been hungry for centuries. There was never enough to eat. Even when I was growing up, forty-five years back, not that long ago, fat babies were the best. Chubby fat babies that laughed a lot. They kept feeding 'em—"

His words trail away wistfully. "It's something new," says Goldberg, "that you're supposed to be thin."

While Larry Goldberg doesn't believe in psychotherapy, Elaine Kaufman, another famous restaurateur, believes in it five times a week. She differs from Goldberg in other ways too; his weakness has been grease, and he never touched liquor; her weakness has been sugar, and she used to drink "a quart of booze between 12:00 and 4:00 A.M. every night."

But Elaine Kaufman, like Larry Goldberg, has lost a whole person—207 pounds. She lost the weight in less than two years, although twenty-five years of therapy went into giving her the strength to do it.

She sits at a table in her Second Avenue restaurant, which has been at the same address for seventeen years, and which she sometimes has painted, but refuses to change—"The essence of it is an old Greenwich Village place"—and laughs about the sightseers who come "looking for posh and velvet. And they see this"—gesturing toward the blue-checked tablecloths, red napkins, little carafes holding flowers, the plastic grapes hanging between bar and dining room, the faded murals, the old wood—"and they say, 'That's it?'"

Elaine's has a reputation for exclusivity—if you're not a famous writer, or a friend of hers, you can cool your heels, or leave hungry—that she says is exaggerated. "Everybody gets a table. Sometimes the place is filled up, and you have to wait till the people leave, but we don't turn people away. They come in with that idea, and in the meantime, I'm seating people all night long."

Seating herself is one of the things that delights her more than it used to. The old fat Elaine couldn't cross her legs, now she does it easily; the old fat Elaine used to spill over a barstool, now acquaintances wander into the place, and don't recognize its trim proprietor when her back is turned.

"The changes have been wrought by no miracle cures, gimmick diets, enzyme injections, or any other ostensible magic," wrote Leslie Bennetts, in a 1979 profile. All of the weight was shed "on a simple low calorie, high protein diet."

But fate also had a hand in the metamorphosis of Elaine Kaufman.

"I fell into the thing," she says, puffing at a Kool cigarette. "I had torn cartilages in both knees, which amounts to a form of arthritis. I went into the hospital for that operation the athletes have where they put some artificial thing in your knees. It would have meant six months in a wheelchair, crutches, being immobile, and the immobility was more threatening to me than anything else. In the hospital, I was lucky to find a doctor who said, 'We'll try to get you to lose weight, so we don't have to operate. You're not going to be an athlete, and anyway, even if we operated, if you kept the weight on, the operation wouldn't hold.'"

The doctors at the hospital helped her, swimming helped her, and

Elaine helped herself. Even pared to the bone, she isn't fragile and she makes the point that your frame determines your minimum weight. "America's idea of fat is not the world's idea of fat."

Unlike Larry Goldberg, Elaine had not been a heavy kid. "I was a little chunky, but okay. I see the pictures now, and I was fine. I wasn't a model, but I wasn't looking to be a model. I have a typical European build."

She was a spirited child, she remembers, "and they couldn't put me in a slot. I was bright, and I read very young. My sisters and my brothers would take me to the library when I was three, four years old. I learned fast. My mother didn't know how to deal with my spirit, she was always trying to bang it down."

Unwilling to be disciplined, even by herself, Elaine grew up "the infant still controlling the adult. I want, I want, I want. Instant gratification. I see it in people in the restaurant, people like alcoholics, who are compulsive. Tell somebody who drinks that they can't have their martini, and you'll see somebody hysterical."

The pounds piled on, as ventures failed. "I had a lot of jobs, and they never worked. Until I walked into this business, and I never walked out of it again. It was like it was waiting here for me. All of the facets of my personality that I couldn't use in other places, I was able to use here."

Elaine first got interested in running a restaurant because of a lover. The lover didn't last, but Elaine still has most of the rest of the staff with whom she started. "Which is," she says, "extraordinary."

In the beginning, she had no thought of creating a special kind of place, she was just trying to make a living. "I liked it, it came easy to me."

If her working life had begun to bring rewards, her emotional life was something else again. "I was always grateful to anybody who would be nice to me—that's the childlike approach, right there—and when I got involved with anybody, I would feel all this anxiety and fear."

The restaurant provided a kind of extended family without the emotional drain of unhappy romantic attachments. Food surrounded her, and Elaine grew ever fatter. "It was easier to eat than get involved."

Now she looks back and says fat people use their fatness as the excuse for everything. "Nothing is right, because you're fat. You think if you were only thin, everything would fall in your lap." She laughs. "It doesn't. When you lose the weight, you find out the world hasn't changed. It's all excuses, blaming the fat for your problems doesn't solve the problems."

Although she's been thin for more than a year, Elaine, like Larry Goldberg, is fearful of the weight's creeping back. "I'm still at a point where I have to watch it all the time. It's a habit to watch it."

Over the 1979 Christmas and New Year's holidays, she backslid, partly because she went to parties at people's houses where "the purpose of being there was to eat," and partly because an old boyfriend reappeared.

"It took me four years to get over this one," she says, "and he still came into the restaurant, and every time he came in, it took me weeks to get over it. Even with therapy. His con is a con I'm very susceptible to, and I never understood a lot of things about it. I realize now that I gave him the power. He's the same as he always was, I gave him the right—"

She shakes off the memory, and the weakness with it. "I would have gone through the holidays, dealt with them very well, if I hadn't seen this guy. As it was, I messed up."

But she didn't stay messed up. When she's feeling all right, Elaine says, she is seldom hungry anymore. "I have to remember to eat something, because the body needs a certain amount."

Elaine's diet, under strict medical supervision, during the almost two-year period it took her to drop from 357 pounds to 150 pounds, contained no fats, starches, or sugars.

Now she can have one dessert a day, but doesn't always eat it. On a typical day, "I'll have some cottage cheese and tuna fish. And then I'll have some broiled chicken, if I feel like it. Or I may not. And then I'll have a piece of melon later. And I take supplementary vitamins."

Diet food doesn't have to be unpleasant, she says. "You can eat skinned, broiled chicken, fish, veal, vegetables. You can have things like puréed squash, with a little cinnamon. It's sensational. There are a lot of dishes like that which most people don't think about."

Elaine is against the Goldberg style of cheating two days a week. "That's feeding the baby," she says, "making the hot fudge sundae more important than yourself, the self you aren't pacifying in other ways. You have to deal with the way you live. What I did was take the focus of my life off food, the pacifier."

It's interesting that being surrounded by food—pizzas, in Goldberg's case, wonderful pasta specialties in Elaine's—hasn't interfered with the serious dieting of either entrepreneur. "I plan the menus," Elaine says, "but in the restaurant business, you taste with your fingers, you put your fingers in and taste the flavors of the sauces, you don't have to eat the whole thing to find out what it's like."

She still has a problem with sugar, even though "I know when I'm craving it, it's not the sugar I want, it's some form of pacifying," and she has stopped drinking entirely. She points to her cigarette. "I'll eventually stop this too. Because I don't like what it does to your voice."

Being thinner, she says, has altered her personality somewhat. "I'm less defensive. The point is, fat or thin, you have to have a feeling for yourself. The fat comes because you don't have a good self-concept."

She exercises ("I have a stationary bike at home, I do about fifteen minutes twice a day, and I'm getting a rowing machine because it takes care of the upper part of the body"), she's thrilled to be wearing a reasonable dress size, but she doesn't believe, as once she may have done, that there are amazing external rewards offered to those who grow thin. "That's the baby, looking," she says. "The reward is yourself. That's hard to accept. But the streets are not going to turn to gold."

She tries, Elaine says, "to avoid anger, and anxious positions. I find it's very important for me to feel free, to be able to come and go as I please. I prefer to go home to my apartment, which is peaceful and calm, rather than to be running around all the time. I do a lot of things, I feel compelled to do more, but I'm learning to slow up. It works, and it's well worth it."

Even love doesn't scare her so much now. On Christmas Eve, 1980, Elaine got married—for the first time—to a man named Henry Ball, who manages the restaurants at the new Helmsley Palace Hotel. She didn't tell anybody. She just went and did it.

Elaine Kaufman, brown-eyed, brown-haired hostess to New York's inkiest, stubs out her Kool, and stands up. "You have to learn that you have a choice," she says, and turns to deal with a greengrocer who's been waiting at the bar to take an order for vegetables.

TAKING IT OFF:
Over the counter and through the mails, we chase the Bluebird of Skinniness.

18 Diet Pills, Diet Potions, and Addiction, Which Is "Socially Acceptable"

And what can we expect if we haven't any dinner
But to lose our teeth and eyelashes and keep on growing thinner?
—EDWARD LEAR

THE ANCIENT Egyptians thought all disease originated in food, and purged their bodies every month.

The Greek father of medicine, Hippocrates, prescribed meats, undiluted wine, and bread in the winter, soft foods, vegetables, and "copious" amounts of diluted drink in the summer. Hippocrates also believed "our natures are the physicians of our diseases," and treated patients not with religion, but with fresh air and changed eating habits. Honey was among his favorite restoratives—"The drink to be employed should there be any pain is vinegar and honey. If there be great thirst, give water and honey"—and he often suggested barley gruel for the ailing.

Addressing himself to fat ("Corpulence is not only a disease itself, but the harbinger of others"), Hippocrates offered the following bits of wisdom (from a translation by W. H. S. Jones, published in 1931):

"Fleshy people should work faster, thin people slower. . . .

"Fat people who wish to become thin should always fast when they undertake exertion, and take their food while they are panting and before they have cooled, drinking beforehand diluted wine that is not very cold. Their meats should be seasoned with sesame, sweet spices, and things of that sort. Let them also be rich. For so the appetite will be satisfied with a minimum. They should take only one full meal a day, refrain from bathing, lie on a hard bed, and walk lightly clad as much as is possible."

The Hippocratic Oath began with the words, "I swear by Apollo, the physician, and Asclepius and Health and All-Heal and all the gods and goddesses," and included the promise to "follow that system or regimen which, according to my ability and judgment, I consider for the benefit of my patients, and abstain from whatever is deleterious and mischievous. I will give no deadly medicine to anyone if asked, nor suggest such counsel . . ."

In modern times, numbers of doctors have not shared Hippocrates' rectitude. The amount of deadly (and nondeadly but ineffectual) medicine pumped into fat patients in order to shear off their poundage is mind-bending. Shots of "enzymes" that aren't enzymes at all, shots of hormones that don't harm but don't help either, shots of amphetamines that *do* harm, all are routinely given. Because of amphetamine abuse, there are countless citizens—and the word countless is not used carelessly—who are speed freaks, drug addicts, chemical dependents.

Amphetamines came to light in the 1930s, as a treatment for depression. But the drugs were found also to have an anorexic effect, which led doctors to begin prescribing them for fat patients. When many of these patients became nervous and irritable, and some even suffered delusions, the sedative phenobarbital was added to the formulas, and the pill pushing went forward.

The dangers of amphetamine usage were observed throughout the 40s and the 50s, but diet doctors kept on dispensing the pills and the shots that fed drug dependency in their patients. The alarm didn't go off until the children of pill poppers began their own destructive flirtations with speed because they liked the way uppers made them feel.

Suddenly, we seemed to be a nation of junkies.

Hilde Bruch, in *Eating Disorders*, points an accusing finger at "certain 'reducing doctors' who together with drug houses created a whole industry devoted to 'treating' obesity with 'rainbow pills,' various combinations of drugs which were offered in different colors, to be used at different times of day."

These combination drugs, which fad doctors across the country commended, most often consisted of amphetamines (for the suppression of the appetite) along with thyroid pills and digitalis. A large number of the doctors ran their own pill businesses out of their offices, and while they didn't agree on everything—some said you had to diet, along with the pills, some said you could eat whatever you liked, some said you should exercise, some said you should drink lots of water—all were afloat on a river of gold.

"Many experts considered amphetamines far more dangerous than heroin," wrote James Trager in *The Belly Book*, "yet the drugs enjoyed a quasi-innocent, quasi-legitimate status that deceived many people into thinking they were harmless."

In the summer of 1970, says Trager, "about 8 percent of all prescriptions being filled were for amphetamine drugs, with as many as ten billion pills—fifty-eight for each American man, woman, and child—being legally produced."

It wasn't too long afterward that the government got into the game. The FDA forced drug manufacturers to stop making false claims guaranteeing weight loss on their labels, the Department of Justice took steps against methamphetamine (taken by injection), and Congress, after listening to testimony from college students who'd bought pills through the mail and wound up in mental hospitals, empowered the government to set production quotas for the drugs. In 1972, domestic production of amphetamine and methamphetamine was cut by 82 percent, irritating the drug industry, and incurring warnings from diet doctors that bootleggers with a little knowledge would just whip the stuff up in their basements.

Amphetamine users have been cautioned about the possibility of severe side effects—central nervous system stimulation, physiological dependency, and the buildup of tolerance levels—while they're on the pills, and sleepiness and paranoid depression when they come off, but Dexedrine, Benzedrine, and Methedrine are still being sold, and there are still doctors willing to prescribe them, though the traffic is a bit more secret than it once was. (In a few states—New Jersey, Maryland, Wisconsin—the use of amphetamines for weight control has been banned.)

"There shouldn't be doctors who give amphetamine shots," says Dr. Martin Katz, a Manhattan cardiologist, internist, teacher, and gourmet cook, "but as long as there's a demand for them, there will be. Everybody's looking for the fountain of youth, nobody has the patience to understand you have to learn a way of life which will help you stay at a reasonable weight."

After a while, amphetamines don't even suppress your appetite anymore, but you're hooked. This is a fact. A couple of weeks, and you're hungry again, so you step up your dosage, expecting that more pills will do the trick.

"I've got patients who've been to diet doctors and who are amphetamine junkies," says Dr. Katz. "They come to me because they have other illnesses, but I find out they're taking a drug like Dexamyl. Offhand, I can think of five patients who have been to diet doctors and are hooked. I can't get them off the drug, they're emotionally and physically dependent on it. I have a patient who's been on amphetamines for seventeen years."

One of the problems, observes Dr. Katz, is that amphetamine addiction is "socially acceptable." These patients, he says, "live within the framework of their addiction, and they take the pills just to keep them from going into withdrawal. You see, there's a difference between this kind of addiction, which is personally destructive, and the kind of addiction which is socially destructive.

"I'm not a psychiatrist, but I think fat people are overeating out of anxiety and unfulfillment. So when you take food away from them, you must supply something else. The diet doctor offers two things. One, he charges them. That's very important. They're paying by the pound to lose weight. Two, he's giving them magic in a sealed envelope. They don't know what it is—of course, it's a diuretic, it's an amphetamine, it's thyroid medication, along with something like Valium or Librium to control the side effects of the other drugs—but they hope it will help. What you're dealing with is people who will pay anything not to have to deprive themselves."

Larry Goldberg, who did eventually learn to deprive himself, recalls a brief encounter with amphetamines when he was sixteen. He visited a diet doctor who "weighed you, gave you a bag of pills, shook your hand, smiled, and said good-bye. You were supposed to come back every week to be weighed and get your new bag of pills. The pills were Dexedrine—uppers. The doctor charged ten bucks for the weigh-in and the pills. After being high for three days and giggling a lot, I flushed those little honeys away."

A slender young magazine editor who wanted to lose another ten pounds had a more frightening experience on Eskatrol (which is the same as Dexedrine). If she'd known the street names—eye openers, lid poppers, rippers, ups, wedges, brain pills—for the drugs, she might have thought twice.

As it was, she swallowed her first pills ("I couldn't sleep for a week afterward") and found her heartbeat had not only accelerated wildly, but was behaving erratically. "I was terrified," she says. "I wanted to call my mother and ask her to come and help me, but I couldn't even remember her phone number. I was sure I was dying. I stumbled downstairs and asked my landlord to find me a doctor."

It was a doctor, of course, who had dispensed the stuff in the first place. To a patient who was obviously not overweight. And what he did was absolutely within the law.

(Between 1974 and 1975, 450,000 prescriptions for amphetamines were dispensed every month, reports the Drug Abuse Staff of the Bureau of Drugs in the FDA. Between 1977 and 1978, only 300,000 similar prescriptions were dispensed monthly, so it would appear that the traffic—the legal traffic, at least—in amphetamines is on the decline in the United States.

Oddly enough, a 1978 survey shows that only 4.7 percent of adults twenty-six years or older who were polled would admit to having "ever used" stimulant prescription drugs, and of these same adults, only six tenths of one percent would admit to being a "current" user. Stimulant prescription drugs include drugs other than amphetamines, but most drugs in this category are amphetamines, according to Dr. Joan Rittenhouse and Dr. Barry Brown of the National Institute for Drug Abuse, which conducted the survey.)

Outside the law, traffic in uppers flourishes (most city kids know where to go to buy any drug you can mention), but amphetamines can no longer be sold without a prescription, over the counter.

Plenty of other—nonamphetamine—diet pills are in trouble now too.

"Magical diet potions are being promoted in a new and, according to some doctors, alarming form," reported *Time* magazine in September of 1979. "These widely advertised nonprescription products contain two familiar ingredients, benzocaine and phenylpropanolamine (PPA). Benzocaine is a local anesthetic . . . it presumably dulls the taste buds and discourages eating. PPA, a drug related to the amphetamines, has enjoyed a long history as a nasal decongestant in cold remedies. In such popular diet pills as Dexatrim, Prolamine, Spantrol, and Appedrine (which also contain caffeine), manufacturers say that it depresses the brain's 'appetite center' in the hypothalamus."

PPA appeared to have some mild effect as an appetite suppressant, but its potential for good was no greater than its potential for harm. Even the drug companies who made it admitted that PPA could raise blood pressure, and would be bad for a patient with prostate trouble, heart disease, diabetes, or an overactive thyroid gland. In 1979, a special advisory panel to the FDA expressed the tentative finding that benzocaine and PPA appeared to be "safe and effective"—if taken as directed—but critics countered that the panel had been working with data supplied, and paid for, by the drug companies.

By the spring of 1980, the FDA changed its collective mind. Phenylpropanolamine was *not* all that safe, and the government would like the companies that made diet products to stop selling Dietac Diet Aid Drops, Extra Strength Appedrine Tablets, Vita-Slim Capsules, Power-Slim Packets, and New Improved Super Strength Hungrex Plus Tablets. To name just a few. Some of these were new, some like Vita-Slim Capsules, had been on the market for more than four years.

Joanna Wolper, who produced, wrote, and appeared in an ABC television special about weight loss (called *Take It All Off*) reported buying "a pile" of diet pills, both through the mail and over the counter. "The prices varied, but the mail-order brands cost a lot more than the drugstore variety."

Included with some of the drugs were low-calorie diets for the fat person to follow if he really wanted to get thinner.

Wolper had, she told her television audience, taken a number of the diet pills to Dr. Fotios Plakogiannis, at Long Island University, for analysis, and the doctor had put the pills "into an acid solution similar to the one found in the stomach."

Dr. Plakogiannis' testimony:

"This pill for two hours did not dissolve. That means that within two hours, they will leave the stomach, they will go to the small intestines without even being dissolved. That means that that is not active; doesn't do anything it's supposed to do."

The main ingredient of the stash Miss Wolper had brought to the lab was phenylpropanolamine, but since, as she observed, these particular pills would "streak through your stomach like a silver bullet," they wouldn't relieve you of any weight except the weight of your money.

The heartbreak of obesity (like the heartbreak of psoriasis, but more prevalent) has been making snake oil salesmen rich for a hundred years. In 1878, the Botanic Medicine Co., Proprietors, of Buffalo, New York, advertised something called Allan's Anti-Fat with a picture of a rotund lady, stuck behind a small turnstile, saying, piteously, "How am I going to get through?" To which her willowy companion answers, "Take Anti-Fat, as I did."

Anti-Fat, declared its makers, was "purely vegetable and perfectly harmless. It acts upon the food in the stomach, preventing its being converted into fat. Taken in accordance with directions, it will reduce a fat person from two to five pounds per week."

When pressed to divulge the nature of Anti-Fat's mystery ingredient, the Botanic Medicine Co. confessed that it was a "concentrated fluid extract of sea lichens."

"While this preposterous claim would fool few people today," says a 1967 book called *Food and Nutrition* (from the Time-Life science series), "modern Americans spend $100 million each year on . . . fad diets, tonics, and 'reducing aids' that are no more effective than Anti-Fat."

By the 1920s, dieters had been introduced to a product called Rengo, "Nature's Remedy for Obesity. Eat It Like You Would Fruit or Candy. Rengo is the only remedy for obesity which builds up your strength while it reduces your superfluous flesh."

The secrets of what really went into Rengo and Anti-Fat died with their inventors, and nobody knows what was in Kellogg's Obesity Food ("Will Reduce Your Weight to Normal, Free You From Suffering, and Turn Your Fat Into Muscle") either.

While you're laughing at the innocence of a bygone age, consider a guy calling himself John Andre (he'd been born John Andreadis) who came along in the late 40s. The Post Office had stopped him—once—from using the mails to defraud by misrepresenting the properties of a certain Hollywood Beauty Cream (about which more later), but you can't keep a good con man down.

Andre bounced back with Propex, an appetite suppressant that he packaged along with a "recommended" 1,000 calorie a day diet. The

Post Office decided that if you lost weight with Propex, it was because you'd cut your calories to 1,000 a day, not because of the appetite suppressant, and once again, took away Andre's stamp machine.

He didn't sulk, he went straight out and hatched Regimen. Regimen consisted of a "recommended" low-calorie diet, along with green pills (our old friend, benzocaine, the anesthetic), pink pills (ammonium chloride, a diuretic for water loss), and yellow pills (PPA, the appetite suppressant), none of the drugs in quantities large enough to be effective.

But the hype was first-class. "AMAZING NEW MEDICAL RELEASE (Available Now Without Doctor's Prescription)," blared a Regimen ad. "NO-DIET REDUCING with New Wonder Drug for Fat People CAUSES YOUR BODY TO LOSE WEIGHT THE FASTEST ACTING WAY!"

And the fakery was total. Andre paid the doctors who gave him his endorsements, Andre and his associates invented the "clinical evidence," patients who had never lived except in Andre's imagination appeared on the Regimen charts losing weight by the ton, and patients who lived, but were accomplished liars, went on television. In 1959, Dave Garroway, then the host of the *Today* show, welcomed a group of hefty housewives to his bosom, promising that they could come back each week, weigh in, and explain to the world how much they'd lost on their Regimen regimen.

The public was fascinated. Every seven days, the ladies showed up, ever more slender, even though they said they were continuing to eat desserts and bread and potatoes.

Regimen made the difference.

To Andre, too. Regimen was raking in $4 million a year when the bubble burst, and it was revealed that the "housewives" were actresses (Andre had advertised in various show business newspapers for fat girls who had once been thin) losing weight because they were living on 500 calories a day, and getting bonuses for every pound they dropped.

"Interestingly enough," reports Edwin Bayrd, "Andre himself never prescribed any sort of diet for his recruits. The cash inducements that he offered, in combination with the implicit understanding that failure to lose twenty pounds during the first month of the diet would mean termination of their contracts and an end to the lucrative television appearances, was the only inducement that any of these women needed to put themselves on near-starvation diets of the most dramatic and debilitating sort."

The Federal Trade Commission went after John Andre, so did the Better Business Bureau, the FDA, the Justice Department, and his nemesis, the Post Office, but it took six years before they could put him out of business. In May of 1965, Andre was fined fifty thousand dollars and sentenced to eighteen months in jail.

"By that time," says Edwin Bayrd, "overweight Americans had invested $16 million dollars in his sensible little diet and utterly superfluous pills." (Bayrd makes another surprising point. At the time John Andre came to grief, phenylpropanolamine, or propanol, as the drug was also known, "had been largely abandoned by the medical profession after nearly four decades of ineffective experimentation." Nevertheless, fifteen years later, we were told that most of the "new" over-the-counter diet pills were based on phenylpropanolamine.)

I've been tearing diet aid ads out of the papers for the last year or so, ads that mostly feature pictures of twenty-year-old starlet types in bikini bathing suits. You can have your choice—do you want to burn off your fat, or flush it away?—by sending money to the advertiser.

How about Millburn Products, of Maplewood, New Jersey? The Millburn folks say "an amazing diet breakthrough has been developed by a southern California M.D. This breakthrough literally allows you to burn off body fat faster than someone who runs almost 100 miles a week." To be sure, the testing of this diet formula "so far is incomplete," but the doctor who developed it was not only an M.D. but a psychiatrist who had treated "more than 2500 drug addicts" and learned that "overeating is as difficult to deal with as any hard-core addiction."

Welcome to the club, Doctor.

"Of course," confides Millburn Products, "something like this cannot be kept secret. Rumors of this doctor-developed breakthrough are spreading like wildfire. The rush is on. It is easy to imagine that professional actors, actresses, and other celebrities will be going out of their way to get their hands on this wonderful anti-fat weapon."

So that you can avoid being trampled underfoot by the likes of Elizabeth Taylor rushing to storm the factory, the company promises to mail you a ten- (or fifteen- or twenty- or thirty-) day supply, as soon as they receive your check.

After which you just mix a bit of the formula "with a glass of your favorite beverage and drink it every day the first thing in the morning . . . During the rest of the day, you eat a wide selection of tasty foods which is scientifically programmed to maintain a high level of fat burn-off."

What do you bet that the "wide selection of tasty foods" comprises a low-calorie diet?

From Canton, Ohio, the Weight Loss Center volunteers "The Pill to End All Diet Pills! . . . With the new Dyna-Slim Fat Liquidation plan featuring a remarkable One-A-Day Tablet, years of accumulated fat are quickly washed away."

The peddlers of Dyna-Slim say their pill is "as powerful as dynamite, as safe as aspirin," and that it has been "heralded by the medical community, leading newspapers, and weight loss specialists around the country . . . Here is what one New York M.D. said about this sensational diet aid: 'It's the best appetite suppressor I've ever run into, and this is my 49th year of medical practice.'"

Doctors, for the most part nameless, their credentials unspecified, are leaned on heavily in these ads. We're a country that believes in the medical profession (if they weren't smart, would they all be driving Mercedes-Benzes?), the very hint of scientific inquiry fills us with awe, and advertisers play on our superstitions.

From Florida comes the Total Diet Program, which you can order rushed to you "in a plain wrapper" (conjuring up pictures of the kind of covering a fat lady often wears anyway), and its "doctor-tested, medically proven formula" is designed to attack "both excess fat and excess fluids held in the body."

If you don't lose up to five pounds the first day, you can get your money back. (Most of these diet-formula outfits offer refunds, which makes you realize that people must just be too embarrassed to admit their failures.) Say the Total Diet Program people: "Your body's furnace can be turned on to high and your body literally forced to burn away excess fat. Lose as much as a full size the first week as this super fat burner goes to work. Bulging pockets of fat and fluid will be destroyed as you start to look better and feel better. What's more, you lose that gnawing craving for food you always had."

The 3-Way Diet Program, also from Florida, shares a copywriter with Total Diet. Most of what the two ads say is identical, but 3-Way is a tad more violent, declaring that its program turns on your "inner furnace so high it literally melts the fat off your body—like a blow torch would melt butter."

If the mention of melted butter makes you hungry, take five, go have an English muffin, and come back so I can tell you about the HB Hunger Brake Tablet System developed by—here's a doctor who's got a name—William Farrar, M.D. Dr. Farrar "has helped over 200,000 people nationwide" (well, maybe they weren't quite so wide as all that) "lose weight. Dr. Farrar has personally lost 32 pounds by following his system."

The Hunger Brake Tablet is a "100% natural appetite suppressor . . . First, pure honey is obtained from carefully cultivated bee hives. Then, special layers are extracted from whole grain wheat kernels. The honey and 1000 active wheat kernel units are then combined using a special process to form the HB 1000 Hunger Brake Tablet."

Dr. Farrar explains that natural ingredients are better than chemical aids, and that honey and whole grain wheat kernels will "cause fewer calories to be absorbed from the foods" you eat, and will speed up your "fat burning metabolism."

Still, he's got a face, and a name, and eyeglasses; if I were going to send for anybody's "system," I'd lean toward Dr. Farrar's.

After studying these ads, one comes to recognize a bit of—dare I say it?—collusion. Maxi-Slim, for instance, with its "once a day Power Packed Maxi-Slim 1000 capsule," quotes the very same "New York M.D." that Dyna-Slim leaned on. There he is saying Maxi-Slims are "the best appetite suppressor I've ever run into; and this is my 49th year of medical practice." (Either he's the very same New York M.D., or the entire profession is speaking as one.)

With all due respect, Doc, the Maxi-Slim ad and the Dyna-Slim ad ran a full year apart, so you must be in your *fiftieth* year of medical practice by now, and a perfect flibbertigibbet of a guy, at that. Just let some teeny new pill come along, and it gets your vote. Off with the old, on with the new. Whatever happened to the quaint traditions of steadfastness, loyalty, house calls?

But I must stop nattering. Would you like to be stimulated? "An appetite suppressant/stimulant capsule is available through the mail for a limited time." (Why do you suppose there's a time limitation? The hot breath of the authorities on the necks of the vendors? The lab rent being decontrolled?) "These GREEN and CLEAR capsules, with tiny specks of green and white, help DISSIPATE FATIGUE often associated with weight loss," the ad continues.

"There are a substantial number of firms that spend their time going in and out of the weight-loss, mail order, diet pill, diet device business," Karl Lauby, an official of the Better Business Bureau told Joanna Wolper. "In many cases, the promoter is in and out of business before a law enforcement agency has time or is able to gather its resources to act effectively. And even if they do act effectively, and the promoter agrees to discontinue the promotion, he'll go across the street, rent a new post office box, and start a similar promotion with the same product, perhaps under a different name, all over again."

A different name, a different post office box, but the same doctor in his forty-ninth year of medical practice!

The FDA's Al Lavendar says there are presently twenty-two nonprescription appetite suppressants on the market. Besides those previously named, such products as Anorexin, Fastin, Statobex Capsules, Tenuate Dospan, and Varnail are available at your friendly neighborhood drugstore.

But suppose pills and powders and liquids don't ring your bell. You can also buy chewing gum, cookies, or candy, and tell yourself they're diet aids.

Slim-Mint Flavored Chewing Gum is made of benzocaine (taste-bud anesthetizer, remember?) and essential oils and methylcellulose (a noncaloric indigestible vegetable product that, mixed with water, gives a feeling of fullness). The gum comes packaged with a diet plan.

Pillsbury's Figurines *are* a diet plan. "Just 275 calories in two crunchy bars."

If you ate nothing else, two Figurines, four times a day, would provide you with 1100 calories and enough protein, vitamins, and minerals to satisfy the U.S. recommended daily allowance but, asks the *New York Times*, "is this a good way to eat, let alone diet? . . . are two cookies . . . a satisfying meal that will assuage your hunger for four or more hours?"

Fifty-two percent of Figurines' calories are fat calories (from coconut and palm kernel oil), and the cookies also contain sugar. There is no clue on the Figurines label, the *Times* reporter observes, as "to how much dietary fiber, an important factor in proper bowel function, is contained."

Anyone who would rather chew on Figurines than fix himself a balanced meal might lose up to three pounds a week. And his temper, depending on whether or not he is bored easily.

The diet candy called Ayds is just that—candy. Each Ayd (made of sugar, benzocaine, flavoring, vitamins, and minerals) contains 25 calories.

What's most amazing about Ayds is that the Campana Company (now a subsidiary of the Purex Corporation) has been marketing them successfully since 1937, with present sales of more than $7 million a year.

Old ad collectors (lovers of "I was a 97-pound weakling," and "They laughed when I sat down to play" qualify) cherish memories of the "I was a 325-pound creampuff until I met Ayds" kind of testimonial, and the company's tales of movie greats nibbling their way to contentment were socko too.

"Today's screen stars now eat candy," confided one ad. "Oh, not ordinary candy, but a special low-calorie, vitamin and mineral enriched candy, called Ayds. Taken as directed before meals, it curbs the appetite, so you automatically eat less and lose weight naturally."

In 1945, the Federal Trade Commission protested that candy wasn't a diet food, and Campana sprang into action. "The manufacturer, understanding full well that the only real difference between its product and, say, Hershey's bars," writes Edwin Bayrd, "was that Ayds were being bought almost exclusively by the very people who had sworn off candy bars—rightly saw the F.T.C.'s complaint action as a threat to Ayds' continued existence and fought back in court."

What happened then sounds like a Woody Allen movie. The judge found for Ayds. "If you believe eating candy before dinner will make you lose your appetite," he ruled, "then you can use candy, any candy, as a therapeutic remedy."

P.S. In the Ayds package is a low-calorie diet. Follow that diet, says the manufacturer, and you'll get thin even faster than those who put their faith in candy alone.

While Ayds may have been the first diet candy, it certainly wasn't the last. Writing in *Diet Times*, a lady named Dorothy Livaudais was extremely laudatory about a candy called Arlington Nuggets. (*Diet Times* is a publication that doesn't always know that Jean Mayer is a man—sometimes a piece will refer to him as "she"—but it has a refreshing modesty about its own limitations. "*Diet Times* is in no way an authority on diet, health, beauty, or medical matters," the publisher confides in a paragraph printed right under the list of editors and diet, health, beauty, and medical columnists.)

Telling of the Paul-Christian Arlington Appetite Control Method,

Dorothy Livaudais said, "Everybody is talking about it. Because it works with and conquers one of the principal causes of obesity—the *oral syndrome*.

"Perpetual snackers. This is the best way to describe people who suffer from the oral syndrome. They rarely eat large meals and often skip them entirely. They have difficulty distinguishing between hunger and boredom, fatigue, depression, etc., and therefore 'feed' rather than recognize their emotions. Millions of people experience the symptoms of the oral syndrome. Women are particularly susceptible."

Oh, Dot, you're boring and depressing me, and I want to feed right now! What have you got to offer?

"A hard nugget made of glucose, benzocaine, caffeine, and vitamins, whenever the urge to snack is present. The candies are taken fifteen to thirty minutes before meals and immediately following meals if there is a desire for 'seconds.' Up to fifteen nuggets are allowed each day at ten calories each."

All together, let's sing it. We got glucose to elevate our blood sugar level, and satisfy our sweet cravings. We got benzocaine to numb our teeny taste buds. We got caffeine to "combat fatigue" and vitamins to "supplement the reduced calorie intake diet."

But soft, what light through my poor thick head breaks?

A reduced calorie intake diet?

Only a minute ago, Dorothy was saying that the Arlington Appetite Control Method worked "without stringent traditional dieting."

I knew it was too good to be true. In that same issue of *Health & Diet Times*, the Arlington Method took a nice ad for its classes. Instead of "limited time," Arlington featured "limited Clientele." Limited, I'd guess, to people willing to get up the $120 for four sessions (one a week for a month). More than fifteen pounds overweight? You'd need the $295 three-month drill. "Medical research has found that at least twelve sessions are required to redesign eating and drinking habits sufficiently to enable persons to maintain the ideal figure indefinitely."

The Paul-Christian Arlington Method was dedicated, said the ad, "to the private overweight person (the perfectionist who dreams of attaining the ideal figure, yet has tried everything and failed)."

Private fat folks would get "personalized attention" and "full daily supplies" of the "doctor-developed" nuggets containing "effective and safe ingredients that absolutely quench hunger and thirst."

Furthermore, Paul-Christian's place was a "posh Park Avenue salon where professionals train the 'beautiful' people to take off as much weight as desired. Without exercise. Simply. Easily. And to keep it all off. Forever!"

Forever is a long time, but dieters are terrific at the suspension of disbelief.

Take this clipping I've had filed away for months now. It's from a paper called *Midnight/Globe,* and right here on page 19 is a warranty of heaven, pie in the sky turned into pie on the plate.

"Soon you can eat that double fudge sundae with whipped cream and stop counting your calories," pledges one article. "That's the word from scientists who say they are on the verge of developing several safe and painless diet medicines which may eventually take all the worry out of being gross!"

Dr. Sarfarez Niazi had told *Midnight/Globe* about a drug called perfluoctyl bromide that, taken before meals, "travels to the intestines and coats them before the food has time to reach them and be broken down into calories and nutrients that would then, normally, be absorbed by the body."

Perfluoctyl, said Dr. Niazi, acted like "a teflon coating on pots and pans." He'd already tested it on rats, he was going to go ahead with dogs and monkeys, and then, whoopee! on humans.

"We're very encouraged by our experiments with the rodents," he said.

On the same page, *Midnight/Globe* broke the news of a pill (BAY g 5421) that would "eagerly eat up the fat already accumulated" in a person's body.

"West German researchers explained that the pill absorbs starch and sugar directly from the bloodstream, and these are the main culprits when it comes to putting on the pounds. Dr. William Frommer, one of the pill's discoverers, said tests on six humans proved successful."

Aren't these the tidings we've been waiting for?

I'd mail my money tomorrow, but neither perfluoctyl bromide nor BAY g 5421 has a box number yet.

TAKING IT OFF:
No thingamajig or widget made for diet is so bizarre that somebody won't buy it.

19 Diet Gimmicks, Diet Gadgets, and Creams to Melt Your Fat Away

Oh! My name is John Wellington Wells,
I'm a dealer in magic and spells
—W. S. GILBERT

IF YOU WANT to lose weight, but you don't want to swallow a diet aid, you can wear one made of rubber.

Or you can go to a cellulite therapist who wraps you in parrafin and attacks you with an air hose.

Or you can be hooked up to a machine that sends electrical currents through your muscles.

Or you can be hypnotized, or acupunctured, or acupressured.

Or you can buy a battery-operated voice that berates you when you open your refrigerator. I am not making this up. At the crack of a door hinge, the "Diet Conscience" starts spewing out vituperation—"Are you eating again? Shame on you! No wonder you look the way you do! Ha! Ha! Ha! You'll be sorry, Fatty! Do yourself a favor. Shut the door!"—and keeps on repeating this message until you shut the damn door.

(Some scientists think the insulin in thin people's brains may be responsible for their moderate food intake, and that fat people's brains don't have a high enough level of insulin to signal them to quit eating. "Diet Conscience" does the job an insulin-soaked brain would do, and for a mere thirteen dollars.)

A sensitive soul who can't cope with being bawled out in a loud voice might investigate the noiseless persuasions of engineer Hal Becker, who invented a "little black box" that works by subliminal pressure. In department stores, shoplifters have put back goods they were about to walk away with when exposed to "I am honest, I will not steal" repeated fast and low—9,000 times an hour at a volume the human ear can scarcely make out—and Becker foresees a time when we will have "audio-conditioning the same we now have air conditioning."

Becker's box, reports *Time* magazine, "is also being used by psychologists to help people lose weight, stop smoking, and overcome phobias like the fear of flying. If subliminals were put on TV, explains Becker, they could be directed specifically at such killers as obesity, drugs, and bad driving. Says he, 'We could eliminate weight problems in one generation.'"

Progress. You can't knock progress. There you'd be, flat on your back, beer in hand, watching Mike Wallace or Morley Safer exposing some miscreant, when through the public air waves a message too soft to be heard would plug itself into your gray matter, chivying, "Lay that bottle down, Pig."

No longer safe in the kitchen, no longer safe in the bedroom, from the hounding of inanimate objects, you might be forced out of the house and onto the streets, where the exercise of wandering lonely as a cloud would help you to drop a great number of calories.

Unless you headed straight for a frozen custard stand. The guy at the stand might own a black box, too, programmed to beam the subliminal message, "Frozen custard is good for you, frozen custard tastes swell, frozen custard is sweet and gooey, and pardon my language, ladies and gents, but the hell with wheat germ."

For the person who has more money than brains (one of my mother's favorite phrases), Hammacher Schlemmer proposes an Electronic Diet Fork that looks pretty much like any other fork, except it has lights on the handle. "New, an eating utensil designed with built-in lights which automatically signal you when to eat and when to stop," says the ad copy. "Induces weight loss through behavior modification. The green light signals to eat, the red light how long to chew and stop. Ideal for dieters and those who must watch their weight. Dishwasher safe"; $12.95 will take it away.

And when all else fails, you can stand on a scale in an elevator. A "former physics major" wrote to Craig Claiborne about it. "Take an express elevator down from an upper floor of a tall building while standing on an ordinary scale. As the elevator begins to descend, you will notice that your measured weight decreases a trifle."

Here's a note from the EYE column of *Women's Wear Daily*, dated August 27, 1979. "'I drank so much champagne last night,' said Régine, 'that my husband had to sit on my stomach this morning to get rid of the bubbles.' Régine has other ways of exercising, including one now popular in Monte Carlo—wrapping oneself in plastic. Albert Ropossi plays tennis in plastic pants. 'I lost two litres of water today, it makes you feel wonderful,' he proudly announced."

You kids who have been following closely know that water loss doesn't mean diddly squat, which puts you one up on the jet set.

But plenty of us in the great middle class trust in flimflam too.

Pursuing the facts for her TV special on weight loss, Joanna Wolper went to the Pennsylvania Medical Society, which had surveyed 500 national publications, and found that a quarter of them ran "sure-cure diet and health ads."

The Medical Society's Dr. Steven Barrett told Wolper that "not one single product lived up to the claims in its advertisement. Quite a shocking thing. You look at health ads in a magazine, and the products are for sale by mail, and not one single product lives up to its claims. The claim that you can lose weight without ever being hungry, that you can lose two pounds a day, that pounds melt away, that they go away while you're sleeping—all of these are false or misleading claims. 'Sauna suit,' the ad says. 'Melts away pounds and inches.' That's completely false. You can't melt away pounds. There's another problem with a sauna suit and that is, if you exercise vigorously on a hot day, it could be dangerous because it interferes with the body mechanism to keep cool."

The mail-order traffic in reducing gadgets may not be as brisk as the mail-order traffic in pills, but sometimes it's even more ingenious. Take Slim-Skins. For $9.95 plus postage and handling, you get a pair of plastic pants, Bermuda-shorts length, with a built-in hose. The hose attaches to your vacuum cleaner, and when you turn the vacuum on, "the Slim-Skins seem to come alive with a delightful reducing action on every single inch of your body from beltline to knees."

A lovely creature called Cheri Drake took "2½ inches off my waist, 4 inches off my tummy, more than 2 inches off my hips, and nearly 3 inches off each thigh" the day that "someone gave me a pair of Slim-Skins and told me to try them. I zipped into them, did the 10 minutes of rhythmic motions, and the 15 minutes of lovely relaxing. Then, after just 25 total minutes, I popped out of the Slim-Skins—suddenly, sensationally, over 14 inches slimmer. Who needs a magic wand as long as Slim-Skins are around?"

Fourteen inches, Cheri? For ten minutes' work, and fifteen minutes stewing in your own juices? I believe you, thousands wouldn't, as the lady said in *Saturday Night and Sunday Morning*.

Haven't got a vacuum cleaner? How about rubber thigh slimmers to "massage away your fat"?

Or Slim Sleepers reducing pajamas? A fabric called Tyvek "seals in body heat, and while you're blissfully asleep, works to rid you of unwanted, excess tissue moisture. Wake up thinner, more rested, and ready to go!" In the illustration, Slim Sleepers look like long underwear; you may buy two pairs for $18.95, so you and your mate can pass the nights in twin pools of sweat.

Waist-Trimmer, Touch-and-Stay, Waist Away, and Trimline are all girdles, wide belts that squeeze your middle. Even if your middle measures 50 inches, you can bind it up in nylon and Spandex (Trimline, $7.98), or a "rubberized material the athletes use" (Waist Away, $19.99), or "powerhold s-t-r-e-t-c-h fabric with comfortable quilted support panel for lower back, and infinitely adjustable Velcro fastener" (Waist-Trimmer, $7.99). Touch-and-Stay doesn't say what it's made of, but it suggests tightening it before meals to "help boost your will power." It costs twelve dollars.

The companies that sell these belts explain that they are so comfortable you can wear them playing tennis, or doing your housework, and only Touch-and-Stay suggests that you might want to couple your wearing of the "shaper" with a reducing program. The others offer loveliness without dieting.

The gratification-without-pain pitch is hardly new. For those around the turn of the century who weren't willing to cut down on their feasting, there was Howard Obesity Ointment.

"It removes fat from that part of the body to which it is applied, restoring the natural bloom of youth, leaving no wrinkles or flabbiness," the Howard ad promised. "No nauseous drugs that ruin the stomach, no dieting, no change of habits whatever. The application is simplicity itself. You merely apply the *ointment* to the part you wish reduced, then literally 'wash the fat away' without injury to the most delicate skin."

In 1948, John Andre (the Regimen king whose fairy-tale reign was discussed in Chapter Eighteen) updated the Howard Obesity Cream scam. He sold Hollywood Beauty Cream, guaranteed to "melt away" fifteen pounds in thirty days, although it was subsequently revealed that Hollywood Beauty Cream was nothing but Vaseline, wintergreen, and water.

There's an old joke about a *nouveau riche* lady who goes into the lobby of a resort hotel waving a fistful of cash and asks for a couple of porters to come out and carry her son in from the car. "Ah," says a sympathetic desk clerk. "The poor boy can't walk?"

"Of course he can walk," says the mother. "Thank God he doesn't have to."

When it comes to taking off poundage, most of us are like that mother, searching for some salve, some system, some machine that will do the hard part for us.

The Disco-Shaper ($9.95, "not available in stores") is a kind of machine. Resembling a lazy Susan turntable, it's an eleven-inch-round steel plate upon which the user stands or sits in order to "change fat and flab for a new, leaner, trimmer body." According to an "independent test lab," twisting on a Disco-Shaper would burn up more calories per hour (1240) than playing tennis (591) would.

Exercise is half of any decent weight loss program, and at least the Disco-Shaper compels its manipulator to move, no matter how languidly. Not so the Relax-a-Cizor.

During the 1960s, the Relax-a-Cizor, a machine that made your muscles leap while you lay there listening to music or thinking about your income tax, was bought by 350,000 people, at more than $300 apiece.

The machines were advertised widely, and became so popular that you could rent one by the month. The action—low-level electrical impulses fed through rubberized cords into little round pads strapped onto the body—spooked some people, didn't bother others at all, and left the scientific community unimpressed.

The machine was doing the work, but it wasn't the machine that needed to tone up.

Early in the 70s, cellulite (pronounced cell-you-leet) therapy arrived from France, and women who had always known about the crinkly fat suddenly had a new name for it. Actually, the dimpling of thigh and buttock, explains Edwin Bayrd in *The Thin Game,* "is a result of aging rather than overindulgence. It manifests itself when the subdermal connective tissue that forms a sort of honeycomb around the body's adipose cells begins to lose its elasticity and shrinks with age. When this happens, the overlying skin also contracts—and if the encased fat cells cannot shrink, they cannot help but pucker."

Wrapping hips and thighs in cheesecloth soaked in paraffin will *not* cause the breakdown and reabsorption of "fatty globules," says Bayrd, no matter what the cellulite therapists tell you. And the warm air hoses used in cellulite treatment not only don't break down subcutaneous fat, but can cause "bruising and hemorrhaging." If massage were good for breaking up adipose tissue, reasons Bayrd, we'd all have dainty thighs and backsides, "for no part of the body is more frequently massaged by sedentary Americans than the part they sit on."

An electrical machine, cousin to the Relax-a-Cizor, and to the Diapulse machine (which can no longer be shipped interstate since the FDA took its makers to court, claiming Diapulse was "ineffective and mislabeled"), is used on cellulite too, but again, it's the machine that's getting the workout.

Some people attempt to lose weight through hypnosis. A friend told me about a gentleman of her acquaintance who had gone to a little old lady hypnotist and said he wanted to give up cookies and ice cream.

"We can't do both at once," the little old lady said, with some asperity.

"Okay," the fellow said. "Ice cream."

All he recalls of the session is the little old lady going away and reappearing with a dish of ice cream that she waved under his nose. "Isn't this disgusting?" she said.

My friend who told me the story said she didn't think the cure had taken. "The last time I saw him, he was eating an ice-cream cone."

"Creative hypnosis" is advertised in *Diet Times,* and a *Diet Times* columnist talked to the creative hypnotist, Dr. Gene Baron, who teaches his clients "that you can eat anything you want, as long as you *really* want it and are not just feeding an *emotional* hunger." Dr. Baron believes, said the reporter, "that diets are negative and cause more stress, which leads one back to food for comfort."

I'll go along with him on that one.

Have you ever thought of bellowing off the pounds? A woman named Linda Burns directs a workshop called The Singing Experience. She says singing is especially helpful for people who want to lose weight. "They are orally oriented and this is the perfect way to release tension and get in touch with their bodies."

Linda dropped thirty pounds by opening her mouth to warble, not to chew, and "worked out my divorce" the same way.

You'd rather not sing? Then how about an enema? I just read a dissertation that said an enema could "prevent or relieve overweight." And a fancier enema, an irrigation known as a high colonic, involving "twenty to thirty gallons of warm water mixed with a special solution of natural herbs slowly pumped throughout the seven to twelve feet of large intestine" would be better still, for flushing out "months and years of built-up, encrusted bile, acid, mucus, and gas." After the high colonic, the doctor puts you on a vegetarian diet, and not only do you get skinny, but your prostate trouble, bad eyesight, and hearing loss disappear. You can't believe it? Don't tell me, tell the doctor who's warming up all that water.

Other days, other ways. In the China of 5,000 years ago, at the court of Emperor Huang Ti, physicians healed by means of gold and silver needles that pierced a patient's body at carefully selected points.

Here is the way acupuncture works (from a book called *Dr. Bahr's Acu-Diet,* written in German by Frank Bahr, and translated by Paula Arno): "Free nerve endings are located under the skin at acupuncture points. Stimulation of these points by needle pricks releases impulses that travel via the respective nerve pathways and the spine into the brain stem and on to the midbrain. There, in a netlike brain structure and in the nonspecific nuclei of the midbrain, the impulses are processed and release corresponding effects through neurophysiological reflexes and neurochemical substances that serve as transmitters of information."

If that's Chinese—or German—to you, don't feel bad. Even a scientific researcher like me who knows how to check a fact (go to the library and grovel at the feet of the librarian) gets a bit bogged down in nonspecific nuclei, and even a genuine Oriental doctor like Dr. Er Yi

Ting says the mechanics of acupuncture are a mystery. "We know it works, but we don't know how it works."

The Chinese use acupuncture in place of anesthesia—somebody's always showing us a picture of a Chinese lady drinking tea and smiling while three men in white coats remove her appendix—and also for all kinds of medical complaints that don't require surgery. But a few years ago, Americans were told that acupuncture was useful in controlling weight, and suddenly the therapy became chic. Numbers of doctors and clinics got into the act.

An outfit called the Acupuncture Treatment Group, in New York, tells why a needle in the ear may act as an enemy of fat:

"For centuries, the Chinese have known that the ear is an important nexus, or 'switchboard' for acupuncture points controlling many body functions . . . When used for obesity, ear acupuncture (auriculotherapy) cuts down on the craving for food . . . The most commonly accepted conclusion is that acupuncture blocks certain 'messages' which are sent from the body to the brain . . . Overeaters often blame their excessive intake on a variety of rationalizations such as, 'I'm unhappy at home,' 'I lost my job,' 'Nobody loves me,' etc. Many nutritional experts agree that these thoughts trigger the stomach to send messages to the brain saying, 'Satisfy my hunger.' Acupuncture seems to reduce the frequency and urgency of these self-pampering hunger messages, thereby removing the compulsion and enabling the individual to more easily cut down on caloric intake."

From a 1977 *Vogue* magazine comes this description of the auriculotherapy:

"Tiny open-end circlets of stainless steel—called press needles and made in China—are inserted at auricular pressure points (in the ear) that are believed to communicate with the mouth, the stomach, Shenman ('God's Door,' or the cerebral cortex of the brain), the hunger point, and the spleen . . . After insertion (done in an instant with sterile cotton and tweezers), each press needle is neatly taped over, and the patient is instructed to press each one for thirty to sixty seconds four times a day whenever there is a craving for food between meals.

"The traditional theory is that this blocks the messages from stomach, et cetera, to the brain. In a recent book, *The Acupuncture Diet* by Frank Z. Warren, M.D., and Theodore Berland, the theory is advanced that the blockage occurs in the vagus nerve in the cranium that travels to the esophagus and stomach as well as to the external ear. No matter which version you choose, you still will be taking the mechanism on faith."

Besides the needles, there are also tiny metal balls that go *inside* the ear, as a literary agent, who wasn't familiar with God's Door, but went for acupuncture because a friend had tried it, was kind enough to explain.

"I've never been fat fat," she said. "I think God intended me to be healthy. My mother grew up on a farm, and I was always rewarded with food. But I got a little more healthy than I cared to, and I'm categorically opposed to drugs, so I went to this doctor.

"I hardly saw the doctor. He didn't pay much attention to you, just sort of watched while you had your blood pressure taken, and were weighed in. Five minutes of basic stuff. Since he wasn't giving you anything, he knew he wasn't going to kill you. There was a Chinese lady doctor who did the actual acupuncture. She was so Chinese we couldn't understand each other, but she was very gung ho. If you lost weight, she was very enthusiastic. 'Oh, oh, oh, nice,' she would say. She didn't believe anyone should drink, and you couldn't ask her anything very serious. It wasn't a great problem. I couldn't think of a serious question anyhow.

"In addition to the tiny tiny tiny needle that looks almost like a thumb tack inserted in the front of your ear, there's a tiny tiny tiny silver ball kept in place inside your ear with pieces of Scotch tape.

"In addition to manipulating the thumb tack, you manipulated that little round ball. The theory is that those points control certain oral problems we have with food and alcohol; they curb your need to ingest.

"Anyway, I went to the doctor's office once a week, and the Chinese doctor would remove the pins and clean out my ears with alcohol and put the pins back and cover them up with tape again. So that they would stay in all week. You were to manipulate them several times a day if you thought about it, and naturally you would think about it.

"I never drank while I was undergoing acupuncture. Part of it was because I knew I wasn't supposed to. At one point, the doctor gave his patients two diets. You did one or the other. One was a calorie-counting diet, and one was a vegetarian diet. Since I'm a vegetarian, I opted for the second.

"People think vegetarians don't have weight problems, but they eat pasta a lot when they go out to lunch. You think, shall I have an omelet or pasta? And I love pasta.

"With the acupuncture, I lost a lot of weight. All I wanted to, and more. For me, it was probably behavior modification. I had to get in a cab and go up there on my lunch hour. I had to pay six weeks in advance. And I think if you're committed enough to do that, you're committed enough to lose weight, you're basically psyched up to do it.

"I went out and bought a whole new wardrobe, and it was wonderful for about a year. But after a year or so, I started slipping back, a little bit here and a little bit there. I don't know whether I'm weak-minded or strong-willed, but I can only do it if I do it all out.

"It doesn't matter what the diet is—Stillman, Atkins—they temporarily change your eating habits, and while you're on the diet, it works. Then, bingo, we're right back to, 'Well, I'll just be my own sensible self,' and it doesn't work anymore. Most of us won't change our eating habits. I'm sitting here right now having a drink and thinking of tacos.

"I had two clients who went to acupuncturists for bad backs. The acupuncture gave them a sense of well-being. I didn't particularly notice that acupuncture for my weight loss gave me a sense of well-being. Except that if you lose weight, then of course you feel terrific about yourself because that's what you wanted to do in the first place."

Another woman I know went for acupuncture to the same doctor, but didn't have the same luck. "It was pretty much a fiasco for me," she says. "It hurt so much when I went to press my ear, it was like pressing an infection. My mother went too. And she took off weight. On the other hand, she had taken off weight before. Without things in her ears."

For those who can't abide being stuck, acupressure is like acupuncture, but without needles. An acupuncture needle "is not an instrument that can be handed to just anyone to play around with indiscriminately," says Frank Bahr in *Acupressure Weight Loss Program* (the paperback version of the aforementioned *Dr. Bahr's Acu-Diet*). "The situation is different in the case of acupressure. The fingertip pressure exerted here only massages a point on the body, and could never injure organs situated close to subcutaneous tissue."

Acupressure is "especially beneficial for the curbing of the compulsive-eating center," says Dr. Bahr, who prides himself on having found the overeater's acupressure point (inside the upper lip), a point he describes as having been "well hidden, indeed. That is why the Chinese never discovered it and could not include it in their acupuncture charts.

I found this point only by chance, while systematically investigating the whole mouth area of one of my patients."

Five thousand years of Chinese searching put to shame as Teutonic thoroughness carries the day.

Dr. Bahr instructs his readers about which pressure points to massage, shows pictures of these points on the human body, and gives the Chinese names of these points ("In case of restlessness during depression, make use of the point tsu-san-li—'Asiatic calm,' or 'heavenly equanimity'—and massage it downward"), but in the end, he tells us what we have suspected all along: We must eat less, even while massaging our upper lips, and our little fingers, and our belly buttons.

"Diet alone does not help," says Dr. Bahr. "It removes the pounds but not the craving for food. Conversely, acupressure eliminates the craving but not the pounds . . . To reduce—made easy by acupressure—you need a diet."

Darn ole fishtail, foiled again.

Anyhow, dieting with acupressure doesn't always sound that "easy," either. Here among my massive research materials is a bit of information on G-Jo (it means "first aid" in Chinese), a version of acupressure that a psychotherapist named Michael Blate says "can be an important weapon . . . in the constant battle against fat. While not a complete therapy in itself, G-Jo techniques will give you up to several hours of relief from gnawing hunger, if you apply them properly."

You have to probe your legs, Michael Blate says, "until the right point announces itself with a 'loud' twinge of sensitivity. It will feel like a sharp toothache or a pinched nerve."

Thanks, Mike. I'm grateful for the tip, but I think I'll just go with gnawing hunger.

TAKING IT OFF:
Shutting your mouth is only half the secret; bending, leaping, running, tumbling, stretching, gasping, and sweating are the rest.

20 Exercise: Shake That Thing

"You are old, Father William," the young man said,
"And your hair has become very white;
And yet you incessantly stand on your head—
Do you think, at your age, it is right?"
—LEWIS CARROLL

I KNOW WHY Fred Astaire married that lady jockey. Besides love, I mean. She can make the weight.

An interview with Fred Astaire in *TV Guide* is what tipped me off. Fred gave the interviewer a cup of coffee, but didn't have one himself. He said a cup of bouillon and a boiled egg pretty much summed up his day's rations. I may be wrong about the bouillon, it could have been tomato soup or something, I can't find the *TV Guide*, but the gist of the encounter was as I have relayed it. Fred weighs 135 pounds. He has always weighed 135 pounds, and he told the interviewer he didn't like to work when he was feeling stuffed.

Well, where's a guy like him going to find a woman who will put up with that kind of discipline? A movie star takes a regular date out, she most likely orders shrimp cocktail, steak, fried zucchini, apricot tart, and Irish coffee. When she's with a movie star, she expects to live like in the movies. But this would be very tedious for Fred. He would probably be looking at his watch from the second shrimp on.

No wonder he's hooked on a jockey. I imagined their wedding breakfast was *two* boiled eggs apiece—people splurge at a celebration, time to cut back tomorrow—on a really pretty platter.

It was Barbara Walters who uncovered the news about Fred and Robyn Smith when she asked Fred straight out—on television—if his intentions were honorable. All right, Barbara may have scooped me on the what, but when it comes to the why, kindly remember who figured the whole thing out for you.

In another magazine article, I read about another dancer, Leslie Browne who made a hit in *Turning Point,* and went on to play Nijinsky's wife in *Nijinsky*. After finishing *Nijinsky,* she was miserable because of the work it was going to take for her to get back to "dance weight." Leslie wore a warm-up suit "to hide a slightly voluptuous figure that horrifies her," wrote the reporter.

Would you like to know how much *avoirdupois* old voluptuous Leslie was hauling around? A hundred and eight pounds. She wanted to drop down to 100 pounds. Maybe she hasn't heard that Fred Astaire is taken.

Dancers are a special case anyway. Astaire used to work ten hours a day when he and choreographer Hermes Pan were plotting the numbers for the old Astaire-Ginger Rogers movies, but he insists he's "never exercised. Have you noticed," he asks, "joggers don't look happy?"

What's to look happy about?

Pound, pound, thud, thud over the pavements while your arches fall. Dr. Christian Barnard, that eminent South African transplanter of human hearts, gave us indolent slobs a boost when he said jogging wasn't all that good for you. Particularly if you ran on the roads where you would encounter "a sewer of noxious gases from car exhausts stirred up by your pounding feet and dragged into your straining lungs with every breath."

Dr. Barnard said he trotted around his lawn a little, but he didn't expect too much in the way of results. "If the poor overweight jogger only knew how far he had to run to work off the calories in a crust of bread," declared the doctor, "he might find it better in terms of pounds per mile to go to a massage parlor."

Massage parlors. That's what exercise leads to. Massage parlors and divorce. The divorce rate among the 1978 New York marathoners was twice as high as the national average. I got that statistic out of *Vogue,* along with the information that exercise fanatics "oftentimes neglect their families," and that an overly strenuous exercise program could jeopardize one's health.

It certainly can be detrimental to the health of pigs. In May of 1980, at Arizona State University, some humans decided to examine the effects of exercise on the heart by using pigs. The Arizona State researchers studied eighteen porkers. Six jogged from piglethood, six began jogging when they reached what passes for middle age in pigs, and six never jogged at all.

You can lead a pig to the track, but you can't make him hop it. Unless you prod him with a two-pronged fork. "They burn up the track for about the first lap," said one graduate student. "After that, most of them need encouragement."

Would the brave pigs be rewarded for their contributions to science?

Not so's you could notice it, as my grandma used to say. The minute a pig reached a weight of 200 pounds, he was sent off to be slaughtered, and his heart removed and frozen for future study. By August, just four months after the experiments had begun, there were only six pigs left. "Two thirds of them have gone off to piggy heaven," said an assistant professor of agriculture. "The sedentary ones were the first to go. They put on weight very quickly, and were dispatched."

Lousy, right? Gain a little weight, and they cut your heart out.

Some humans, incidentally, can become allergic—literally allergic—to exercise. In the *Journal of Allergy and Clinical Immunology* (August 1980), two doctors from Harvard documented sixteen cases of "anaphylactic attack" brought on by physical activity. All the patients were "well-conditioned athletes." Some of them required shots of Adrenalin to bring their blood pressure back up from almost zero.

This sort of information may be what caused a man named Don Lessem to write a book called *Aerphobics: The Scientific Way to Stop Exercising*.

In the simplest terms, says Mr. Lessem, "Aerphobics . . . is the avoidance of exercise . . . Fitness itself counts for little against the threats of a modern world; your pulse rate before impact is of little import when you kiss a truck at highway speeds."

Lessem promises that his book has "proven strategies with which you can rid yourself, once and for all, of the exercise monkey on your back."

Ours is not the first health-obsessed modern society. The mid-1800s in England saw such a plethora of boxing and riding and bicycling and rowing and croquet and tennis and football and lacrosse that Professor Bruce Haley has described it as "a national mania."

English gentleman writers climbed mountains not because the mountains were there, but because *mens sana in corpore sano* was more likely to produce masterpieces. "The greatest poetry," said Leslie Stephen, "like the greatest morality, is the product of a thoroughly healthy mind," and he looked around for higher peaks to scale.

Yes, but.

In twentieth-century Florida, where old folks throng the golf courses, ambulance sirens pierce the air with regularity as heat-struck octogenarians keel over on the greens. Up North, middle-aged joggers collapse in their tracks, out West, middle-aged tennis players fall dead on the courts, and still, American exercisers keep on trucking, drunk with the romance of physical fitness.

"President Carter has the body and face of a far younger man," sings the ordinarily sober Hugh Sidey in *Time* magazine. "His running has boiled off even the traces of fat, made his stomach almost concave. His muscles and bones have adjusted to the new physical challenge."

Being skinny is better for dodging, whether issues or enemies, so slenderness could offer an advantage to a politician. My encyclopedia hints at this: "More of the obese die of accident," it warns, "probably because fat people are less agile than thin people."

While you're wondering if you're too fat to leap to one side when a safe falls out of a third-story window headed in your direction, more bad news comes your plump way, via Dr. Frank Katch, chairman of the Department of Exercise Science at the University of Massachusetts.

Dr. Katch says if you could take all the excess fat of 50 million American men, 60 million American women, and 10 million American teen-agers and turn it—the entire 1 billion, 444 million pounds—into energy, it could supply the electrical needs of all the homes in Boston, Chicago, San Francisco, and Washington, D.C.

I told a friend about this, and he got very sulky. "Okay, so I could light up Akron, Ohio," he said. "But for how long?"

Dr. Katch has some of the nastiest ideas you'd ever want to hear. "If you're fat, the best place to go and exercise is where it is continually cold," he says. He further suggests exercising naked, because shivering burns off 10 to 15 percent more energy.

Talk about Jack Frost nipping at your nose. I guess the Doc means exercising naked in your house, and not down by the police station, or on the frozen tundra, like a penguin, but that man will never be *my* leader.

Writing about adult toys, journalist Nancy McKeon has observed that "The ultimate toys of the seventies were, of course, our own bodies. These we tortured on Nautilus machines, jolted with jogging, tanned with tennis lessons. Yet even this toy—a free toy!—wound up costing us a fortune. Because jogging didn't become a worthy activity until it was accompanied by $40 Nike running shoes. Meanwhile, the finished basement/playroom of the fifties was fast turning into the home gym of the seventies, chockablock with slantboards and pulleys and weights and Bullworkers—indulging our need for paraphernalia."

The Nautilus machines are expensive equipment, and big city gyms are abloom with them. Unlike the Diapulse and the Relax-a-Cizor (previously discussed), these machines don't do the work for you; they're the plow, but you're the horse. You can adapt them to your own purposes, whether you're a healthy athlete in your prime or a heart patient whose doctor has said, "Shape up, or forget about buying any long-playing records."

Nautilus machines are not for your apartment; they belong in what has come to be known as fitness centers. On East 49th Street in New York City, for instance, there's a place called the Sports Training Center where tennis players, swimmers, basketball stars, and baseball pitchers come to work out on machines and to get stronger and skinnier.

One of the Sports Training Center's clients has been Billie Jean King, who turned to more intensive exercise in 1976, after a knee operation left her less mobile than she wanted to be. She says now that she's in better shape than she was in the 60s "when I was world champion. You only have to look at the old photographs. I was a tank. Gross."

A man named Arthur Jones invented the first Nautilus machines in 1948, in Tulsa, Oklahoma, but he didn't start selling them commercially until 1970. Today, rehabilitation centers and health clubs all over the country feature the equipment against which you push, pull, lift, and stretch.

If you are drawn to machinery, but not to public places, you may furnish your own bedroom or basement with rowing equipment and exercise bikes and treadmills. Eighteen hundred dollars buys you the motorized sort of treadmill doctors use for stress tests, but there are cheaper versions available. There's also a gizmo for jogging at home that tells you how many miles you've come, and how many calories you've burned up along the way, and there are Benchercycles and Portagyms and Bodybars (with attachments called Tummy Trimmers).

I am not going to buy any of these things myself, because I already have an exercise bike. It was sent to me as a gift. Often, I think about using it. Sometimes I glance up from my bed, and I have the distinct impression that the contraption is standing there looking reproachful, unridden, unoiled, unloved. I sincerely hate my exercise bike. I used to try getting on it to watch the evening news, but that made me sincerely hate Walter Cronkite, which was un-American and bad for my marriage.

I have other confessions. Once I joined a health club run by a man with big muscles and thick glasses. He had Nautilus machines and a swimming pool. In spite of my terrors, he taught me to swim—I wore ear plugs and eye goggles and a bathing cap and a little gadget that clamped on my nose, and sometimes people asked if they could take my picture—and a couple of times, he lashed me to the mast of the Nautilus machines.

I paid $300 to this man, but I never go to the health club anymore. I don't like anybody to see me in a bathing suit, and they wouldn't let me swim in a skirt and sweater. As for the Nautilus machines, they're probably a lot of fun, but I never could remember how to use them. With some of them you lie down and pull things. With some of them you kneel down and pull things, and with some of them you sit down and pull things.

Anyway, my mechanical skills are known to be deficient. If I screw in a light bulb, it breaks off at the base, and all those wires stick up out of the lamp and look threatening, so machinery is not the best road to beauty for me.

Neither are calisthenics. "My clients have found they can sculpture their bodies to their liking, bone structure permitting," says Marjorie Craig, the Elizabeth Arden salon's renowned exercise teacher who's sixty-eight years old and looks like Bo Derek on the beach. My bone structure doesn't permit. You gotta be kidding, says my bone structure.

Many jet setters patronize Miss Craig's classes, but you can pick up other slimming tips from the rich if you've got the price of a newspaper. Columnist Eugenia Sheppard reports that Mrs. Clyde Newhouse "climbs the stairs of her townhouse instead of taking the elevator, and often walks from 79th Street to Macy's to keep physically fit . . . Simone Levitt exercises with weights on both arms and legs every day. On the yacht, *La Belle Simone*, she has her own little gym, complete with the weights, a stationary bicycle, and a jumping rope that she uses on deck . . . Standing on her head helps Pauline Trigère keep healthy and happy."

Certain that Miss Craig would reject my peasant bones, and unable to haul my stationary bike onto the Staten Island Ferry, I once attempted to find my perfect body (it's in there someplace) by joining the classes at Nicholas Kounovsky, Inc., lured by a friend who had improved her legs and her social standing in a matter of months. Though she'd had a sticky entry into the world of health. During her first, or test, lesson, the instructor had asked how much she weighed, and after she'd told him, he'd turned aside, looking sick. Anxious to make things better, she'd volunteered some good news. "I play the piano." He wasn't impressed. "And when he told me to get up, I lurched across the floor on my stomach and crawled up his pants leg."

My teacher at Kounovsky was named Ivo, and his accent was Yugoslavian. Once you got used to it, it made perfect sense. "Go with your head on my shoe down, directly bending your elbows," became perfectly clear to me, but I didn't make progress. Ivo, a wonderful teacher, used to watch me sadly. "No strengt'," he would say, breaking my heart. It was the only thing I hadn't already broken attempting a backwards "somer-selt."

If machines defeat me, and my bones refuse to be sculpted by calisthenics, perhaps, I've been telling myself lately, aerobics would be a nice way to train my heart.

According to Dr. Gabe Mirkin who, with Marshall Hoffman, wrote *The Sportsmedicine Book,* training your heart is the sole purpose of exercise.

Aerobic exercises, says Dr. Mirkin, "must give you a pulse rate of 120 beats a minute and sustain it. They must last at least thirty minutes. You must do them at least three times a week."

Walking won't train a heart, Dr. Gabe tells us, unless you're in such bad shape that walking will bring your heart rate up to 120 beats. Forget bowling, and golf and tennis too.

"Besides running, other good aerobic sports are roller skating, cross-country skiing, aerobic dancing."

Aerobic dancing was put on the map by a lady named Jacki Sorenson who realized that millions of women despised exercise, and who worked out a system of leaping, kicking, and bouncing around like a cheerleader to lively music. "Most of us don't have the discipline to stick to a regular exercise program unless it's fun," says Mrs. Sorenson, for whom part of the fun has been to watch the money roll in, as her Aerobic Dancing, Inc., spread across the country, classes sprouting in thirty-six states. "Why exercise only part of your body as you do with jogging, when you can tone all the muscles and burn off 300 calories in a 45-minute routine to the latest discs?" she asks.

"Controlling your weight is mostly a matter of balancing your food intake with your exercise output," states a booklet issued by the President's Council on Physical Fitness and Sports. "Inactivity is often as critical as overeating in creeping overweight. To the degree that physical activity helps control your weight, it will also aid in preventing degenerative diseases."

Dr. Jean Mayer concurs. "Lack of exercise," he says, "may be of critical importance in predisposing to heart disease."

After naming high-saturated fat diets, cigarette smoking, and untreated hypertension as contributing factors to atherosclerosis, Mayer comes down hard on sloth. Hard enough to make an impresson on us layabouts, despite our mocking ways. "Inactivity is a paramount reason for obesity," Mayer writes. Since 1900, the average caloric intake in the United States has decreased, "but the incidence of obesity has increased . . . the only possible explanation for this seeming paradox is that the energy expenditure ascribed to physical activity has decreased faster than food intake, and this ratio difference has become physically visible in the form of fat."

If a man walks two hours a day, we classify him as moderately active. "At the turn of the century," says Dr. Mayer, "this same man would have been considered sedentary."

Studies have shown that London bus drivers suffered more heart disease than London bus conductors (because the conductors were on their feet, running back and forth, collecting fares) and that mailmen who walked the streets had less coronary trouble than mailmen who sat in the post office.

Physical activity lowers the serum cholesterol level, says Dr. Mayer, "even in subjects consuming a high fat diet. In Finland, the food consumption of lumberjacks in five camps in the eastern part of the country were studied. These men had an extremely large average daily intake: more than 4,700 calories, of which no less than 45 percent was derived from fat. Yet their serum cholesterol levels were no higher than that of the average Finnish man who had a much lower caloric intake, only 35 percent of which was derived from fat."

On this point, Dr. Richard Remington, dean of the University of Michigan School of Public Health (who once declared, "Someone who thinks he's protecting his heart by running around the track several times a week but continues to eat a high-fat diet or smoke two packs a day is just kidding himself"), appears to be in disagreement with Dr. Mayer. In an article in the *New York Times,* Jane Brody quotes Dr. Remington as saying that even though the Finnish lumberjacks expended "many thousands of calories a week in their work," their diet was so heavy with saturated animal fats and cholesterol that their death rate from heart disease was "the highest of any population yet studied.

"Physical activity probably does have a protective effect, but it has to be integrated into a healthful life style," says Dr. Remington.

Exercise not only improves the blood's circulation, but may also help the body dissolve blood clots. Even after people have had heart attacks, exercise is prescribed, and some European countries have reconditioning centers where workers "judged to be prone to heart disease" are sent for four to six weeks.

"In the absence of such facilities in the United States," says Jean Mayer, "it would seem that general practitioners should be much more directive about a patient's schedule of activity, and give close periodic attention to the patient's cardiovascular function during and after exercise."

Mayer also debunks (in an article written with Dr. Johanna Dwyer) the theory "that exercise burns up so few calories it is not worth considering as a means of weight control. This myth is very appealing from the vantage point of a soft armchair before the fire. But it's simply not true . . . If you walk at a brisk rate for an hour, you use 300 to 400 calories."

In an experiment with rats, Dr. Mayer gave the animals one hour of exercise a day. The rats ate only as much as they needed to maintain their body weight. Then the doctor prevented the rats from exercising, and they got fat. They seemed to have lost the ability to judge the amount of fuel required for their daily activity.

In this regard, fat human beings behave very like rats.

Even without a terribly restrictive diet, we are assured that exercise can help us maintain—or lose—weight. With a diet, results come faster. Once we start exercising regularly, the experts promise that we'll start experiencing a loss of appetite too.

But be advised. It takes sixty-nine minutes of walking to burn up the calories in a piece of strawberry shortcake, and ninety minutes to walk off a five-ounce sirloin.

We're told not to punish ourselves, to find exercise we like, but if eating is the only exercise you've ever enjoyed, you're a hard case, and probably should not enter a six-day bike race. (For the terminally slothful, a book called *Autocize* might help. It offers simple "flab reduction exercises" to practice while sitting in a car, stopped at a red light.)

An observer of the social scene, Rhoda Koenig wrote in *New York* magazine that during the 70s, there was an "obsession with Olympic-class fitness by people who get paid to sit at desks all day—the runners who would rather be knocked off by a Central Park mugger than have their arteries harden quietly in bed, the people who don't know you are supposed to give up jumping rope at age six. . . . [they] scrutinized the nice old American dinner plate of meat and two veg and proclaimed it a mass of carcinogens and ugly fats."

It got so bad, said Rhoda, that you couldn't have the "fitness" people to dinner with the "cream" people. "The fitness people preened and smirked about how much longer they were going to live. The cream people said they were happier making better use of less time, and made nasty inferences about the fitness people's incapacity to experience sensual pleasure."

For those whose muscles and heads ached from trying to be fitness people when they were more naturally drawn to rich desserts, Rhoda Koenig held out a ray of hope. "I think," she said, "the fitness people have had their day, and the future belongs to the world of cream."

She was reckoning without Nathan Pritikin.

TAKING IT OFF:
Health can weigh heavier than beauty.

21 Nathan Pritikin: A Promise of Longer Life

They found that even the Belly, in its dull quiet way, was doing necessary work for the Body, and that all must work together or the Body will go to pieces.
—AESOP

NATHAN PRITIKIN's future does *not* belong to the world of cream.

Neither do the futures of the people who spend twenty-six days and about four thousand dollars apiece at one of his Longevity Centers in California or Florida.

Long ago, Nathan Pritikin put cream behind him.

He also abandoned simple carbohydrates such as sugar and honey, along with white flour, alcohol, caffeine (which means tea, coffee, colas), whole milk, butter, oil and other fats, egg yolks, most cheeses, nuts (except for roasted chestnuts and diced water chestnuts), mayonnaise, pastries, chocolate, jams, jellies, bacon, pork, well marbled beef, and salt.

What *does* he eat?

Whole grains, fresh fruits, vegetables (except avocados and olives), legumes (except soybeans and peanuts), tubers, some fish, chicken, turkey, and a tiny bit of very lean meat.

If you are not a student of best-seller lists, you may be asking, who is Nathan Pritikin? And why is he pushing complex carbohydrates?

The answer cometh, but first a word or two about other grain and berry fanciers, because Nathan Pritikin doesn't pretend to have invented the fat-free diet, he simply took it and—literally—ran with it.

Most of us have been vaguely aware, particularly since the communal-living-brown-rice-whole-earth-movement spread among the middle class, of a growing belief that vegetables and fruits, rather than animal fats would make one healthier. But most of us kept right on ordering rare steaks, and slathering our potatoes with butter and sour cream.

All the nuts don't have shells on them, we told ourselves in 1968, when Tiny Tim, that singer of 1920s songs, touted a diet he said had done wonders for him. "I eat one meal a day at six o'clock in the morning. A raw onion, prune juice, grape juice, half a pound of peanuts, mangoes, and three bananas. Every day."

Twelve years later, such a repast—saltless, sugarless, meatless, but still full of vitamins, protein, and bulk—would be commended by many nutritionists. And, except for the peanuts, by Nathan Pritikin. Pritikin thinks the aflatoxins in peanuts cause liver cancer.

Diets once considered eccentric are now reported to be excellent for the health.

The Dani of New Guinea get 90 percent of their nourishment from steamed sweet potatoes (they have seventy varieties of sweet potato in their gardens) and they thrive.

The prehistoric people of the American Southwest were plant fanciers too. Dr. Vaughn Bryant, Jr., of Texas A&M, went on a caveman diet a while ago. "Cavemen ate almost everything in the way of plants, nuts, birds, lizards, snakes, fish, rabbits, pack rats, and mice," he said. "In the spring, they ate a great deal of flowers."

Chickening out, Dr. Bryant didn't eat rats or snakes or little birds, but he did cut down on fats, built up his fruit, whole grain bread, and fish intake, and lost forty pounds.

The last decade's emphasis (remembering Dr. Kellogg, and Battle Creek, we can't call it a new emphasis, though it's certainly been born again) on foods that have roots, rather than hooves, led to jokes like, "See America before Euell Gibbons eats it," and to a more serious interest in Chinese cooking.

Chinese cooking doesn't use a lot of meat—for centuries, most of the people in China couldn't afford meat—and has no truck with butter or cheese or cream, but features vegetables mixed with small amounts of chicken, fish, or pork. Even the rice isn't fattening—half a cup has 100 calories—and bean curd is one of the best sources of protein available.

The Japanese, who also eat rice, vegetables, and fish, are not fat either; they only get fat after they come to America, and start eating like us.

Dr. Julian Whitaker, of the LEAN Treatment Center in Southern California, tells us the Bantu Africans are slender too. The Bantus eat "primarily vegetable foods, high in carbohydrates and fiber, low in fat."

The Hunzas in Pakistan and the Vicambas in Ecuador eat like the Bantus and live long. Their diets have one fourth the fat of the average American's diet, and only half the protein.

In our own country, poor Southerners who lived to be old heard their longevity credited to a diet of mustard greens, collards, and fish.

Nathan Pritikin will tell you all—or most—of this, if you'll listen.

Which brings us back to, who is Nathan Pritikin? and why is he carrying on such a ferocious campaign against pigs and peanuts and other delicious substances?

First off, Pritikin is concerned with health, not beauty. You do lose weight on his program, but, says Pritikin, his system of diet and exercise was designed to help people suffering from heart trouble, diabetes, and hypertension.

Nathan Pritikin is a sixty-four-year-old maverick. At the age of thirteen, he had memorized the names of all 206 bones in the human body. "I thought if I was so interested in the mechanism, I ought to know what the parts were."

He dropped out of the University of Chicago (even though he had a tuition scholarship) when he couldn't raise the five dollars a week he needed for his room and board, and proceeded to become an inventor. (He holds patents in physics, chemistry, and electronics, which he leases to big companies such as Corning Glass, General Electric, and Bendix Aviation.) This prompts him to say that he's never held a job, and it's probably too late to begin now.

More than twenty years ago, he was told he had "substantial coronary heart disease." His doctor suggested an end to walking, and the beginning of long naps.

Pritikin, not a man to take anything—including long naps—lying down, questioned the doctor's advice.

He recalled a research project he'd worked on during World War II, and some of the astonishing information he had gleaned concerning death and disease rates in European countries where food had been rationed.

Although stress was then thought to be the main cause of heart disease, in 1944, the death rates from heart disease in England, France, and Holland dropped to half their prewar levels. And this was among populations being subjected to fire bombings, suffocation in air-raid shelters, and fears for the lives of their children.

"It was that way in all countries under food rationing," Pritikin says, "where the diets had been greatly reduced in fat and cholesterol. But a year or so after rationing was lifted, the death rates from heart disease began to rise again, and to exceed prewar levels."

Remembering this data, and faced now with a doctor who wanted him to stop all physical activity, Pritikin decided to take his treatment into his own hands and experiment with changing his diet.

He went to UCLA, and tried to hire a nutritionist to guide him.

The people in UCLA's nutrition department said cholesterol levels were inherited, and diet couldn't change them. "Besides, the best foods, eggs, cheeses, are high in cholesterol, and your body needs them."

Pritikin tried other places, and got the same answer. "Nobody would take responsibility for anything so abnormal as trying to change a cholesterol level."

So he did it himself. He altered his eating habits, and his cholesterol count dropped from 300 to between 100 and 120. It took him three years.

(For the sake of argument, it should be mentioned here that the National Research Council's Food and Nutrition Board thinks fear of cholesterol—Pritikin's and everyone else's—has grown excessive. As recently as June of 1980, after reviewing more than a dozen studies, the board said none had proved that cutting fats out of the diet protected people against heart disease. There *was* certain circumstantial evidence—animals fed high-fat diets developed atherosclerosis, and in areas of the world where humans ate quantities of saturated fats, heart disease *did* flourish—but even in groups where diets had been modified, and cholesterol levels lowered, there had been "no effect on over-all mortality." One report pondered by the Board showed that men with cholesterol counts lower than 180 seemed actually to run a higher risk of dying of cancer.)

Anyway, by 1961, says Nathan Pritikin, "I'd solved my cholesterol problem, but what about my coronary arteries?"

He'd seen an animal study that showed that dogs who walked on treadmills had 50 percent more blood vessels in their legs than sedentary dogs. This sent Pritikin off to find a capillary expert.

"I want to grow new capillaries," said Nathan Pritikin.

"You can't," said the capillary expert. "You only have what you're born with."

Pritikin whipped out the animal study. The doctor was unimpressed. "First of all, this is about dogs, not humans," he said, and pointed to a wall of books. "All of those books will tell you that you can't grow capillaries."

Pritikin persisted. "How about when people have heart attacks? They grow collaterals, right in the coronary care ward."

"That's the only exception," the doctor said. "When the body is dying, it will grow small collaterals to try to save itself—"

It took Pritikin five years of cautious dissent. First he walked six blocks a day, then eight blocks, then ten blocks, always frightened he might die. And when he didn't die, he began running, still cautiously. But by 1966, he'd proved his point. He took a stress test, and "there was not a single heartbeat with coronary insufficiency, though my heartbeat got up to 177 beats a minute and stayed there."

Elated, he went forth to convert the world.

For the most part, the world didn't listen. "I wasn't a doctor, I had no credibility."

Still, Santa Barbara, where he was then living, is a small town, and at one medical meeting to which he'd been invited (he was a medical buff, read all the medical journals, went to conferences), Pritikin managed to convert a psychiatrist to his theory.

The psychiatrist had brought a lunch basket to the meeting, and was chewing on a chicken leg. "You must like chicken legs," observed Pritikin, idly.

"I hate chicken legs," the psychiatrist said.

Pritikin was baffled. "But you've got about ten chicken legs in your basket."

"That's because I have hypoglycemia," the psychiatrist said. "I have to eat chicken legs. High protein is the diet for hypoglycemia."

"The wrong diet," said Pritikin. "You should be on a high-carbohydrate diet."

The psychiatrist was fascinated. He came around to Pritikin's house, looked at some data Pritikin had collected, and decided to try the new diet. Ten days later, he telephoned, worried. "I can't take my afternoon nap."

"You're cured," Pritikin said. "Go out and play tennis."

The fatigue that is one of the symptoms of hypoglycemia had disappeared.

Slowly, Pritikin's reputation grew. A lady named Mrs. Eula Weaver, eighty-one years old, with congestive heart failure, angina, and hypertension, came to him. When she was eighty-five, she entered the senior Olympics in Irvine, California, and won two gold medals, the first for running the mile, the second for running the half mile. As this is written, she's ninety, still running, lifting weights, and free of the drugs she used to take for her heart, her arthritis, her high blood pressure, and her intestines.

Medical doctors, says Pritikin, knew everything about vitamins and minerals and low-salt diets and the American Heart Association diet and the American Diabetic Association diet, but they were oblivious "to the nutritional factors that caused degenerative diseases."

Nevertheless, in 1974, Pritikin was invited by a doctor at California's Long Beach Hospital to cooperate on a study with heart-diseased patients. For his part, Pritikin rented a house, outfitted a kitchen, and took in nineteen men who "despised each other."

He set them to exercising, and served them carefully supervised meals, but he couldn't make them behave. They acted like children, he says. "Two of them in their sixties, one with congestive heart failure, the other with serious angina, got into a fist fight. They were hanging on to each other, both in such pain they couldn't move their arms."

Despite the emotional immaturity of his wards, Pritikin prevailed. After five months of the regimen, new angiograms (X rays of blood vessels treated to show their shape) revealed openings in arteries that had once been largely closed.

Word spread, and letters came to Long Beach. "Where is it possible to get this nutritional therapy?"

"No place," Pritikin says wryly, thinking back. "If I'd waited for the medical community to do something, it would have taken two hundred years. So in 1976, our first center opened with nine patients. Since then, we've had over three thousand people come, and there's been lots of investigation to check whether or not we're doing what we claim to be doing.

"In the beginning, we had zero credibility. Now, many doctors are writing for information. I never had a vision of what this thing would grow into—"

The success of his best-selling book (*The Pritikin Program for Diet and Exercise*, by Nathan Pritikin with Patrick M. McGrady, Jr., published in 1979) must have surprised him too. But he'd have gone right on proselytizing for his ideas even if his audience had been limited to his wife, because Pritikin has the purity of the fanatic; he cannot stop telling the truth as he sees it.

There was a Pritikin seminar at a New York hotel on May 12th, 1979, and I went to see what the shouting was about. What I saw was Nathan Pritikin, standing on a platform, showing us slides, reading us statistics, talking himself hoarse for hours on end.

He said some scientists had fed monkeys a typical American diet, and killed the monkeys.

He said heart disease and diabetes were unknown in New Guinea.

He said three thousand years ago, only royalty got diabetes, and when the doctors fed their royal patients grain and fruit, the diabetes disappeared.

He said anyone who ran without first changing his diet was committing suicide. "Jolting breaks off plaques. Joggers drop dead on the track."

He said plaques (deposits of fatlike matter) caused progressive artery closure, and too much cholesterol would cause you to grow plaques, and plaques could kill you.

He needled the medical establishment ("It cost one group $42 million to find out that no drug lowered cholesterol, and the drugs they tested produced side effects of blindness, cancer, and phlebitis; a placebo worked better"), called the Scarsdale diet "a blight," said colon cancer was "one benefit of the American diet," and had no good word for polyunsaturated fats. "Israel's big on polyunsaturated fats. They even fry eggs in them. They have a big cholesterol problem there."

Fats, said Nathan Pritikin, are worse than sugar for diabetics, because high fat in the blood acts as a shield between the body's natural insulin and glucose.

Like an Old Testament prophet, Pritikin warned of the future unless we changed our ways. "There was a study of 22 million teen-agers. Their blood pressure is rising so fast we're going to have 90 million hypertensives in the next fifteen years. There are no twenty-year-olds with clean arteries anymore."

And:

Cheese has more cholesterol than meat. Mineral oil coats the stomach and allows no vitamins to get into the blood. Seventy-five percent of the calories in nuts and seeds is fat; 48 percent of the calories in whole milk is fat. No to French fries. No to oils, which are 100 percent fat, and block the small blood vessels.

As part of the day-long indoctrination, a Pritikin-prescribed lunch was served in the hotel's dining room. There was carrot soup, which looked like carrots, and tasted sweet, but didn't have much other flavor.

There were chick-peas, and beautiful raw vegetables—scallions, peppers, mushrooms, cauliflower, and broccoli.

There was a rice salad, kind of gummy. There were baked yams (no butter) and fresh fruit and Linden tea, or Postum, to drink.

I sat next to a man who had been to one of Pritikin's Longevity Centers, and was a convert. "I was supposed to have a heart bypass operation. I decided to go to the Center instead. I hated it. I hated all the walking. I went to Pritikin and said I was having terrible pain when I walked. 'What can I do?' I said.

"He said, 'Carry Kleenex, wipe the tears from your eyes, and keep walking!'

"I told him I hated the food too. 'Okay,' he said, 'tell them to warm up the bypass team.'"

The onetime heart patient was pink-cheeked and healthy-looking, as was his wife, who had gone to the Longevity Center with him, and learned how to plan his meals. Each of them had lost more than twenty pounds, and had kept the weight off for more than two years.

"They teach you what to eat there," the man said. "Whole wheat, rolled oats, corn, things found in nature. Did you know that no animal in the world drinks milk after it's weaned? Did you know that, in 1822, the average person ate 8.9 pounds of sugar, and in 1971, the average person was eating 118.6 pounds of sugar?"

His wife nodded. "The body makes all the cholesterol you need. Egg yolks are the worst."

Pritikin is viewed with distaste by the AMA, the American Heart Association, and the National Institutes of Health (some members of these organizations say he's just a clever entrepreneur, others are less critical, but don't believe he has yet amassed enough data on the long-term effects of his treatment), but Pritikin doesn't care.

"The American Heart Association's diet has not produced benefits for those who've been on it," he says. "Their arteries have continued to close. In one of the largest studies in this country, half of 846 men were put on the American Heart Association Diet, and the other half were left on the regular American diet. After eight years, the death rate was almost identical, but those on the American Heart Association's polyunsaturated diet had two to three times as many gallstones. Polyunsaturated fats create gallstones . . . On our diet, you don't have to choose between heart disease and gallstones."

Pritikin also tends to laugh at the behavior modification people who "subject dieters to various contortions of their natural responses to food." In his book, he lists some of the behaviorists' suggestions, then comments on them. Here are a couple of sample gibes:

BEHAVIORAL MODIFICATION SUGGESTION	PRITIKIN RESPONSE
Use a small plate and fork, to make less look like more	. . . and a large table to catch spillovers.
Throw any scraps away right after the meal. If you keep them around, you might eat them.	On the other hand, in time they may become valuable.

Most doctors—and they're probably right—think the average American, unless he's sick, is not strong-willed enough to stick to a diet as strict as Pritikin's. Patients who *are* sick, and frightened, candidates for coronary bypass operations, the obese, the hypertense, may be more ready than you or I to give up our ice cream and our bacon and our coffee in exchange for salads and grains and herbal teas.

Still, it's something to think about. By cutting down on their fat and cholesterol, and making them exercise every day, Nathan Pritikin appears to have helped many victims of gout and angina and hardening of the arteries to throw away their pills, lower their blood pressure, and lose their pains.

Moreover, Pritikin's emphasis on walking and running is increasingly justified as scientific reports from other sources pile up.

In the May 1980 issue of the *New England Journal of Medicine*, the blood-clot-dissolving properties of vigorous physical conditioning were described by a team working at Duke University. And in that same issue of the *Journal*, Dr. Ralph S. Paffenbarger of Stanford University School of Medicine said the Duke study was only one "of a number of investigations" that made the case for exercise having "a direct and favorable association with processes important to cardiovascular health."

As though that weren't sufficient, an anthropologist, Dr. Alan Walker, of Johns Hopkins, now discloses that an examination of teeth of the earliest hominids—ancestors of man—seems to offer evidence that the hominids were fruit eaters, not meat eaters.

Nathan Pritikin must be laughing at that.

TAKING IT OFF:
If you have no will, you can pay others to starve you, take you on forced marches, and pummel off your pounds. It only costs about $20 an ounce.

22 Spas: How the Rich Get Thinner and Poorer

I eat the air, promise crammed.
—WILLIAM SHAKESPEARE

YOU DON'T have to be sick to go to a Pritikin Center, but it probably helps. Because fun is not the goal. Nathan Pritikin is a health crusader, as was our old friend, Dr. Kellogg, in the 1800s.

From Dale Brown's book, *American Cooking* (part of the Time-Life Foods of the World series), comes an account of that last-century American spa, Dr. Kellogg's Battle Creek Sanitarium:

"Here the sick and the neurotic, the underweight and the overweight went for complete overhauling. 'Bran does not irritate,' said the good doctor. 'It titillates!' And bran was on every tongue. In addition to being titillated, his patients were put on strange diets, suited, the doctor assured them, to their own special needs. The skinny were plied with twenty-six feedings a day, forced to remain motionless in bed with sandbags on their bellies to increase absorption of nourishment, and not allowed even to brush their teeth, since any expenditure of energy might deprive them of a valuable calorie or two. Patients suffering from high blood pressure were served nothing but grapes; they were obliged to swallow 10 to 14 pounds of grapes a day."

In our time, for anyone who is just fat, not unhealthy (assuming such a condition exists), there are spas that offer pleasures you could not have got from Dr. Kellogg, and still can't get from Mr. Pritikin.

In some spas, a lady may have a daily massage, facial, manicure, pedicure, and flowers on her breakfast tray.

Which is nice, because there is nothing resembling breakfast there.

Actress Peggy Cass once tried a spa where the morning began when a waitress brought her a tray bearing half a grapefruit, a cup of black coffee, and a rose. The first day, Miss Cass admired the beauty of the arrangement. The second day, she was slightly less appreciative. The third day, she says, "I ate the rose."

Starving for the sake of beauty was modish in Europe before we imported the idea. Even A. J. Liebling, the American poet of the taste buds, once fell victim to the lure of potential slenderness, and signed himself into a spa in Switzerland, an experience he later recounted in the book, *Between Meals*. He wrote about drinking rose hip tea and eating "muck made of apple cores and wheat germ," and being mentally tortured by a sadistic masseur who always tendered reports of what he, the masseur, had eaten the day before.

"'Good morning,'" he would say. 'Calves' hocks have I yesterday at lunch to home eaten, with potato dumplings, and to dinner spring chicken with another time dumplings.' Then he would laugh."

Liebling declared that the dieting had so destroyed his health that he'd had to go to friends in France to recover. And when he parted from those friends, "I left . . . like Mother after her reducing tours long ago, pounds heavier than when I flew to Zurich to get weight off. This episode has remained unique in my life: it is the only time I yielded to the temptation to give myself pain."

Despite such cautionary words, ever-increasing numbers of Americans are flocking to ever-increasing numbers of spas. (For treatments still considered too radical by the American medical profession, and the Food and Drug Administration, seekers after beauty and long life have to leave the country. Devotees of clinics in Switzerland and Spain and Germany and Romania and Nassau in the Bahamas claim to have discovered the fountain of youth in such therapies as sheep-cell injections, shots of buffered procaine, and the swallowing of chicken embryos. Pope Pius XII was given the sheep cells; other injectees are alleged to have included Merle Oberon, Greta Garbo, Marlene Dietrich, and Charlie Chaplin, while the procaine formula—called Gerovital—was tried by politicians John F. Kennedy, Nikita Khrushchev, and Konrad Adenauer.)

"A billion-dollar-a-year business in the United States, fat farms prosper because Americans are leading lives of diet desperation," wrote Kitty Kelley in her funny, gossipy book called *The Glamour Spas*. Kelley said it cost a spa client an average of $350 to lose one pound.

But the ladies who elect to go to Maine Chance (it's ladies only) aren't worried about where they're going to get the rent.

Elizabeth Arden, the late queen of beauty products, started Maine Chance in 1934—there were still some people in the Social Register whose husbands hadn't lost everything in the crash—and although the original place, in Waterville, Maine, was closed down in 1970, its sister spa in Phoenix, Arizona, lives.

Maine Chance is a paradise of bone china, Aubusson carpets, good paintings, fine gardens, and crystal chandeliers, and many clients come back again and again, requesting the same room each year.

Most of them are what used to be called "society women," because those women were Miss Arden's friends. "Certain people would not be happy here," a reservation clerk told Kitty Kelley. "Peroxide starlets, divorcées, neurotic film stars—these types of people go to one of those *nouveau riche* spas in California."

Another Maine Chance worker confided to Kitty that Miss Arden hadn't known too much about politics. "She hated Democrats on principle because they were so poor, but for many years she thought Henry Cabot Lodge was a New England motel."

Pink beds, fresh lemonade, acupressure for the feet, paraffin baths (warm, melted wax poured over the naked body), scalp massages—these are a few of the ways a Maine Chance client is pampered. For a price.

When the essayist Jessica Mitford went to Maine Chance in 1966 (she was writing a magazine piece), the price of a week's room and board, if you wanted a bathtub, started at $750. Today, that figure has almost doubled.

Another minor note about inflation: Mitford assessed the free Arden preparations adorning her dressing table (prices marked on the packages) at "a total retail value of about eleven dollars." Ten years later, Kelley said the "free" merchandise was worth fifty dollars.

Over the years, women who have gone there pronounce the Maine

Chance food delicious but sparse. Four-ounce steaks, no liquids with the meal. The honor system obtains. You serve yourself from silver trays passed by waitresses; there is no portion control except the kind you exercise yourself.

Jessica Mitford met a lady who stole steak to take to her dog—for the two weeks of her stay at Maine Chance, she'd rented an apartment in Phoenix, ensconced the dog and a maid, and went to visit them every day. And Kitty Kelley met a lady who swiped the sterling silver coffee spoons for *her* dogs, boarding in a kennel in Scottsdale while their mistress was at the Arden spa. "It might sound silly," this lady told Kelley, "but I just *know* their custard tastes better from these little spoons than from the cheap plastic utensils they use at the poodle parlor."

Once upon a time, the story goes, Maine Chance ladies' bags were searched, not for silver spoons, but for booze, which wasn't permitted on the premises. That kind of supervision is a thing of the past. And there are phones in the rooms now, where once they were prohibited. "Why court bad news from out there?" Miss Arden used to say.

Kelley called the calisthenics at Maine Chance "extremely gentle," Mitford compared them to a class at the YWCA, and Emily Wilkins, in a book called *Secrets from the Super Spas*, steered a middle course. The exercise program, she said diplomatically, was "vigorous as any high school gym class" but a participant would be "less prone to strain a muscle or pull a ligament."

Mitford lost five pounds in one week; Wilkins and Kelley didn't report their losses.

Other spas, other ways.

The Golden Door, created by Deborah Szekely Mazzanti, in Escondido, California, is so tough in the exercise department that the genteel speak of the exertions as "vigorous," while the less euphemistic compare the routines to boot camp. Again, there's much herbal wrapping and massage and facial sculpturing, but the emphasis is on fitness. Some people might pay "to stay out of this body-beating fat farm," observed Kitty Kelley, adding that Marlon Brando had once checked in, looked around, and left. (Eight weeks of the year are set aside for men; Brando wasn't crashing a women's party.)

The dinners are accompanied by candlelight at The Golden Door, but they don't take long to eat. Eight hundred and fifty calories a day is all you get for your $1,250 a week.

About an hour's drive south from San Diego, The Golden Door's owner runs another place, founded by her first husband who, like Dr. Kellogg, believed in a grape cure. This Mexican spa, Rancho La Puerta, in Tecate, Baja California, is cheaper (as low as $345 a week) than spas in the States, the food is vegetarian, and dieters are expected to keep their intake down to 1,000 calories a day.

In July of 1980, Joan Kennedy, taking a two-week break from campaigning for her husband, checked into the Mexican spa, but Joan didn't go the bargain route. She rented Deborah Mazzanti's own casita, complete with swimming-pool-sized Jacuzzi, and enough rooms for several Secret Service agents.

At Rancho La Puerta, the exercises, including hiking up and down mountains, are as rugged as those at The Golden Door, but overweight people who come there have a good time. One employee says it's because "Mexicans like acres of flesh. The fat girls always have dates."

About as far north of San Diego as Rancho La Puerta is south, you find La Costa, a health spa the Teamsters' union more or less owns, since it holds the mortgages on the property. In 1979, hair stylists, masseurs, weight reduction technicians, beauticians, and cosmetologists went on strike for more money. A La Costa masseuse who'd been massaging people like Mary Tyler Moore, Bette Midler, and Cheryl Ladd pointed out that her customers were spending $165 a day to lose weight, while she, after four years of hard work, was still earning $140 a week.

La Costa's mix of show biz with an overlay of mobsters is glittery. There, if they have it, a lot of them flaunt it. Arriving at La Costa in chauffeured limousines, they flash their jewels, and bellboys sometimes get hundred-dollar tips.

Men and women can fraternize at La Costa. The spa programs are separate, but a husband and wife—or any other combination that makes a couple, for that matter—may eat together, sleep together, play backgammon together of an evening, or be bussed together into Tijuana for the jai alai games.

Dieters are offered food with the calorie count of each course listed on the menu, and are advised to stick to 600 calories a day.

Movie stars go to La Costa; so do people hoping to see movie stars.

Southern women are more likely to prefer The Greenhouse, a Texas fat farm operated in part by Neiman-Marcus. Stanley Marcus once called The Greenhouse "a hothouse for wilted ladies."

The Greenhouse draws a certain amount of wilted royalty, along with plain, untitled rich folks, and it actually simulates a greenhouse. No good for claustrophobics, it's spread out under a great glass roof, with the temperature, the humidity, the light, all controlled. Plants are everywhere, meals measure 850 calories a day, and most guests lose about two pounds a week. For this they pay $1,800, plus a 15 percent service charge.

Consensus has it that The Greenhouse is the most luxurious and elegant of all the spas. The least elegant may be the Bermuda Inn, which is not in Bermuda, but in California's Mojave Desert. It's cheap and casual, and in the 1960s it put its fat customers—it used to get 400- and 500-pounders—on fasts. Now under different management, the Bermuda Inn offers diets ranging from 200 to 400 calories a day, and close medical supervision. Dieters take water pills, walk, and play cards. They aren't even allowed fresh fruit, because of the high natural sugar content. They eat bouillon, green salads, cooked vegetables, and Jell-O; their evening snack is celery. "We're a nuts-and-bolts fat farm devoted to grizzly dieting," the owner once said.

Some spas operate on the "Do as I say, not as I do" system, as journalist Blair Sabol discovered back in 1978 when she went out to try Minden, at Hampton Court, on New York's Long Island.

Minden, once the mansion of a coal magnate named John Berwind, had recently been converted into a "reconditioning center" by Dr. E. Hugh Luckey, who permitted his guests no drugs, no liquor, no cigarettes, put some of his clientele on a "300-calorie a day Optifast liquid-protein diet," and kept the rest on 850 calories a day. (Sabol said one cook was terrific, but another made soup taste like gasoline.)

Dr. Luckey himself smoked *and* drank—though not in front of the guests—and he felt that he and his wife were the perfect team to be running a spa. "See, I'm strongly medical and Veronica goes for all that metaphysical stuff like food allergies and yoga fastings. I'm open to that. After all, we met through our astrologer."

Spas die, spas are born, spas lose their employees to other spas. Chris Silkwood, who used to labor at The Golden Door, was recently lured away to be physical fitness director for The Phoenix, a new spa in Houston, Texas, that opened in June of 1980.

The Phoenix was developed by Frances Baxter and Judy Fatjo who, after looking over all the other available facilities in the country, decided they could improve on them.

Besides The Phoenix's ladies having access to a *carpeted* jogging track (a mile long, and bouncy underfoot), they would have privacy. The spa would book only thirteen women a week, at a cost of $1,850 apiece, for which the women would get board, health food, and first crack at a couple of brand-new gimmicks. "We have a new way of measuring the weight of bones, muscle, and fat in a human body," Frances Baxter told journalist Eugenia Sheppard. "We put the results into a computer and it gives the exact weight he or she should be. This could put a stop to some of the boring talk about diets."

There's no way to cover all of America's fat farms in a few pages, or even to cover a few of them—adequately—in a lot of pages. But in the interests of science, and also because I was hoping to melt away my thighs, I personally checked out one spa.

It was Palm-Aire, in Pompano Beach, Florida.

It cost $1,082.90 for seven nights in the hotel (on the spa plan), and my friend Bobbie elected to come with me. (It also cost her $1,082.90 for seven nights in the hotel on the spa plan; I don't mean to imply that she just crept past the concierge when he wasn't looking.)

I have to tell you up front that my friend Bobbie was a poor choice of companion.

To begin with, she has a very pretty, slender shape, so when she walked around in a bikini, the other ladies tended to snarl, "What's *she* doing here?"

Then she refused to stay on 600 calories a day, but got us moved over into the heavy feeders' part of the dining room, where she could order an ice-cream sundae.

Then she wouldn't take all the exercise classes listed on our locker doors, and she wouldn't take any of the dance classes listed on our locker doors, and she wouldn't take any of the walks or jogs that the hard-core body punishers embarked on first thing in the mornings. She would only take water classes, and not too many of them. And she always cut the last class, whatever it was, on the grounds that it would tire her. Little by little, she eliminated whirlpool baths and herbal wraps in favor of more time in the boutique.

But I am getting ahead of my story. I just wanted to tell you about my trouble with Bobbie, so you will be sympathetic if I missed some of Palm-Aire's salient features, and can't report on them the way a fearless journalist should do.

To begin with, we took an airplane from New York to Fort

Lauderdale, and a cab from Fort Lauderdale to Palm-Aire. "You know who goes to the spa?" our driver asked, and then answered himself. "Elizabeth Taylor. Jackie Kennedy. You're in for a week of seaweed."

He was not being accurate. Our week was marked by a complete absence of seaweed. Jackie and Elizabeth were missing too.

Palm-Aire isn't only a spa, the hotel also houses non-spa guests who have come to play golf and tennis and swim and eat whatever they please, and drink too, if the truth were known. The brochure of March 1980 promises that "the additional hotel pool will have a wet bar which we are certain will be well received by guests."

The wet bar begins to sound more entertaining when you take a look at the other entertainment. A sign in the lounge says that on Monday night, a car will take us to a shopping center where we will find a Saks, and on Tuesday night, a bunch of high school kids will come and sing to us.

Our first dinner—we tried the diet menu, we really did—was less than thrilling. Half a cup of watery chicken soup. Fresh asparagus so overcooked it had lost its color. Zucchini and carrot salad. On each table, Vegit, a low-sodium vegetable seasoning, and Sugar Twin, which, the packet says, "looks and tastes like sugar." (Sugar Twin is made of dextrose, soluble saccharin, and silicon dioxide.)

Here is a sample diet menu for a Sunday dinner at Palm-Aire:

APPETIZER

Choose One

	PORTION SIZE	CALORIES
☐ VEGETABLE BROTH	6 oz.	20
or		
☐ FRESH GARDEN SALAD LEMON DRESSING	1 Cup	20

ENTREE
Choose One

☐ BROILED FLORIDA FISH	4 oz.	150
or		
☐ ROAST TURKEY • FIBER DRESSING	4 oz.	150
or		
☐ PALM-AIRE "CLEANSING" SALAD	2 Cups	150
WITH YOGURT	½ Cup	

VEGETABLE

☐ GREEN BEANS WITH WATER CHESTNUTS AND MUSHROOMS	½ Cup	25

DESSERT
Choose One

☐ PUMPKIN TART	2½ oz.	45
or		
☐ FRESH SEASONAL FRUIT	½ Cup	40

BEVERAGES

☐ ROSEHIP TEA or ☐ DECAFFEINATED COFFEE

Any changes or alterations must meet with the approval of the Dietitian.

The sign in the lounge had suggested that when we were finished dining, on our first night, we should walk down the hall and "Meet Your Dictician."

Bobbie didn't want to meet her dietician. I dragged her. Our dietician was skinny, I'll say that for him. He was this little dark-haired guy; in another life, he'd have been an Apache dancer, and he was smug with sinews.

He flicked us spa guests a glance in which was mixed ennui and despair, but when he got down to cases, he sounded very sensible. I suppose it's hard to be charmed by an influx of brand-new fat people (brand-new to him, anyway) week in, week out, for nine years, which is how long he said he'd been at Palm-Aire.

He said fasting—eating fewer than 500 calories a day—isn't good, because it makes you lose lean body mass. He said the diet at Palm-Aire was high in protein and undigested fiber—wheat, bran, vegetables, fruit—and low in fat and oils.

He said we all consumed less fiber than we should, and that most Americans ate a diet that was 40 percent fat—fat is added for flavor in frozen food entrees, in restaurant vegetables, in places we don't suspect—and that one tablespoon of fat equals 150 calories.

He said there was no caffeine available on the spa menu because caffeine is a pancreatic stimulant that releases insulin, and makes you hungry. (Due to my arduous research on this book, I already knew that. I didn't understand it, I just knew it.)

He told us how hard it was to avoid sugar. "It's in corn bread, it's in spaghetti sauce." He said if our blood sugar was low, we could have protein snacks—"Don't grab peanuts, or a candy bar"—and he said we should drink two quarts of fluids—mineral water, herbal tea, decaffeinated coffee—every day, and take potassium tablets if our fingers tingled. (You lose potassium through sweat and urine.)

He said we wouldn't get salt because salt caused one to retain fluids, he said our protein portions would be limited to four ounces (although a restaurant steak is ordinarily twelve ounces), and he said most diets were nonsense. "If anyone puts a diet in front of you and says, 'You're gonna lose X amount of weight,' you know he's a charlatan. A five-foot woman won't lose the same amount as a six-foot man."

He also warned us against health food stores—"I see people go in, say, 'I'm tired, what should I take?' and the proprietor tells 'em"—and against the oils, creams, and scrubs with which we would be anointed and laved at the spa. "If you don't rinse off the soap, you'll get an allergy rash. Every week, four or five people break out."

He said, finally, that we should try to get our minds off food. "I circulate in the dining room. Everybody's talking about chocolate sundaes, restaurants, food, food, food. Well, sure we're gonna deprive you, but you're gonna be happy when you leave."

Then he gave each of us a recipe book full of dishes to be made with skim milk and Vege-Sal and low-cal commercial French dressing and artificial bacon bits and artificial sweetener and low-calorie D-Zerta and Sugar Twin and safflower oil and frozen vegetables and Dream Whip.

That night, in our splendid room—we had two big double beds, two bathrooms, comfortable couches, color TV—Bobbie and I studied our recipe books. "I'd rather have an allergy rash than jellied spring salad and sherry custard," Bobbie said thoughtfully.

I tried to cheer her up. "He said you'd be happy when you leave."

"I want to leave now," she said.

In the morning, we had breakfast served in our room. Bobbie faced a Double Egg-White omelet (35 calories). With no yolks to give it color, the omelet was odd to behold, all white and dimpled.

"It looks like a washcloth," I said.

Bobbie took her fork down from her mouth. "It tastes like a washcloth," she said.

We spread our ½ slice of 7-grain toast (35 calories) with imitation cherry flavor diet jelly, choked it down, and mushed out to our first class.

I can't remember the classes in order, but everyone's first session was warm-up exercises. Then there were dance classes, spot reducing classes, gym classes, everybody-into-the-pool-for-volleyball classes, interspersed with whirlpools and massages and facials and loofah baths.

A beautiful Peruvian lady—she said she was a grandmother—who taught both yoga and belly dancing, tried to explain to us the right way to breathe. In her accent, it came out as "the morning bread" and "the evening bread."

"Don't say bread to a starving woman," muttered Bobbie (under her bread) as she attempted the cobra position.

There was another instructor, very young, a dancer and actress who was just waiting for her big break. Some of her breaks had already been big, but bad. She'd lived through a plane crash, and remembered stumbling along in the snow, bleeding, and telling herself, "As an actor, I'll use this experience."

There was also an elderly instructor with lined tan skin and a Dutch accent. She was rumored to be seventy, was built like a tank, and had the energy of the Oakland Raiders.

"Stretz! Stretz!" she would cry. Sometimes this lady took people on a hike up the beach at 7:00 A.M. The people were transported to the beach in a car. The Dutch lady got there on her bike. Then, after the hike and some exercises, she biked back to the spa.

The spa featured a hostess (she drove guests to shopping centers, signed them up for boat trips, beach trips, etc.) who said she'd lost weight by staying on the spa diet, but she'd had help from a hypnotist too. She believed in hypnosis. "My fourteen-year-old son went in to have two teeth pulled. He had no pain, no bleeding, and half an hour later, he ate two tacos."

The hostess had stopped drinking coffee, and smoking as well. Many of her charges were also trying to kick nicotine, but it was hard. Being deprived of food and coffee, they tended to cling to tobacco as the only comfort left them. Coming back from shopping in the Palm-Aire bus one night, a woman bragged that she'd made it. "I quit smoking."

"Did you find it hard?" someone asked.

"No," said the woman.

"When did you quit?"

"Today."

Gallows humor flourished. When the hostess told us about a nightclub where she sometimes took people, one listener, aware that we weren't supposed to eat or drink anything unprescribed by the dietician, looked nonplussed. "What in God's name do you *do* there?"

The ladies talked about men ("My first husband told me he wanted a divorce at breakfast one morning. I almost dropped the coffeepot. I was so dumb I said okay. That was on a Monday. I was divorced by Friday."). They talked about plastic surgery ("You see that woman? She's just had a face-lift, boob job, and tummy job, they had to give her a new belly button"). They talked about other spas. One said Palm-Aire was better than La Costa. "The people are friendlier." One said Maine Chance cost thousands of dollars a week, but you got lots of individual attention. One said she'd been to a spa run by a fat snobbish woman who said, if you'd ever been a Maine Chance girl, or a Greenhouse girl, "that's the kind of girl we want."

But mostly, the ladies talked about food.

A woman with a friend living forty miles away got a phone call. The friend wanted to come visit. The Palm-Aire inmate said okay. "But if you don't bring me a hot corned beef sandwich, you can go to hell."

Sitting around the pool, sitting in the bus on the way to shop, sitting at a table facing spinach salad and decaf coffee, they talked about food.

The dietician hadn't just been whistling Dixie.

One tall young girl (she said she'd weighed 195 pounds, but had lost 65 of them on some kind of shots) complained about the spa's inability to prevent temptation. "If we have non-spa guests, we sit at a table with salt and sugar instead of Sugar Twin. That's hard on the willpower."

Her companion rejected the complaint. "We *have* no willpower. If we had any willpower we wouldn't be here."

Poundage haunts every waking hour. A woman who has paid $125 to a behavioral modification doctor for one week's sessions—he promised she would lose eight pounds—tells why she'd signed up. "I couldn't wait to lose eight pounds, so I could go out and eat."

A seventy-year-old woman with still brown—undyed—hair says, "I never weighed over a hundred until I hit sixty-nine."

A much younger woman hoots. "I never weighed *under* a hundred since I was ten."

Tips are traded. "Fill up with as much water as possible before a meal. When you're eating, take a sip, eat, take a sip . . . Chew each bite a long time . . . Put down your fork when your food is only half gone, and ask yourself, 'Am I still hungry?'"

Unfortunately, the answer most people give to that question is, 'Yes, indeed," if the testimony of a Palm-Aire busboy is to be trusted. He told Bobbie and me he'd gone to a soda fountain down the road, "and there were fifteen people from Palm-Aire pigging out on ice cream. Listen, I've seen ladies after their first spa dinner, wandering down the halls of the hotel, checking out room service trays the regular [non-spa] customers leave outside their doors. It's a big find if they come across half a baked potato."

One woman who'd checked in with her husband the same day Bobbie and I arrived was holding up better than he. After two days of spartan meals and furious exercising (in the gentlemen's wing of the spa), he was beaten. "I feel like a hostage," he cried. "Let me out."

Bobbie sympathized. She was ready to make a break for it too. Which is why, after two days of spartan meals and furious exercising (in the ladies' wing of the spa), we moved away from the dieters' section of the dining room. At dinner on that third night, Bobbie leaped into the bread and butter, the potatoes, the hot fudge, the coffee with cream, in a shameless display of weakness. I pointed out to her the valor of the dieters we'd left behind, only a few feet away in terms of space, but in terms of pluck, grit, determination, separated from us by infinity.

Bobbie pointed out that the valorous, plucky, gritty, determined dieters were fat, and she was not.

Still, most of the people who managed to get through the first couple of days of deprivation seemed to start enjoying themselves. There's a camaraderie with your fellow sufferers, there's the knowledge that every tough class is followed by some coddling treatment of face, foot, body. And hope never dies.

One woman was standing by the pool, expounding—"Exercise is against my religion, I haven't exercised this much in five years"—when a passerby interrupted her. "You're in luck. A ladybug just landed on your butt. That means your butt will be gone in the morning."

The exercise-hater brightened. "From your mouth to God's ear," she said.

At the end of a week, most of the ladies still had their butts, though several of them were a few pounds lighter, and most of them—including Bobbie and me—were saying how much they'd like to come back again.

Because there's something about being curried, scrubbed, fussed over, fed (or half-fed) that cools out the brain and the bones. At home, most of us don't have the leisure to be totally self-absorbed, even for a day. At home, we'd be too guilty anyway. At the spa, the narcissist in you, the child, the weary homemaker yearning to breathe Chloe instead of Clorox, is tended. And a whole week of the world's appearing to revolve around your backside, no matter how ample that rumble seat may be, leaves you feeling smooth and loved and kept and decadent, like a concubine from the *Arabian Nights*, all oiled and perfumed for a king.

TAKING IT OFF:
There are people too scared to bake a cake, because they'll eat the whole thing. They buy their dinners ready-cooked, one day at a time.

23 The Cheapest Health Resort: Your Own Apartment

Sigh much, drink little, eat less.
—WILLIAM CONGREVE

YOU AREN'T in a position to spend six months' pay on a week at a spa? Never mind. There are places you can go for less.

On the East Coast, *New York Times* columnist Enid Nemy checked out three weight-reducing farms for her readers. First, she went to the Englewood Cliffs Spa in New Jersey. Englewood Cliffs limited its guests to 1,000 calories a day, and imposed no other rules. If you wanted to take exercise classes, you could, but it was your body and your business.

At the New Age Health Farm in Neversink, New York, life wasn't that simple. Anyone fasting there had to take a daily enema. "It's dangerous to fast without an enema," one of the farm's proprietors, Elza Graydon, told Nemy. "Toxins are not released properly and go back into the bloodstream." Mrs. Graydon and her husband, boosters of holistic health (integrated care for body, mind, and soul), offered clients lectures on topics ranging from "You and Your Colon" to astrology.

(Anyone not wishing to lose weight, but looking for peace and fresh air, was fed fruits, vegetables, cheeses, and herb teas.)

Nemy also researched the Pawling Health Manor at Hyde Park, New York. Fasting again. Five days on water, before working one's way up to salads and cottage cheese. (At Pawling Manor, vegetarian meals were also available for the not-so-fatties.)

Nemy said accommodations in these three places cost anywhere from $175 to $350 a week, but that was back in the summer of '79. They're probably more expensive now.

In March of 1980, Janet Froelich, an employee of the *Daily News* (staked by the paper, at the behest of food editor Suzanne Hamlin), embarked on the cheapest spa plan of all. She had fifty dollars' worth of carefully planned low-calorie meals delivered to her by a store called Skinny Dip. At the end of what her editor called "a five-day, in-town fat farm week," Froelich had lost five pounds.

"I've always wanted a week at The Golden Door," she said, "and this is the closest I've ever come to it." (To be sure, there are low-calorie meals available in supermarkets, notably those sold under the Weight Watchers label, but the Skinny Dip concept is different, because each day's menus are figured out for the customer. "Being told I could eat just this and no more was an enormous relief," Froelich said.)

The Skinny Dip five-day diet is a service provided by Barbara Haroche, whose low-calorie food emporium on Second Avenue between 72nd and 73rd streets came into existence in July of 1979.

Barbara Haroche has always had a weight problem ("I understand what the customers go through") and she still is not a sylph. After all, she works right next to the low-cal-ice-cream machine, and besides, she likes junk food. "Twinkies," she says. "Oreos. If I eat one Oreo, the whole box goes. This is true of most compulsive eaters."

To interview Barbara Haroche on the premises of Skinny Dip, a small, cheerful shop with a long, hot kitchen behind it, is to get a nervous stomach. She's up and down twenty times a minute, taking phone calls ("Mrs. Davis didn't get her breakfast," "Miss Hamburger is missing an ice-cream cake"), trying to explain to a pretty young assistant how to wrap an outgoing order (if you're afraid to keep a week's worth of food in the house, you can have your meals delivered daily), and dealing with the traffic off the street.

One browser is wandering around with a bottle of salad dressing in her hand. "How many calories is this?"

"It says on the back of the bottle," says Haroche.

Another customer orders six cookies. "They're seven calories each?"

"Seven and a half," says Haroche.

"Oh," says the customer, "I don't think I'll take them."

The difference comes to a total of three calories, but the customer still rejects the cookies.

Haroche is patient, because she has shared many of the problems of weight-obsessed people, and she still isn't home free. "I'm an elevator. I go up and down. I have clothes from a size four. The small ones I keep, the big ones I throw out."

Haroche put in her time as a Westchester housewife—"In my day, you stayed home with your children"—and turned into a closet eater. "I never eat in front of anybody. A closet eater is worse than an alcoholic. You don't have to walk into a liquor store, but you must buy food, or you'll die. You go to check out of a supermarket, and that's where all the candy is. If I'd been buying for myself, I wouldn't have shopped in supermarkets, but I was buying for my kids. Only they never got near the stuff. I finished it all at night. Between two and six in the morning, by myself.

"If I take home a quart of ice cream, that quart is going to be gone in one sitting. It won't get put back in the refrigerator. My kids take ice cream and put it in dishes, like normal people. I don't, I eat it right out of the container.

"I don't eat sitting down at a table. Because standing up, you don't realize you're eating."

But didn't she share meals with her family, in the old days? No, she didn't. "I would sit there with a cup of coffee while they ate. I went after the food when nobody was watching. Sick. Very sick."

When her children were no longer small, Haroche went back to work, a move that didn't help her shape. "I had a terrible job. I got very depressed. When people are depressed, either they stop eating, or they overeat. My mother, she doesn't eat when she gets upset. I'm the eater."

Diets? Barbara Haroche tried them all. "On the Stillman Diet, I lost about sixty-five pounds. I looked like I came out of Auschwitz, but I thought I was gorgeous."

Stillman was abandoned because "I just couldn't face those eight glasses of water every day," and the weight came back.

Heavy again, Haroche joined Overeaters Anonymous, a group that tries to help its members stop compulsive overeating.

For Haroche, it didn't work. "You can't say 'candy' or 'popcorn' at a meeting. You're supposed to say 'carbohydrates.' It's ridiculous. I went to OA with my girlfriend once, they were having some sort of party, and halfway there, we said, 'What do we want to go for? There won't be anything to eat, what fun is that?'

"When I belonged to OA, I still lived in Westchester. If you get an urge to eat, like a piece of chocolate cake, you're supposed to call your sponsor. But this woman had a husband and a baby. I'm not gonna call her at three in the morning and say I feel like having a piece of chocolate cake. How can you disturb a whole family for your own vanity?

"So Overeaters Anonymous didn't work for me. Furthermore, I'm the kind that lies to myself. All of us here do that. I wouldn't have anybody working in the store who didn't have some sort of mental problem because they wouldn't know how to talk to the people who come in. I'll show you how sick we are—"

Haroche interrupts herself to go and get a tiny paper cup. It's fluted, the kind used for tartar sauce in one-arm joints. "We inherited these from the Chicken Delight place that used to be here," she says. "We fill up this size with ice cream, and we think we're not eating. But we fill it up a hundred times a day."

Stillman and Overeaters Anonymous were followed by a stint on liquid protein. "I took off about a pound a day. But because I couldn't eat any solid food, food became a total obsession.

"I'd never cooked in my life, except what I had to do for the kids so they wouldn't starve, a lamb chop, or a steak, but now I started cooking.

"I was fooling around with recipes, buying low-calorie books, thinking about starting a business with homemade foods. But I wanted diet foods that wouldn't taste like diet foods.

"For a year, I cooked at home and gave the food away. I had about twenty friends, most of whom had never dieted. *I* wouldn't know what a real Pepsi-Cola tastes like, I only know from Diet Pepsi, but I wanted to test my food on people who were used to high-calorie cooking."

Did they like it? She says yes, but mockingly, reminding the listener that the price was right. "For nothing, they liked it."

And that's how Skinny Dip was born.

Divorced and on her own, Barbara Haroche sold the house in Westchester to get money for the store. Her first idea had been to have women in their own homes cooking Haroche-devised recipes, the resulting dishes to be sold in the store. That turned out to be illegal. The Board of Health doesn't permit such cottage industries, because there's no control over the cleanliness of the operation. "Also," says Haroche, "you have no control over the cost of it."

Her next thought was to hire churchwomen—the kind who put on bake sales and chicken dinner socials. "Find women who like to cook, and have them come into the store and do it. I talked to a caterer. He said forget it. I was afraid of a chef, though, afraid he'd fool around with the recipes. So I got this cook, and she couldn't cook. I couldn't deal with it."

Skinny Dip wound up with a chef, Roger Loose, trained in Europe, who does most of the food in the kitchen behind the store—entrées like Chicken Cordon Bleu (173 calories, $4.25), Tournedos Bordelaise (180 calories, $7.25), Filet of Flounder stuffed with Crab Meat (185 calories, $5.25) are cooked, packed in foil containers, and frozen—and Haroche explains the way the chef keeps the calories down. "We use low-fat cheeses, skim milk, egg whites instead of cream, vinegar rather than oil on the salads, whipped diet butter. And instead of sugar substitutes, we just use less sugar."

Daily News food editor Hamlin sampled some of the foods and found they "tasted more real and civilized than dietetic. Perhaps too civilized. Those portions are small."

Right, says Haroche. "The controlled portions appeal to people who can't limit themselves."

Less than a year after Skinny Dip opened, it began to break even financially, which made its owner very happy. "Because you know, your landlord doesn't care if you're new, and Con Edison doesn't care if you're new."

Mimi Sheraton didn't care either. Barbara Haroche says the *New York Times* critic almost put her out of business.

It happened after the first summer. Haroche spent ten thousand dollars to run an advertising supplement in the *New York Times*, and hired extra help. "Because we expected a response. Which we got. Then Mimi Sheraton did a review."

The Sheraton notice, printed on October 17, 1979, said in part, "It would be gratifying to be able to report that a new source of low-calorie diet foods offers food as delectable as what has gone before in this report. Unfortunately, this is not quite the case." (What had gone before in Sheraton's report was, among other things, a rave review of a non-diet food shop called Word of Mouth.) Sheraton went on to say that Skinny Dip promised eaters that only their scales would know they were chomping low-calorie fare, but it wasn't true. "Your taste buds will get wind of it at the very first bite."

The critic talked of "pasty sauce," "dreadful duck," "steam table-type chicken cacciatore," "insipid chocolate mousse," added that the shop itself had "a stained carpet" and "untidy counters," and summed up by saying that Skinny Dip "leaves virtually everything to be desired."

Haroche grants Sheraton the carpeting and counters ("I had a girl working here who was a slob. Fair is fair. Though I wonder what would have happened if Mimi Sheraton walked in when we had the explosion with the yogurt machine, and there was ice cream hanging from the ceiling."), and she says she isn't even mad anymore, because she feels she evened the score. After Skinny Dip got the good review from Suzanne Hamlin, Haroche took a newspaper ad quoting both food experts. In the ad, Hamlin comes first, saying, "food which is cut-rate in calories, but a pleasure to the palate." Sheraton follows, saying, "gratifying to be able to report . . . a new source of low-calorie diet foods . . . everything to be desired . . ."

"It's perfectly legal," Haroche says triumphantly. "Just like theater reviews. I got the dots there and everything."

Haroche's contention is that Sheraton had no right to compare Skinny Dip to Word of Mouth. "Compare us to Weight Watchers, compare us to Diet Plan, but not to Word of Mouth, and not to Zabar's. A fifty-dollar bottle of wine is going to taste different from a five-dollar bottle of wine, although they both might be good for what they are.

"Our quiche is made out of cottage cheese and skim milk. It's not going to taste like quiche that's made with heavy cream, but for what it is, it's good. But if somebody in the media doesn't like it, and gets on television and says so, or prints that they don't like it in the newspapers, I'm in a lot of trouble.

"Until Mimi Sheraton, I was very much afraid of the media. But after her review, I figured what the hell, and I sent out menus with a press release and little bags of cookies to all the food editors, and that's when Suzanne Hamlin contacted me."

The idea of providing a whole week's diet came to Haroche when she started noticing signs in restaurant windows that said, "We have the Scarsdale Diet today."

"I thought, why not the Skinny Dip Diet? A new place has to have some gimmick to get known. Nobody advertises, 'Our Food Tastes Terrible,' so how are you going to tell people that the food tastes good? You have to find a gimmick to make the people come in and get it.

"I figured out a week's worth of food, had a nutritionist go over it—she said add a vitamin pill and 18 milligrams of iron every day—but it's better balanced than the Stillman Diet or the Atkins Diet, which are limited to protein. And I added up the prices of everything, and it came out to $56, so I rounded it out to an even $50." (Haroche is not overly impressed by nutritionists. She says "proper nutrition" is too many calories for most people. "If you eat what the nutrition charts say is proper, you'll put on weight. If you have eggs and cereal and toast for breakfast, and then you eat lunch and dinner, no woman is going to maintain her weight. As far as nutrition goes, nobody's going to drop dead in this area of New York. We're not Cambodia.")

Here's a sample menu from the Skinny Dip Diet:

WEDNESDAY		CALORIES
Breakfast		
TOMATO JUICE		28
BLUEBERRY MUFFIN		58
		86
Lunch		
¼ lb. GREEN BEAN SALAD		20
¼ lb. RA-TA-TUI SALAD		37
¼ lb. BROCCOLI OR CAULIFLOWER		35
1 FRUIT MOUSSE		60
		152
Dinner		
CHICKEN CORDON BLEU		173
ZUCCHINI DELIGHT		35
ICE CREAM CAKE		108
		316
Snack		
1 CHOCOLATE CREAM CHEESE PIE		145
	Total	699

Now a customer is asking about the calories in a container of yogurt. Barbara Haroche tells her 200. "Yogurt is higher in calories than our ice cream."

Nearby, a young girl in a woolly hat is studying some cookies that are 7½ calories each. "I've lost forty pounds," she says. "I have twenty more to go. I'm doing it on my own, I can't afford Weight Watchers, but I did buy their books, and I use a lot of their recipes. I'm not going to their classes or anything, but I figure out calories. For breakfast, an egg is 80 calories, half a grapefruit is 60 calories, a teabag is 2 calories—"

The girl goes on and on, reciting the details of the year she's spent taming her wayward flesh. "Before, I'd try crash diets, and gain it right back. Now I've learned to eat fresh fruits. After a while I began to like the stuff. Once a week, I cheat. Every Sunday I let myself go out to a restaurant, buy one piece of cake. I never make it at home because if I made it at home, I'd eat the whole thing—"

Gently, Barbara Haroche offers the girl one of the cookies she's been mulling over. "Here, taste it."

The batter for these cookies has been dropped onto cookie sheets with a demitasse spoon, rather than the usual teaspoon. "At 40 or 50 calories, they won't buy, at 7½ calories, they will."

A tall, skinny woman is ordering salads to eat at one of the little tables in the store. She wants bits of three kinds of salad, all on one plate, total weight one quarter of a pound, not a fraction of an ounce more.

Haroche says many of the customers are gaunt. "We deal with anorexics here too. A lot of them. Really emaciated. There are men anorexics too, which I never knew.

"Some of the thin people count every single calorie because they say they used to be fat. They bring me before and after pictures. We have one girl who comes in, buys like twenty-five dollars' worth a day, mostly desserts. Maybe two salads, and the rest are desserts. She claims she throws it out, she doesn't eat it all. I don't know. She walked in once about twenty pounds lighter, she'd been on a fast. We have another one that bicycles up here from 23rd Street and buys thirty dozen cookies. Twice a day, she buys fifteen dozen. She bicycles up in the snow, in the rain.

"Another thing. Every second person who walks in here has hypoglycemia. That's the fashionable disease today." (Many scientists agree with Haroche that hypoglycemia—or low blood sugar—is indeed being diagnosed by too many doctors, and self-diagnosed by too many laymen. In April of 1980, *Time* magazine called it the "in" condition, and said it was "largely illusory." Dr. Leonard Madison of Southwestern Medical School in Dallas, was quoted as having said, "It is a lot easier to say that you have hypoglycemia than to admit you have an emotional disorder," and Columbia University's Dr. Donald Holub pointed the finger at "a few M.D.'s who have espoused hypoglycemia much as some others have become 'weight doctors.'")

Pondering "all these hypoglycemics," Barbara Haroche shrugs. "They drink themselves under the table, they eat honey, which is the same as sugar, but you can't tell them, because everybody's got their own mishegaas."

Other people's craziness is part of Haroche's daily scene. "I had some girls in here one day. They bought ice cream. They had French fries with them, and they wanted to sit down and eat the ice cream. I said fine, provided you throw the French fries out. I can't have a place that smells of deep frying. They said they wanted to eat the French fries, so I said, why don't you go back to where you bought them, and eat the ice cream there? 'We can't,' they said. 'It's too dirty there.' I said, you mean you'd put it in your stomachs, but you won't put your asses in the seats? That absolutely killed me."

If she can keep Mimi Sheraton and girls with French fries out of the store, things are looking good for Barbara Haroche. Although she's lived through some other crises, en route to the place where she finds herself now. "The chef had to go out of town one week, so his wife came in and cooked. With a newborn baby! It was a three-ring circus, the kid was crying, the chef's wife was rocking the carriage with her foot, and chopping onions with her hands. And I hired a girl to help out, and she took the string beans that are marinated in onions and garlic and vinegar, and put the beans in a container and threw the marinade out. And the chicken salad got screwed up—"

The chicken salad's fine again (just enough oregano, not too much) and the string beans are once more bathing in their spicy broth, and in the kitchen, the chef is making tiny chocolate cream cheese pies, and Barbara Haroche is moaning because "there are only twenty-four hours in a day."

Observing her customers has made Haroche a bit less hard on herself. She sees the ones with anorexia, the ones who claim hypoglycemia, the ones who can't handle a 7½ calorie cookie, and says she wouldn't swap her own looniness for anyone else's. "I'll stick with the food thing."

It isn't that she wouldn't prefer to be slender, it's just that Twinkies are always there, beckoning to her in the night. "My theory is," she says, "that if you're content with an apple or cantaloupe for dessert, you're not going to be overweight to begin with. All these diets—people fall off them because they're dying to have the sweets."

About the gourmet dishes whipped up on her premises, she's of two minds. "I don't like half of them. I don't like the fillet of flounder stuffed with seafood." She repeats an earlier confession: "I like junk food."

Anyway, torturing herself doesn't make sense to Haroche. "If you're so hungry, my theory is, go have another piece of cheese. Thirty-five calories is not going to make that much difference in anyone's life."

And yet the idea of getting back into those size 4s sometimes sets up a clatter in her head, and then Barbara Haroche, despite her love of junk food, despite her philosophic willingness to "stick with the food thing" goes on still another diet.

Once in a while she's helped (or hindered) by outside forces. "If I'm busy in the store, I don't eat all day long, and I don't get hungry. But when things get slow here, I get upset, and I can't stop eating."

The only exception to this rule seems to have occurred after the Mimi Sheraton review. Then, depressed in spades, Barbara Haroche still did not eat. "I didn't eat for a week. But I was so tired that the only way I could fall asleep was to drink, so the calories were still there."

In the end, she knows that the only way to diet is to take responsibility and stop blaming fate. "You just have to decide. You just have to say, day by day, I'm going to do it. Until the weight comes off.

"One of these days," Barbara Haroche says, and then flicks a hand in the direction of the shiny equipment standing on a counter. "Those damn ice-cream machines," she says. "That's what kills me."

TAKING IT OFF:
Among their nonjudgmental peers, fat people find the company that misery loves . . .

24 Groups: Friends in Need

Praising the lean and sallow abstinence
—JOHN MILTON

"IF YOU EAT food for pleasure, then you are a food pervert," says Dr. H. L. Newbold, a medical nutritionist, in his book, *Dr. Newbold's Revolutionary New Discoveries About Weight Loss*. "Unlike some perversions," Newbold continues darkly, "food perversions are dangerous because they make you fat and thus cut down on the length of your life."

You said a mouthful, Doc. John Calvin couldn't have put it better. To be sure, a lot of us perverts flat-out don't care (it's on with the orgy, bring us our chestnut-purée-filled crepes, and if we die, we die), but Dr. Newbold is talking to folks who *are* concerned. And it's this second crowd that seeks in groups relief from fatness. In a group, one can learn behavior modification, or how to Take Off Pounds Sensibly (TOPS), or how to watch one's weight, or how to stop (anonymously) overeating.

The group that has become the most famous and has had the most commercial success is surely Weight Watchers.

Jean Nidetch, the self-proclaimed formerly fat housewife who started Weight Watchers, could now refer to herself as a medium-sized millionaire. In one of her books *(The Story of Weight Watchers)*, Mrs. Nidetch documented the ways in which fat people lie to themselves. They've "inherited" their fat, they're "big-boned," they're "glandular," they're "retaining water," they're "cursed."

If Mrs. Nidetch was cursed, she says, it was with a lust for cookies. From a fat baby, she grew into a fat child and then a fat woman, so once she'd taken off her excess weight, it was hard for another fat person to con her.

At one early Weight Watchers session, an elderly woman told Nidetch she was gaining weight because of her grandchildren. Nidetch said nobody got fat from happiness. "Are you sure it isn't because you're eating the wrong foods?"

"No," the woman said, "when I look at my grandchildren, I gain weight."

Nidetch could not be moved. "Madam," she said, "unless you *eat* them, you're not going to gain weight from your grandchildren."

Nidetch herself weighed 214 pounds in 1961, at which time "desperation drove me to the New York City Department of Obesity Clinic." She had gone on and off many diets, and when she was dieting, she was "irritable, high-strung, and cried for no reason at all." She came to the Obesity Clinic looking for a miracle, "a miracle that was going to make me look at a cupcake and say, 'I hate it!'"

There was no miracle available. The clinic was dispensing copies of a diet worked out by Dr. Norman Joliffe many years before. Nothing flaky, very basic. In updated form, that diet is still being circulated by Weight Watchers and other groups. (A dieter is not permitted bacon, fatty meats, sausage, beer, liquor, wine, butter, cakes, cookies, crackers, doughnuts, pastries, pies, candy, chocolates, nuts, cream, french fries, potato chips, popcorn, pretzels, sugar-sweetened puddings, gelatin desserts, gravies, sauces, honey, jams, jellies, sugar and syrup, ice cream, ices, ice milk, muffins, pancakes, waffles, olives, sugar-sweetened sodas, fruit-flavored yogurt. A dieter *is* permitted lean beef, pork, or lamb—one pound a week—four eggs a week, fruits, vegetables, a certain amount of corn, potatoes, beans, rice, spaghetti, fish, some kinds of cheeses, whole grain bread, small amounts of vegetable oil, margarine, and mayonnaise. A dieter may drink coffee, tea, water, club soda, bouillon, consommé, skim milk, and buttermilk.)

Jean Nidetch, thirty-eight years old, "making one last effort to dig myself out of all that fat," took the diet home. She wasn't impressed. It wasn't very different from diets she'd tried before. Except that "I wasn't allowed to substitute anything. I wasn't allowed to cut out anything. I had to go along with the entire program or I wouldn't be permitted to stay with the clinic." Unwilling to face the humiliation of being "terminated" (the clinic was, after all, a public facility with long lists of people waiting for places), Nidetch struggled with herself and the diet, and in ten weeks had lost twenty pounds. She did cheat a little. She gave up cake, pizza, ice cream. She ate vegetables, fish, and drank "miserable" skim milk. She didn't skip breakfast or lunch (regular meals were required), but she still sneaked cookies.

One day, she telephoned six fat friends and invited them over to her house to talk about the cookie problem. "Someone who had never been fat couldn't understand what I was going through."

The six who came understood all too well. (Among them was a woman Nidetch had first met in the waiting room of a doctor who prescribed appetite suppressants. "She and I got to talking and, after our first visit to the doctor, we went to the delicatessen across the street for a corned beef sandwich and french fries.") Now all the ladies shared their miseries, and began to wonder if they might be able to help encourage one another to lose weight.

Further meetings took place. More and fatter people came, hoping to stop their midnight binges, hoping to find in union the strength to keep them dieting.

"I've found," Nidetch has written, "that all overweight people have this tremendous desire to talk. Maybe we're all oral types, we have to eat or talk. We have to talk about our problems and what we're trying to do about them."

So, to the diet she had been given at the Obesity Clinic, Nidetch added talk. That was her secret. The biggest reason for Weight Watchers' success, she believes, is that fat people could finally "reveal our real feelings to other people and those other people will understand. I can say to a Weight Watchers class, 'I remember sitting in a bathtub watching my fat floating,' and there isn't a person there who can't relate to me at that moment."

In 1963, a group member named Al Lippert (he had lost forty pounds, his wife had lost fifty) convinced Nidetch to stop giving away her time and effort and to charge a fee for classes. Eventually, Lippert became

Nidetch's partner, and his marketing genius was responsible for the corporation's expansion.

Groups such as Weight Watchers, says Edwin Bayrd, in an effort to explain the phenomenon further, "offer a highly public system of punishments and rewards for their members, who are openly castigated for each pound gained and warmly applauded for each pound lost. The resultant mix of camaraderie and competitiveness works with great success in most cases, and professional medical men have nothing but praise for the clubs' achievements."

Achievements, in the case of Weight Watchers, is the operative word. In 1968, Weight Watchers became a public corporation, and a share of common stock sold for $11.25. Ten years later, when H. J. Heinz bought the company, each share was worth $72. (Jean Nidetch, like Colonel Sanders, was put on a lifetime retainer, and continues to act as a figurehead, lecturing all over the world.)

H. J. Heinz doesn't publish sales figures, but its Annual Report for 1979 broke down income from Weight Watchers this way: 63 percent of gross revenues came from classroom operations (both foreign and domestic); the rest came from franchise operations, sales of Weight Watchers foods, and such enterprises as *Weight Watchers Magazine* (circulation 800,000), Weight Watchers scales, and Weight Watchers cookbooks.

The Heinz report said that the latest edition of the *Weight Watchers Cookbook* (first introduced in 1966) had sold 275,000 copies in 1979. According to Jean Nidetch, 16,000 Weight Watchers classes are held every week (in the United States alone, 500,000 people are going at any one time), and no voyeurs are permitted. If you don't need to lose at least ten pounds, you're turned away.

A new member of the group gets a copy of the rules, a food plan, a menu plan, a nutrition booklet. You pay your fee at the door each week, then go to be weighed, and to take part in a meeting with a lecturer who leads a group discussion.

Since 1973, when a psychological director was added to the staff, members have also been given behavior modification booklets called "modules." These modules, says Mrs. Nidetch, deal "with moods that trigger eating, keeping track of what, when and *how* you eat, so you can pinpoint trouble areas; getting the *right* kind of help from friends and families; learning to survive the 'eating traps' we encounter at parties and restaurants and other places; learning to keep tempting foods out of sight (and out of mind!)."

Weight Watchers asks its members to weigh every morsel of food before eating it, and not to keep sweets in the house, and not to touch alcohol or diet pills, and not to skip meals.

In 1979, the company, which had been running summer camps for fat children (since 1969, about 1,200 kiddies a year had been dispatched for streamlining), opened half a dozen summer camps for plump adults.

The one in Tarrytown, New York, on the campus of Marymount College (tariff: $400 a week) was visited by Judy Klemesrud of the *New York Times* during its first summer. Klemesrud found one camper ecstatic ("It's a mracle of God that I came here, I had tried everything before this, drinking water for seven months, liquid protein, taking pills, and I didn't lose weight. Here I'm eating three meals a day plus milk and fruit snacks, and I'm finally losing") and a couple of campers inclined to carp. The place had no air conditioning in the dorms, there was no maid service, bathrooms had to be shared. But most of the clients were pleased. "A spa is too posh for me," said one woman. "Here you can wear what you want."

The camp, reported Klemesrud, was run "under standard Weight Watchers principles. Measured portions of three nutritionally balanced meals a day, exercise, and weekly 'encouragement meetings.'" A weigh-in was held every Sunday, "accompanied by much cheering and applause, even if the camper had only a very small weight loss that week."

Since the majority of campers were not 140-pounders trying to get down to 125, but really obese people (Klemesrud interviewed one 274-pound nurse who had weighed 300 pounds five weeks earlier, and one 248-pound schoolteacher who was hoping to shed fifty pounds), many of them did not take part in exercise classes or tennis clinics, but they were still hopeful about losing through diet.

Recently (in August of 1980), I bought a bunch of Weight Watchers frozen dinners to test at home. I bought seven, and tested four. The other three are still in the freezer, waiting for me to suffer a new onslaught of good character. Someday. Meanwhile, I will tell what I believe.

Veal Parmigiana (Chopped and Formed) and Zucchini In Sauce seemed to me delicious. It cost $1.79 in the supermarket, and furnished

230 calories. It wasn't enough food, but it tasted good. Chicken Breast Parmigiana—Spinach was something else again. The chicken "breast" was chicken roll of some sort, little paper-thin slices of cardboard flavored stuff, and the spinach was, of course, plain spinach, no sauce. It cost $1.89, and I hated it.

I also hated the Sole, Peas, and Mushrooms, Lobster Sauce ($1.79 for 200 calories). So far as I could make out, the only place lobster appeared was in the printed list of ingredients on the package—you couldn't see any or taste any—and the fish was fishy and flabby both.

Chicken Creole was the last dish I tried. This was pretty good, spicy with peppers, onion, and garlic, but there was a lot of sauce left after the chicken and vegetables were eaten. (Under non-diet conditions, such a dish would be served over rice.) Chicken Creole cost $1.99, and contained 250 calories.

Obviously, mine was a most superficial experiment. Weight Watchers puts its label on such a variety of foods it would take weeks to try them all. For instance, there are "Three-Compartment Meals" such as Stuffed Greenland Turbot with Zucchini, Tomato Sauce, and Crinkle-Cut Carrots, not to be confused with "Two-Compartment Meals" such as Greenland Turbot with Peas and Carrots and Lemon Flavored Bread Crumbs. There are also "Casseroles," or "One Dish Meals," such as Turkey Tetrazzini Au Gratin, Mushrooms, and Red Peppers.

And more meals are being created, even as you read this. Because Weight Watchers' test cooks never sleep. Right now, Heinz is test-marketing a frozen dessert called Chocolate Treat, a carbonated lemonade, an imitation cream cheese, a Russian dressing, an imitation mayonnaise, a bread, a cooking spray, and several dry mix gravies.

If you don't live in a test-market area, you can still buy Weight Watchers' hard ice cream in flavors such as Alpine Mint and Lemon Chiffon, not to mention more ordinary flavors. You can also buy snack cups of frozen dessert, and a dairy product called Frosted Treat. Weight Watchers puts out fruit snacks that taste of cinnamon, or peach, or strawberry, it distributes "19 pure extracts" (including almond, banana, papaya, and maple), and there are Weight Watchers soft drinks, Weight Watchers skim milk, Weight Watchers cottage cheese.

Weight Watchers is the best-known fat group, but it is not the only fat group. TOPS, The Diet Workshop, Appetite Control Centers, Diet Control Centers, Weigh of Life, Compulsive Eating Reeducation Group, Dieters Counseling Service are the names of just a few outfits offering group therapy for the overweight. In Manhattan alone, there are more than eighty weight-loss programs listed in a booklet called The Dieters Referral Service. Some of these also offer one-to-one treatment (a doctor will plant acupuncture needles in your ears, or hypnotize you, or put you on a fast, or try to raise your self-esteem), but group counseling abounds. If you want to study nutritional ignorance, or the psychological and social causes of overeating, if you'd like to delve into psychodrama, or investigate "gestalt methods," there's a group to help you do it. One program director puts everybody on a diet for hypoglycemia (he forbids all refined sugar, starch, and fat which he regards as poison), another offers "eighty-two behavior modification strategies to cover any problem situation."

Medical men who are experts in the field of obesity often give group efforts high praise. Dr. Albert Stunkard has said that TOPS members get results "superior to that achieved by routine medical management," and Dr. George Mann agrees that while the "modeling of ill-fitting old clothing may seem schmaltzy," TOPS members demonstrate weight losses that have persisted for sixteen months or more, thereby matching any "available medical treatment."

On the other hand, Dr. Hilde Bruch has reservations. Patients who came to Bruch after having tried Weight Watchers had found the Weight Watchers meetings "too unsophisticated and had felt turned off. Some who had attended for a period and had regained the lost weight would speak with a certain embarrassment about having taken part in the meetings and their childish ways of praise and blame."

(Admitting that her experience came "mainly from dealing with obese people with complex psychological problems," Dr. Bruch says for people "with a more secure self-concept," a group might offer "a helpful solution.")

The problem with organizations such as Weight Watchers or TOPS, in the opinion of Edwin Bayrd, is that people lose weight only so long as they remain active members of the clubs. "Without the weekly reinforcement—the threat of humiliation and the prospect of felicitation—they fare no better on the diet and exercise programs promoted by their clubs than do the followers of plans sponsored by other organizations of professional groups."

Bayrd is a booster of behavior modification as the only serious answer to the fat question because "it is not dependent on some outside agent for reinforcement . . . the scope is limited, the specific demands readily met, and the ends attainable. Here as nowhere else the mechanism of control is in the hands of the dieter whose task is to monitor his behavior, not his caloric intake. He need know nothing about the mechanics of fat, the effects of ketosis, the regulation of hunger and satiety, or the food value of specific nutrients to do this. Instead, the less he thinks about such matters and the more he thinks about setting his fork down after every other bite, the better off he will be."

Dr. Alfred Rimm is a scientist whose files contain documentary evidence of group members falling off the wagon, once they strayed from the group. TOPS referred 175 obese women to Dr. Rimm for a study he was doing at the Medical College of Wisconsin, in Milwaukee. Under his direction, the ladies spent three weeks in the hospital and averaged a weight loss of fifteen pounds apiece.

Two years afterward, 60 percent of them had put the weight back on, some having gained more than forty pounds.

What about the 40 percent who'd stayed thin, or got thinner?

"When Dr. Rimm compared the eating habits, medical histories, family backgrounds, and psychological profiles of the women who maintained their weight loss with those who failed to do so," wrote reporter David R. Zimmerman, in the May 1980 issue of *Ladies' Home Journal*, "he found that only two factors out of the eighty-nine he analyzed were of any self-help value. He sums them up as vanity. His psychological tests show that women who feel responsible for themselves, but who also care a great deal about what others think of them, have a tendency to stay slim."

Jean Nidetch ratifies this thesis. "A desire for cupcakes can be replaced by a desire to look good," she says in *The Story of Weight Watchers*. "In other words, vanity. There is no more compelling reason to lose weight. Occasionally, a person comes to our classes because his doctor says he has to have surgery, but must first lose one hundred pounds. Occasionally, someone joins because his blood pressure is so high that he is in danger of having a stroke. But even if it is for a serious, medical reason, I've discovered he really comes because he wants to look better. Vanity is the major reason people want to lose weight. I, for one, could never get all choked up about the health benefits of proper eating habits. I never cared about nutrition. But I did care about how I looked."

Unfortunately, the desire to look good can coexist with a desire for cupcakes, rather than replacing it. Many people locked up in prisons of fat cherish fantasies of their own beauty. "Like Cinderella or the Frog Prince," writes sociologist Marcia Millman, in a book called *Such a Pretty Face*, "the fat person lives with a double identity. Her present self-in-the-world may be fat, ugly, despised, or disregarded, but inside, carefully nourished, is a private self that is beautiful, powerful, lovely. The poignancy of the expression 'such a pretty face' derives from the individual's involvement with her magnificence and the tragedy of its entrapment.

"Many fat women wistfully remark, 'I've been told that I'm so beautiful that if I were thin I would stop traffic when I walked down the street.' The need to be extraordinarily beautiful is related to the need for unconditional love. So severe was the original rejection and injury, that it is not enough to be average."

One of the places where wounded souls (with fat bodies) can find unconditional love is Overeaters Anonymous.

Overeaters Anonymous declares that it is not a diet club, but a "fellowship" offering a program of recovery from compulsive overeating. OA is based on the principles of Alcoholics Anonymous. AA's serenity prayer ("God grant me the serenity to accept the things I cannot change; the courage to change the things I can, and the wisdom to know the difference"), AA's use of the word "abstinence," AA's Twelve Steps, its Twelve Traditions, and its slogans like "One Day At a Time" have all been adopted, with obvious minor changes. (In Overeaters Anonymous, a member admits he's powerless over food, not alcohol.)

OA was started in 1960 by three housewives in Los Angeles. There are no fees, no dues, but after a meeting, a hat is passed, and the collection goes to help with expenses, like printing the OA literature.

Following are passages from that literature:

"We believe that we have a progressive, three-fold illness affecting us physically, emotionally, and spiritually. Over a considerable length of time it gets worse, never better."

"Our primary purpose is to stop eating compulsively . . . and we welcome in fellowship and friendly understanding all those who share our common problem."

"A diet is a diet. We've all been on them. Some of us have tried grapefruit, eggs, protein, water, and fasting. Some of us have also gone the diet pill route. All of these methods seemed to say, 'If you'd only eat a special way, the desire to overeat compulsively would leave.' But somehow it didn't. It never was the food. We were using the food as the alcoholic uses alcohol and the drug addict uses drugs. Early on, we had chosen food as a solution. It helped block out the feelings. OA offers us a different solution. OA's solution is a program of action and service. We abstain from compulsive overeating and offer service by reaching out the hand of help to each other and to those outside our fellowship who are still suffering. If we abstain from compulsive overeating, we can get on with our recovery. Once the symptom is brought under control, we can get at the underlying problems."

OA presents its members with a choice of food plans (suggesting that you see a doctor before embarking on any diet), and a maintenance program, and asks members to abstain from eating between meals and to avoid "binge" foods. (One man's binge food is another man's celery; some crave peanut butter, some go weak when faced with sweets.)

At OA, a new member may ask a more experienced member (one with a record of at least thirty days' abstinence) to be his sponsor. The sponsor helps the new member with his eating plan, and is available by telephone. The new member is supposed to call his sponsor every day, and discuss every bite the new member plans to swallow during the next twenty-four hours.

An Overeaters Anonymous group meets near my house, and I went to my first OA meeting there, in the basement of an old church. It was a dark, shabby place, the night was wet and snowy, and several of us wandered around stamping our boots on the floor, trying to dry our hair, while waiting for the session to begin.

I eavesdropped on two women discussing food hang-ups. Both women were thin. "I used to eat everything in the house," one said. "Then I would go out. I would never live anywhere there wasn't a 24-hour delicatessen. I would eat the world, then go outside and eat more."

A man came up to me and complained that since he'd stopped smoking, he'd gained thirty pounds. "I can't lose. I want help. But I don't like all this spiritual business. I don't want to find God, I want to lose weight."

(Like Alcoholics Anonymous, Overeaters Anonymous refers to a Higher Power, and turning one's will and one's life over to the care of "God as we understand Him," but the OA literature says OA is *not* a religious organization. Some overeaters, says one OA pamphlet, "choose to consider the group itself as the Power greater than themselves.")

Marcia Millman says that most of the patients who go to diet doctors or diet groups are women, but the group in the basement of the church was well mixed, and on that stormy night I heard three different men testify as to how OA had changed their lives.

Because anonymity is of the essence ("By its practice, members insure that egotism and self-glorification will not be the undoing of the OA fellowship"), I'll call these men Tom, Dick, and Harry.

Tom, handsome, athletic-looking, about thirty-five, and anything but fat, talked specifically for the benefit of the beginners who were present:

"I weighed 100 pounds when I was in the fourth grade. I weighed 180 pounds in the eighth grade. In high school and college, I played sports, got thin, got married, got fat again. The marriage was in trouble. While my wife was away on a trip, I started to take off weight. When she came home, I met her at the airport. 'Look, it's a new me.' Nine months later, I was back up to 240 pounds, and divorced.

"My second marriage also had problems. I realized I had the same problems thin or fat. I was a slave to the goddamn food.

"But I wasn't going to get help. No group, no pills, no doctor. I had to do it myself.

"I was a salesman. One day, after I finished work, I went to the movies. Since I'd had no breakfast or lunch, I thought I could have a candy bar. I bought popcorn, a drink, a candy bar, and ate them. Then I went back to the candy counter and did it all over again. When I came out of the movies, I said to myself, that was a sick thing you just did.

"I came to OA, lost fifty pounds, and have maintained the weight loss for two and a half years. I'm grateful every day. I still have problems, but I'm not enslaved by food.

"At first, I didn't like the meetings. They took place in a church, and I'm Jewish. And I heard people talking about emotional and spiritual recovery, and I'm thinking, what is that? I want to lose weight, I don't have any emotional problems. Still, for four months, I went to meetings every night. I walked through the doors at six, and walked out again at ten. A lot of things that bothered me then still bother me. I have to find another way of solving them, or I'll start shoving food in my mouth. But this thing saved my life. Weight can kill you."

Having sketched in his own background, Tom offered advice to first-timers scattered around the room.

"Write down everything you eat. Anything you don't write down is the first compulsive bite. To avoid the first compulsive bite, go to a meeting, call your sponsor. If you don't like OA after thirty days, we give you back your misery. But as long as you feel you're a compulsive eater, you're welcome in these rooms."

The second man, Dick, was a little guy with dyed hair, a well-worn suit coat, an aura of seediness, but he was as spellbinding as the first man had been.

Dick:

"I'm hypoglycemic. I used to have six soda pops, six candy bars, and a sugar hangover before noon every day.

"I was the fattest kid in seventh grade. I knew how to give directions by grocery stores and restaurants. 'It's two blocks from the Dairy Queen, make a left at the corner of the White Rose Delicatessen.' If anybody was eating, I would eat. I could eat ten times a day."

Then, to the beginners: "You don't have to give up chocolate bars forever. Just for today. And then make the same promise again tomorrow. You have to play straight, be strict with yourself. It's emotional. Any upset can make an overeater go on a binge. In the old days, a long line at the bank could make me splurge. So easy does it. And turn to the literature for strength when you think there's no strength around."

Harry, the third speaker, was fat, a fat man wearing a down vest, and apparently still in the midst of a dire struggle with himself.

Harry:

"I was a writer in an advertising agency once. Then I got fat, and lost confidence, and lost my work. I used to send letters to people to try and get work again. If they wrote back, at least they were interested. I didn't have the nerve to phone. The other day, after several years of this, I finally found the nerve to call somebody direct about a job.

"I used to stand in front of a mirror, in a blue blazer, about to go and look for work, and I couldn't leave the apartment. 'You're fat,' I'd think, and I'd give up. Tonight, after an hour and a half trip to get to this meeting, I stepped off the bus in all the storm and the slush, and there were two stores on the corner. One was the store where I binge, and the other was the store where I knew I should get the food for my dinner. And I thought about Walter Raleigh, caught in a storm on the Thames River, saying to himself that thing about, 'Have I sailed the great and stormy oceans of the world, and survived, only to die in this puddle?' The binge store was my puddle. I went to the other store and got my food."

Anyone who could hear that man bearing witness and not be moved is made of sterner stuff than I.

There *are* funny things about OA to a first-time participant. OA members *are* asked to say "food," not "candy" or "popcorn" or "soda," though the depositions of Tom, Dick, and Harry show this to be a convention more honored in the breach than in the observance. Specific words like "chocolate bar" are proscribed because they make seductive pictures in the mind. In the same way that a Catholic in the confessional will admit to having had impure thoughts, an OA member will admit, "I had food thoughts."

But in the main, a newcomer marvels more than he laughs, awed by the light of the human spirit blazing through the too too solid flesh.

TAKING IT OFF:
You can lose on nuts and bran, or you can try the No-Diet Diet.

25 The Politics of Dieting: In Which Feminists, Kids, a Few Celebrities, and a Doctor Concerned for the Elderly Assume Public Stands . . .

There was an old person of Dean
Who dined on one pea and one bean;
For he said, "More than that,
Would make me too fat,"
That cautious old person of Dean.
—EDWARD LEAR

ARCHIE BUNKER recounted it:

"She went on one of them screwball diets; all the fat come off her behind and went into her fingers."

There's a screwball diet born every minute—the old person of Dean's "one pea and one bean" would scarcely raise an eyebrow nowadays—and some of them will make you thin, some of them will make you sick, some of them will make you crazy.

Since this book is mainly about eating for pleasure, and dieting for looks, we haven't yet touched on diets inspired by religion ("Give God a chance to solve your weight problem," implores the back cover of Evelyn Kliewer's *Freedom From Fat*) and philosophy. But did you know that the Zen macrobiotic diet—mostly cereals—which once spread among the populace—mostly young—left many of them with scurvy?

And did you know there are people who won't eat anything white, but stick to brown rice, and whole grains, while other people won't eat anything brown, but demand that their foods be brightly colored?

And have any of your children refused meat at your table because "I don't eat corpses"? If so, a writer named John Leo has a suggestion for you. "Point out that St. Francis was not a vegetarian, but Hitler was."

There are kids who won't eat steak, and kids who won't eat knishes. Across the face of a receipt acknowledging the delivery of a shipment of lunches for the children of one New York City school, the adult in charge scrawled a message, after his signature. "Please," it said, "stop sending the knishes because the kids doesn't like this. This is not a kosher area, this is basically a black and Haitian area."

A daily diet of knishes might try the digestion of the most rabid heavy food enthusiast, but the deeper one delves into the habits of Americans, the more awestruck one becomes at the sheer variety of ways we eat. And don't eat.

Newspapers and magazines are so full of tales about methods employed by celebrities to lose weight that there's scarcely any room for the news.

Here's a sampling.

Gloria Vanderbilt, jeans queen. She stays skinnier than you by eating stuff you never heard of. Gloria's daily breakfast: one boiled egg, Kava instant, Lahvosh Armenian Cracker Bread, and Willwood spread. *(New York Post.)*

Kitty Carlisle, chairman of New York State's Council on the Arts. She had her behavior modified by her late husband, Moss Hart. Describing herself as "a greedy girl," she says Hart was "always worried" about her getting fat. "If we were at a dinner party, and he couldn't reach my hand, he would pat his own wrist. It was a symbolic gesture, and it meant, 'You've had it,' and I knew I'd better stop eating whatever it was." *(New York Times.)*

Aretha Franklin, singer. She buys diet books, but no cookbooks. This is the don't-tempt-me method of staying straight and narrow. Unfortunately, it doesn't work, because even without cookbooks, Aretha cooks. "Good, plain, fattening stuff like peach cobbler and fried ribs. It's murder on the diet." (*Chicago Sunday News*.)

Allan Carr, movie producer. He tried the fat facilities at Duke University, endured an intestinal bypass (this surgery was later reversed), and once even had his jaws wired shut. (*Life* magazine.)

Vincenzo Buonassisi, Milan-based King of Pasta. He lost weight on pasta. One hundred pounds in two years. He ate pasta with vegetables, but no oil or butter or sauce. When he started getting fat again, he said pasta was not to blame, but rather his life-style, because "often I am part of a jury for cooking contests." *(New York Times.)*

Miss Piggy, star sow. Her secrets are still in galley form, but there *is* going to be a book called *Miss Piggy's Foolproof 14-Day Diet. (Newsweek.)*

Laffit Pincay, Jr., jockey. He breakfasts and dines on unsalted nuts mixed with dry bran, and for lunch, he has a dehydrated food bar. Plus vitamins. This is Pincay's own formulation. A jockey can't weigh more than 116 pounds, and when Pincay, whose winnings in the first fourteen years of his career topped $50 million, first found himself edging up to 120 (pounds, not millions), he started on diet pills. The pills gave him leg cramps and made him nervous, so after trying various other regimens—"lettuce only, sunflower seeds, fish, eggs, skipping meals, liquids only"—he settled on nuts and bran. Pincay loves racing but admitted to interviewer Karen Jackovich that he often thought yearningly of black beans and chicken with rice. He also sounded a bit wistful about the fact that *Mrs*. Pincay had reduced from 135 pounds to 112. "I liked women with meat," he said. (*People* magazine.)

But most women don't like themselves with meat, so the search for the perfect—painless—diet continues.

How about the "World's Easiest Diet," devised by Dr. Neil Solomon, which requires eating an apple and drinking an eight-ounce glass of water before every meal? Dr. Solomon says this diet "tricks the natural mechanism of the stomach."

How about the Conway Diet Institute diet, which advertises "No Fish Required"?

Sleep it off, hypnotize it off, burn it off, pray it off, ask your diet doctor to come to dinner so he can shame it off. Journalist Nadine Brozan wrote an article on diet doctors and what happened when they went out and socialized in the real world. Dr. Howard Shapiro, reported Brozan, once told the woman next to him on a buffet line what he did for a living, and the poor woman tried to gloss over the fact that her plate was piled high by saying the food was "for me and my husband."

"And where is your husband?" asked Dr. Shapiro.

"In Cleveland," said the lady.

Dr. Neil Solomon told Brozan he'd gone to a party where several of the guests were Solomon patients, and the instant he arrived, "One patient immediately gave her food to her husband, the second shoved his cocktail to the other side of the table, and the third . . . told me she had taken all that food to see if she could eat only a little portion of it."

Dr. Morton Glenn agreed that diet experts were killjoys at a banquet. "People never have much food when they're sitting next to me. In fact, some don't eat at all."

A New Jersey outfit called Nutrition Control Clinic, which claims to employ a "multimodal approach" to obesity because "human processes are multileveled," suggests that a person craving a rich dessert can defeat this craving. "If one antidote does not work, the person immediately tries something else." He or she can leave the table, or go for a walk, or reward himself or herself for not eating the dessert "by seeking out some other pleasant sensation such as sex, or listening to music . . . or enjoying a warm shower."

It's all right with me, but that sex and shower act might really upset your hostess. Especially when she's trying to make a good impression on Dr. Shapiro and Dr. Solomon and Dr. Glenn.

Many authority figures who aren't diet doctors also dispense advice to the fat.

A woman writes Ann Landers that her husband's relatives are so fat they "have broken our chairs and damaged our sofa. What can we do about this problem?"

Ann advises the woman to "get some sturdy, inexpensive chairs and tell the obese relatives, 'We bought these chairs especially for you.' Insist that they sit on them—and nowhere else."

A woman writes Dear Abby that she was happily married when she was fat, but the minute she got skinny, she started acting "weak and trampy" and now she can't stand herself.

Abby says get some counseling, and don't worry. "A real tramp wouldn't feel guilty."

The business of female guilt (about fat, not sex) has been dealt with in a serious, in fact, a revolutionary, way by a woman named Susie Orbach, who wrote a book called *Fat Is a Feminist Issue*.

Orbach, a feminist and a psychotherapist, is founder of the Women's Therapy Group. She works with compulsive-eating therapy groups, and the one thing she requires of her group members is that they do *not* diet. Eat what you want, when you want it, she tells them.

For compulsive eaters who have struggled through ordeals with doctors and pills and fasts and shots, this kind of anarchy—no constraints, no rules, no authority but oneself—can be terrifying, but Orbach believes it is a necessary terror that, having been lived through, can set women free.

In 1970, she herself had entered a group for compulsive eaters, a bit embarrassed because she didn't believe a feminist should care how she looked. ("We were ostensibly happy in our blue jeans and work shirts, we were not used to discussing clothes or body size with our female friends.")

But in this group, initiated by therapist Carol Munter, Orbach found answers that had evaded her during ten years of dieting, going on binges, and hating herself.

The truth, Orbach tells us, is that women are afraid to be thin. Getting fat, she says, is a purposeful act, "a challenge to sex-role stereotyping . . . Fat is a social disease, and fat is a feminist issue. Fat is *not* about lack of self-control or lack of will power. Fat *is* about protection, sex, nurturance, strength, boundaries, mothering, substance, assertion, and rage. It is a response to the inequality of the sexes."

Women are not accepted as equals, and yet they're expected to nurture the world, Orbach theorizes, and they feel empty with so much giving, and eat to replenish themselves. Also, the fat is expressing "a rebellion against the powerlessness of the woman . . . We want to take up as much space as the other sex. 'If I get bigger like a man, then maybe I'll get taken seriously as is a man.'"

There are fat women who eat compulsively, as their anorexic sisters-under-the-skin diet compulsively; and for the same reason: in order to avoid becoming sexual objects. "Fat offends Western ideals of female beauty," Orbach contends, "and as such, every 'overweight' woman creates a crack in the popular culture's ability to make us mere products."

Now here is the part of Orbach's thesis that she says is hard to understand. Women come to her hoping to get thin, and yet "compulsive eating is linked to a desire to get fat."

The desire is largely unconscious, since most fat women perceive themselves as miserable, unwilling to dance, or go to the beach, or to try and fit into a seat on a bus. But fat women also feel protected by their flesh; at work, they're more apt to be judged by what they do, not by how they look, and socially they avoid sexual competition with other females. Orbach talks of a woman who gorged before going to a party, so she could "convince herself she was too big to be considered sexual. This allowed her a kind of ease to relate to people at the party—women and men—on her terms rather than on the exchange value of her body."

Women also use their fat as a way to avoid expressing anger, cushioning their "unwomanly" rage behind a protective wall of blubber.

Why do fat women fear being thin? They think of thinness as being cold, unnurturing. They feel they'll be sexually harassed, they feel other women will dislike them, and they feel if they get thin, and *still* don't achieve love and success and absolute happiness, they won't have their fatness to blame anymore.

(The same anxiety appears in anorexia patients. In *Eating Disorders*, Hilde Bruch talks of a girl who had "suffered all her life from the feeling of being 'ugly,' of not being 'a beauty.' She was overweight and started a reducing program, at first rather sensibly, reducing from 140 to 110 pounds between ages thirteen and sixteen. But then, when things were still 'not right,' she went on a starvation regimen, to a low of 67 pounds. She explained it as 'about being fat I could do something, but not about being ugly.' She knew that her skeletonlike appearance was hideous, if not from her own inspection then from the reaction of others. Her argument was, 'What if my weight went back to normal and I were still ugly, what would I do then?'")

Susie Orbach says you have to own something before you can lose it. "You must first accept your body in its largeness before you can give it up." Diets? "Moral straitjackets which confine the compulsive eater. In turning to dieting, all the compulsiveness evident in overeating is now channeled into a new obsession—to staying on the diet. Follow these rules, eat what the authorities tell you. Above all, do what women are so good at—deprive yourself."

Every enforced diet, says Orbach, "disenfranchises the woman from her own body. 'Eat bananas seven times a day; weigh four ounces of fish and three ounces of grated cheese; drink one glass of pulp-free orange juice a day and unlimited cups of black coffee or tea; use one bowl only and eat with chopsticks; always eat in the same place or at the same time; always eat a big breakfast; eat starch, cut out fat; cut out fat but eat high protein; lose weight and get/hold your man.' But never, never let yourself go or find out what you like to eat, when, or how."

Orbach believes that compulsive dieting and compulsive eating are two sides of the same coin. In either case the victim is acting "with little regard for what her body wants and when it wants it."

Compulsive eaters don't allow themselves to enjoy food any more than dieters do; they stuff it in too fast to taste it. The diet-binge syndrome can be broken by the compulsive eater when, Orbach says, "she begins to see herself as a 'normal' person, with fat being nothing more than a descriptive word, connoting neither good nor bad."

Think you're normal, and you'll eat as though you're normal. "The main point is to pamper yourself with food—to allow every eating experience to be a pleasurable one, to see your stomach hunger as a signal for you to enjoy." (Orbach makes a distinction between stomach hunger and mouth hunger.)

Fill the house with foods you love, Orbach suggests. "One woman we worked with was persuaded to keep enough ingredients for seventy-five ice cream sundaes . . . When it was first suggested that she fill the refrigerator with ice cream, sauce, nuts, and cream, she exclaimed, 'But I'll eat it all.' The idea seemed so sinful to her. It was pointed out that if she had enough supplies for a minor army and could prove to herself that she did not want to consume it all at once, she would feel much more powerful and more in control of her food. She learned to love the ice cream and treat it as a friend, to be called on when she wanted it, rather than as an enemy to be conquered."

It's like a prep school kid for whom the rules against smoking make smoking an essential act of rebellion; once he's out of school, and the act is drained of its urgency by the world's indifference, it can be dealt with more rationally; cancer versus the momentary pleasure, game versus candle.

Orbach's route to slenderness is so different from any of the other ways chronicled in this book that they make the head swim. According to her, when their kitchens are full of delicious foods, rather than cottage cheese and skim milk, overweight people begin to feel "safe and protected . . . they even find they have other things to do apart from preparing and eating food. If the food is there, if they know that they are never again going to deprive themselves by their own hands, then they can begin to get on with the business of living, and to start to eat in order to live rather than living in order to eat."

The truth is that many women in compulsive eating therapy gain weight at first. But they also start relating to food in a nonobsessive way, not as a means to destroy themselves.

Eventually, this pays off. "If you are sure that you will allow yourself to eat whenever you feel hungry, and that you will give yourself whatever kind of food it is that you are wanting," Orbach says, "you will find that it is less necessary to stuff yourself. When your body then indicates that it is not wanting much food, it means it is time for you to lose a little weight."

Even then, weight loss will be intermittent, with plateaus, the body "holding still while you do the next level of emotional work, exploring fantasies such as 'Who will I be?' 'Who won't like it if I'm slimmer?' 'How will I protect myself if I am ten pounds lighter?'"

Madeline Lee, an admirer of Orbach, wrote in *Ms.* magazine (February 1980) that Orbach's work had helped her understand herself and her life as a "former food junkie."

Said Lee: "Since nobody makes anyone else eat, I am eating because of things that I *want*. Some of what I want is food, some of it is not. Only that which is food can be satisfied by food. (If what I *want* is a bacon sandwich, settling for melba toast is not going to help.) But if it's pampering, maybe a bubble bath is better than a bagel. If it's revenge, maybe it's time for a temper tantrum. Why take it out on your body?"

There's that bubble bath again. My apologies to the Nutrition Control Clinic.

As fat becomes politicized, more and more feminists are turning to questions of obesity. Dr. Angela Barron McBride (teacher and author of a book called *Living with Contradictions: A Married Feminist*) came to Columbia University in the spring of 1980 to contribute to a forum on the fat problems of women.

She read to an audience of nurses and nutritionists excerpts from her journals and transcripts of tapes she had made while driving to work every day. The revelations were unvarnished. "I am so tired of browbeating, and then stuffing, myself . . . I ooze guilt. To me, sin and a hot fudge sundae are equal."

And, on losing weight: "Will I be able to stand myself reduced, dwindling, negligible, fading, melting? Won't my appetite for life shrink with my size?"

Dr. McBride, who considers herself obese, believes, like Susie Orbach, that obesity is "a fundamental feminist issue . . . If the classic male stance is, 'I will protect you,' the female counterpart is 'I will nourish you and make you feel good,' a sentence that suggests oral gratification, sexuality, satiety, sociability, gift-giving, and the civilizing of raw nature. All these elements associated with food reveal the weight of meaning attached to woman's role as nurturer."

Her diary, said McBride, had helped her to stop hating herself. "When I listened to my tapes, I found that I felt sorry for that poor unhappy woman. For the first time, I realized I would never talk to another human being as cruelly as I do to myself."

If you accept yourself, it's easier to stop the cycle of overeating and self-recrimination, the doctor said, adding that she no longer considered two hot fudge sundaes a mortal sin, "but rather a momentary aberration."

Again, like Orbach, McBride thinks a woman has to recognize "the conflicts that made her fat, and the stresses that keep her that way."

McBride is *not* against dieting, and she thinks psychological help is fine, but she also says a woman has to regain mastery of her own life, and set goals that aren't inflicted on her by doctors or magazines or printed weight charts. "Maybe the person who is 250 pounds should only think of getting over the other side, to 211; maybe it's best to do it in small episodes . . . Who says everyone has to be a size 10?"

McBride's final admonition: "Have sympathy for yourself."

It is not feminists alone, however, who are trying to politicize our understanding of the way we eat.

Dr. Hugh Drummond, a splendid muckraker of a medical man, is angry about health problems of the aged poor. He wrote in *Mother Jones* (in a piece briefly referred to in Chapter Fourteen), that the diet of the poor tended to be high in sugar, low in calcium, and low in fiber.

"Poor people," he continued, "also tend to smoke more and lead more stressful lives. Smoking and stress lead to heart disease. Sugar raises the cholesterol level, increases the likelihood of late onset diabetes, and causes obesity. Obesity itself increases the likelihood and degree of diabetes. Diabetes causes kidney damage which raises the blood pressure (which obesity also exacerbates). The hypertension results in worse heart disease and strokes. The reduced calcium intake also increases the severity of heart disease and diminishes bone density (osteoporosis), which increases the likelihood of fractures—resulting in more stress, the danger of blood clots, and immobilization, which further thins the bones. Calcium reduction also causes loss of teeth, which results in an even worse diet with a greater reliance on processed and cooked foods that are low in fiber. The diminished fiber results in a greater likelihood of bowel cancer, prostate disease, and constipation—

which itself leads to diverticular disease, hemorrhoids, and an increased risk of thrombophlebitis (with its attendant consequences of pulmonary embolism, which further damages the heart and lungs)."

Dr. Drummond advises us that the difference between "relative health and chronic disease a generation from now is a matter of the smallest shrugging off of a habit or two right now. I really do not want you to be hunkering around health food stores counting out chromium tablets. A small reduction in the amount of sugar and fat in your diet is not too much to ask in exchange for ten additional years without chronic illness. Three tablespoons of bran a day—you will not choke on it—is enough fiber to prevent a catastrophe in your gut by the year 2000. And while you may insist that you have a hunger for salt, believe me, there is no such thing: each flick of a salt shaker is an unnecessary nudge to your blood pressure. In place of salt, try flavoring your food with lemon juice and as much garlic as your friends can stand. The garlic actually prevents hypertension, and the more vitamin C you get, the better."

We've come full circle. Back to an authority figure laying down the law about what we should and should not eat. Dr. Drummond is a raw-vegetables-fruits-and-nuts-instead-of-gooey-desserts man, too, but he adds to his recommendation of a frugal diet a warning that the politics of health will be felt by us (citizens who live long enough to grow old) "as a matter of personal experience. It will be *your* scarce dollars counted out for unnecessary and destructive medicines. It will be *your* freedom trivialized in an institution."

I always believe the last person who spoke to me. I was gung ho to try Orbach's 3:00 A.M. chocolate cake method of fat control, right up until I stumbled over Dr. Drummond. Now I'm hauling out the bran, and making a sauce for it, a simple but elegant puree of garlic and raw potatoes.

TAKING IT OFF:
If you're willing to go to extremes, you can usually find a doctor to accommodate you.

26 Radical Solutions: Wiring Your Jaws, Bypassing Your Stomach, and Chomping Down All That Rice...

The stoical scheme of supplying our wants by lopping off our desires is like cutting off our feet when we want shoes.
—JONATHAN SWIFT

THERE IS a consensus that most diets embarked on by most people, whether for a few days or for a few weeks, embody the following problems: the diets are (1) passive; (2) controlled; (3) they cause no basic change in eating habits.

Even a cursory ramble through the literature of fat proves this point.

Dr. Sami Hashim and Dr. Theodore Van Itallie of St. Luke's Hospital in New York fed obese patients as much of a liquid diet as the patients wanted. The experiment showed that grossly overweight people could resist liquids much better than they could resist solid foods. Left to their own devices, and cut off from anything that needed chewing, the obese patients reduced their caloric intake from 3,500 to 500 calories a day.

After eight months in the hospital, one patient had lost 220 pounds. But there was a catch. Most of the patients in the Hashim–Van Itallie study regained most of their weight as soon as they went home again.

Even if their weight loss had been permanent, spending eight months in the hospital (after first having cleared the hurdle of being accepted by such a program) is not an option open to the majority of the obese.

Neither is a $10,000 sojourn in Durham, North Carolina, on the so-called Rice Diet. But Eda LeShan, author, educator, and family counselor, who wrote a book *(Winning the Losing Battle)* about her experience in Durham, says it was worth every penny.

"I lived for three and a half months with some three hundred fat people under the supervision of Dr. Walter Kempner," she writes, after telling us that it took her until she was fifty-four years old to be "ready" to be thin.

(Durham, says Calvin Trillin, is "fat city. That's where all the fat places, all the serious diet places, are. There are four diet places in Durham. One invented the Rice Diet, one of 'em Buddy Hackett goes to all the time.")

Eda LeShan found the Rice Diet to be strictly a medical matter. Dr. Kempner had "no patience with psychology." In the case of obese adolescents, LeShan thought that was too bad. "It was my opinion that they should *not* have been on a diet program that did not include psychological counseling and adult supervision, which they needed desperately."

Because of her background, LeShan could supply her own psychology. "We get fat and stay fat primarily because we hate ourselves."

Some of the fear-of-thinness arguments are familiar. Except for the fact that her emphasis is not a feminist one, LeShan doesn't sound unlike Susie Orbach: if she's thin, she won't be allowed to stay happily married, fat is the price she pays for good fortune; if she's thin, she'll lose control of her libidinal drives and become promiscuous; if she's thin, she won't be kind anymore. (Without hot fudge to coat the anger, she'll attack, assert, antagonize.)

While admitting it's less expensive to diet at home, LeShan says some people will never lose weight and keep it off "unless they completely change the environment in which they diet." Her personal feelings of self-loathing (following bouts of compulsive eating) went back many years. "I'd been a fat child and a fat adolescent and a fat adult . . . There was one time when I was still in my thirties when I lost fifty pounds in the period of a year, and gained it all back in three months . . . I once stayed on a Weight Watchers diet for two weeks and did not lose a pound. On the Atkins diet, I gained five pounds a week. On the Stillman diet, I lost weight, but very slowly. When I went to Durham, I ate nothing but fruit and rice for the first two weeks and I lost fifteen pounds."

In the beginning, LeShan's Rice Diet was two fruits and a bowl of rice at lunch, and the same again at dinner. Eventually, vegetables and chicken and fish were added. For LeShan, salt was discovered to be the enemy. "Salt made me hungry. On a totally salt-free diet, I got over wanting to eat candy and cake."

Sixty-five pounds and three and a half months after she'd gone away, LeShan came home convinced she would "never be fat again."

Although Dr. Kempner had suggested that she bring her weight down to 110 pounds, she never seriously considered this. "When I'm at 148 to 155, which is certainly not thin, I feel marvelous, and that's where I got to . . . I was an incipient diabetic, and I had incipient high blood pressure, and I took care of those things. That was important."

Unwilling to lose as much weight "as American culture would demand," LeShan says she still had something of an identity crisis when faced with her new, thinner self. Before she could enjoy that new self, she had to go through a period of mourning for "Fat Eda . . . who suffered so much and tried so hard."

The fat bone's connected to the head bone, and don't you forget it.

Asked on a television show what she thought of bypass surgery for weight control, LeShan indicated horror. "If a bypass isn't evidence of self-hatred, I don't know what is."

Still, bypass surgery is spreading throughout the Western world. The stomach bypass is said to be "somewhat less hazardous" than the intestinal bypass by Dr. G. Timothy Johnson, who goes on to list in his newspaper column some serious side effects (of *all* bypass operations), including "diarrhea, bone-thinning, and most significantly, a potential for serious liver damage."

The Harvard Medical School Letter also advises caution "about developments such as intestinal bypass surgery. It causes weight reduction, certainly—at the risk of 5 percent surgical mortality, and 40 percent postoperative complications."

Some of the complications are emotional, once a patient has had yards of intestine removed. It's the same old story—the fat was a defense mechanism, it served a purpose. If the fat person isn't psychologically prepared to deal with being thin, tremendous depression may follow the bypass operation.

On the other hand, the medical journal, *Lancet*, published (in its

December 15, 1979, issue) some findings based on a study from Denmark that indicated this drastic form of surgery had many boosters. Danish doctors, wishing to compare the results of the radical treatment with the results of more conventional medication, had operated on 130 obese patients, and given 66 others nonsurgical therapy. Two years later, the nonsurgically treated patients had lost about thirteen pounds apiece, whereas the average bypass patient had lost ninety-four pounds.

"The Danes found a significantly greater weight loss and a much improved quality of life in those who had the operation," *Lancet* conceded.

Almost as extreme as the bypass—though it doesn't entail surgery—is the wired-jaws method of losing weight.

For the magazine *Let's LIVE*, Morton Walker interviewed a 5′, 235-pound Connecticut woman who'd had her teeth banded together with steel wires so that she could not eat. "The idea was to allow her to take nourishment only through a straw—to be able to bite nothing."

The woman told Walker she had felt humiliated by her appearance, was ashamed to go out in public, and was going to keep her teeth clenched until she got down to 115 pounds. If it took a year.

She sipped, she said, "lots of liquids and anything that can be put through a blender. Peas, carrots, string beans, beets, beef, and other pureed baby food." She was also allowed juices, diet soda, and an occasional milk shake.

She couldn't eat fried chicken anymore, she mourned, "and no mashed potatoes or potato chips. No macaroni, no bread, no gravy. I eat none of the real good stuff."

Walker pronounced himself dismayed. "The woman's head is filled with dreams of what she erroneously thinks of as 'the real good stuff.' Despite what may happen to her teeth, her gums, her digestive system, and other body organs, she is willing to shorten her life by putting her whole body under stress."

Walker told of the scissors the lady had to wear around her neck in order to be able to cut the wires in her mouth—fast—if she needed to vomit, so she wouldn't choke to death, and he said he hoped she would spend some time reading and studying correct nutrition, and educating herself "away from reversion to those old, fat eating ways . . ."

Dr. H. L. Newbold is another gentleman who takes exception to America's old, fat eating ways, and who offers what to laymen at least sound like radical solutions.

Ten years ago, Newbold, weighing 232 pounds, had a heart attack, went on a self-devised diet, lost over sixty pounds, and never had another chest pang.

No longer an internist-psychiatrist, but a medical nutritionist, he's written *Dr. Newbold's Revolutionary New Discoveries About Weight Loss: How to Master the Hidden Food and Environmental Allergies That Make You Fat,* and also *Mega-Nutrients for Your Nerves,* and *Vitamin C Against Cancer.*

"I consider obesity only another symptom of improper nutrition," he says, "like pellagra or scurvy."

To Dr. Newbold's way of thinking, obesity is often the result of allergies, and high-protein diets work as well as they do only "because overweight people are most likely to be allergic to carbohydrates rather than to fats and proteins."

He is grimly opposed to processed foods—"If you put yourself at the mercy of the food manufacturers, you're lost"—and sugar and, if you can believe it, grains. "The Primal Foods (back to nature foods) that our ancestors survived on for millions of years," he says, "are the ones to which we are the least likely to be allergic. Our ancestors ate meat and vegetables, roots, and sometimes, depending upon where they lived, fruits. Those who could not thrive on these foods (those people who were allergic to them) died off and failed to pass on as many offspring as those who survived. Thus, natural selection chose people with enzyme systems efficient for metabolizing those primitive foods.

"Only some five to ten thousand years ago did significant amounts of grains, milk, and cheese appear in our diets. Sugar has been added in significant amounts only during the past two hundred years.

"Evolution hasn't had time to equip us to handle these new foods. Many people who eat grains and sweets in large quantities become allergic to these products and suffer from depression, tiredness, irritability, obesity, and early death."

Grains no good?

Nathan Pritikin would faint.

Sugar awful? Pritikin might feel a little better. Newbold blames sugar, wholly or in part, for "diabetes, hypoglycemia, obesity, malnutrition, rotted teeth, shortened lives, hardened arteries, depressions," and other medical liabilities.

Even for patients who are *not* allergic—although Newbold has had them with allergies to wheat, and apples, and cats, and aspirin, and gas fumes, and weather, and dust, and vitamins, and marijuana, and diet drinks—Newbold advises avoidance of processed foods, milk and milk products, nuts, table sugar, grains.

He wants his obese clients to eat meat, seafood, fowl, and vegetables, eventually adding a bit of fruit.

"When I was at 312 on my cholesterol, and 165 on my triglycerides," Newbold writes, "I was eating the 'average American diet.' Some good food and a lot of junk. Today I eat meat (and the fat with it) two or three times a day and all the eggs I want. However, I no longer eat bread or sweets. *I do take nutritional supplements*. These nutritional supplements keep my cholesterol low."

Among the nutritional supplements favored by Dr. Newbold: niacin, vitamin B6, vitamin C, vitamin B12, lecithin, pectin, safflower oil, and calcium, magnesium, chromium, iron, and iodine.

Newbold, who gives the American Medical Association and the Food and Drug Administration equally short shrift for what he considers their obtuseness about good nutrition, says it is extraordinary "that a nation so obsessed with food knows so little about nourishment. Many people dismiss the notion that our diets are inadequate, saying that, if we are so ill-nourished, why aren't people suffering from it all around us? The answer is: They are. We're too fat, too thin, depressed, angry, anxious, sickly. We have a million illnesses—from colds to a world record for heart attacks undreamed of a century ago. If we were to stop people on the street and test them at random for proteins, fats, carbohydrates, vitamins, hormones, and minerals, we would find an astounding number of deficiencies. Most (if not all) of these people could improve their health and well-being immeasurably simply by having their deficiencies corrected."

Nutritionists who base their theories on tests with laboratory animals are anathema to Newbold—"It's like going to a surgeon who has taken many lungs out of rats but has never operated on a human being"—and so are the nutrition departments of most colleges because they fail to "take food allergies into consideration in planning diets."

A dozen or so paragraphs back, I mentioned that Dr. Newbold was against processed foods. He puts the case a little more strongly. He says processed foods contribute "to much that is wrong with the civilized world . . . I speak of problems such as birth defects, crime, unemployment, emotional disorders, violence, a number of illnesses such as headaches, backaches, hypoglycemia, diabetes, arthritis, heart disease, obesity, and high blood pressure."

And probably warts, and a tendency to blush easily.

I'm crazy about Dr. Newbold, he talks so tough, and he wanders Manhattan dressed in blue jeans ("In New York, it pays to look more like a mugger than a muggee," he told *Women's Wear Daily*'s Samuel Feinberg), and he drinks from a hip flask filled with distilled water.

He's convinced me that an allergy to sugar, say, or bug spray, can set a spree-eater off on a bat that would make the lost weekend look like a Sunday school picnic. And that an addictive eater with an addiction to pastry, for instance, is different from a spree-eater, and must abandon his addiction, or remain depressed, hopeless, and fat.

But Dr. Newbold boils his steaks. That's what I said. He talks about an inch-thick steak, and then he tells you to boil it. At first, I thought that was a misprint. I thought it was supposed to read "broil." But no. "Put your steak in a pot," he says, "cover it with water and boil for ten minutes."

It took me back to my childhood and a joke about an American living in London, right after the war. Somehow, in that time and place of scarcity, he had managed to acquire a steak, and he took it to his British landlady. "Would you boil this for me?" he said.

"Certainly," said the landlady.

"That's what I thought, you son of a bitch," said the American.

I took up the subject of boiling steaks with James Beard.

"Why boil a steak?" he asked. "If you're going to boil meat, why don't you get a piece of brisket or something, and boil that?"

He thought a second more. "Boiled steak? Inedible. Forget it. Become a vegetarian."

As was mentioned in an earlier chapter, Beard himself, because of overweight and illness, found he had to change his own life-style. No salt, no sugar, and a calorie count ("which I still think is the most important thing") are the foundation of his medically imposed diet, and he's cut back on beef, too. "Because all the flavor is in the fat. If you cannot have fat, then you might as well eat veal, chicken, lamb. Beef is full of fat, pork is full of fat, and unless you can have some of the fat, what's the use? Fortunately, I never get tired of chicken.

"You see, I think if people have any ability as cooks, and they've cooked a lot before they go on a diet, then their experience is twice as valuable, because they can become creative about food."

Most of the problems touched on in this chapter have been big ones, borne by big people, people too large for the good of their own hearts or their blood pressures or their personal relations. And the solutions they chose, or had urged upon them, have been equally dramatic. But when a huge person does make it, achieves thinness, the satisfaction can be huge too.

I saw a lady on television. She had lost one hundred pounds eight years before, and had kept that weight off. Her name was Helaine Schierer, and she was delighted with herself, eager to share her expertise with the audience.

She didn't counsel operations, or the wiring of jaws—only straight, stringent, constant dieting.

Here are some of her suggestions:

"Have a salad, or a piece of fruit before you go to a party, so you don't walk in and eat everything that isn't moving.

"Don't be discouraged. Make a total commitment to follow your program, a day at a time. And when a nightgown that was tight starts feeling a little looser, you'll feel dignity and pride, and that's an unbelievable feeling.

"When you're so hungry you want to eat the wallpaper, call a friend. But never a friend who's dull. If you call a friend who's dull, and you say to her, 'What's new?', and she says, 'I bought thread,' and goes on to tell you what color, that's no good. But if you call a friend who has a big mouth, and she starts telling you what's doing in the neighborhood, and you swear never to tell, by the time you phone everyone you know, that will keep you busy for four hours, and you won't have to eat.

"If you're going to someone's house for dinner, find out what the food is going to be. If they're serving southern fried chicken, you can't say, look, it's my night for lobster, can I have about a pound and a quarter, but you *can* ask to have your chicken baked."

The host of the TV show on which she was appearing asked Helaine Schierer how people finally become aware that they have slipped over the edge, from stockiness to obesity.

"Well," said Helaine, "if you're walking down the street in a blue and white dress, and you happen to stop and yawn, and four people try to mail a letter in your mouth, that'll tell it to you."

Epilogue

"IF THERE IS a single winning cookbook title of the next decade," writes Mimi Sheraton, "it is likely to be the 'Salt-Free, Fat-Free, Quick, Natural, Easy, Economical, Traditional, Gourmet Diet Cookbook.'"

A further Sheraton prediction for the 80s: "The desire to remain bone-thin and still be seen in the most fashionable restaurants eating the currently 'in' dishes will provide a large serving of conflicts."

Conflicts is what I've kept tripping over in the course of assembling this book.

There are two sides to every question, except when there are three or four sides.

One expert says butter is bad for you, and polyunsaturated fats are good. Another expert—Nathan Pritikin—tells you polyunsaturates are more harmful to you than butter.

One doctor will say that salt is chiefly responsible for America's health problems. A second will say sugar is chiefly responsible. A third will blame cholesterol.

Don't eat much meat, advises a nutritionist, stick to grains and vegetables and you'll stay thin and healthy. But the Pima Indians are fat, and getting fatter, and they live on pinto beans and corn tortillas.

Even "that Cosmopolitan Girl" is worried. A *Cosmo* ad had the lovely creature confessing, "It comes as a shock that after you've given up rum-mocha cake, pecan-ripple ice cream, and pizza, you can still get fat on good-for-you things like yogurt with fruit, whole grain cereals, cheese and sunflower seeds!"

I know how she feels. I haven't given up a thing, but vice isn't fun anymore.

Used to be, I sat down to a fourteen-ounce porterhouse, mushrooms sautéed in butter, a hill of French fries, hot apple pie with whipped cream, and I called it good.

I ate the maraschino cherries, bright with red dye #2, out of all the other high school kids' Manhattans.

Canned fruit was the fruit I fancied because of the thick syrup in which it lolled.

When I first left my father's house, I got up in the morning and ate chocolate-covered cherries, and olives stuffed with anchovies, and washed them down with a Coke. e. e. cummings was right, I thought. Freedom *is* a breakfast food.

Working on this book has robbed me of all pleasure.

These days, every time I swallow an unexamined, undissected, unweighed morsel, I suspect that I am eating up my liver, depriving myself of potassium, clogging my arteries with plaques that will prevent my weary blood from finding its way home.

Not to mention my latest fear, which is that I am despoiling the planet.

My mind is cluttered, heavy with warring opinions. I wish I could close it up, like an apartment condemned by the Board of Health.

But peace is not in the cards. There is no peace for an intrepid reporter, a crack news person on the trail of the answer to the great question of our time: What's for dinner?

Tentatively, I can tell you: Not so much as there used to be.

And not just for reasons of vanity, but because we've been squandering too much food and fuel for too long a time. America's economy and philosophy have been based on consumption. The lightning trip west. Subdue and move on.

But the resources of the planet are finite. Seventy million years ago, the last of the dinosaurs died, and over the centuries, their flesh turned to oil. It takes longer to make oil than to consume it. Food and water resources aren't limitless either.

Apropos of this notion, Doris Lessing, in a science fiction novel, writes of a planet she calls Shikasta, where the people believed too fervently that technology was the key to everything good. "The minerals were ripped out, the fuels wasted, the soils depleted by an improvident and shortsighted agriculture, the animals and plants slaughtered and destroyed, the seas being filled with filth and poison, the atmosphere was corrupted—and always, all the time, the propaganda machines thumped out: more, more, more, drink more, eat more, consume more, discard more—in a frenzy, a mania."

Food was a fixation with Shikastans. There was the man "brought up by a mother who, unexpectedly widowed, consoled herself with food: indulgent, she taught him self-indulgence. He was obsessed with food. This is not an uncommon condition: food has assumed an importance that astonishes every one of us visiting Shikasta . . . So extreme is this situation that it is not thought shocking, in a world where most of the inhabitants starve and half starve, for individuals to travel from one city to another, for the sake of good eating, attracted by places whose cuisine is notable. In describing the attractions of a city, first of all will be listed the food that is available and even the details of the cooking."

You hear that, Gael Greene? Doris got us right between the decadent eyes. I'm so filled with chagrin that I am throwing away a clipping from *Vogue* that tells me I can have fresh white truffles flown in from France.

Still, getting along on—wanting—a little, rather than a lot, is foreign to the American nature. Especially since the Great Depression, which made people determined never to go without again.

That the pursuit of happiness has become the pursuit of excess troubles many American writers and thinkers and politicians too.

Consider these opinions:

"Of all cultural adjustments, the notion of an end to progress seems the most difficult for Americans to accept." (Lance Morrow.)

"America is being pulled apart by selfishness." (Jimmy Carter.)

"The American public . . . needs to be persuaded that the acts of the individual matter, and have an impact on the social and economic well-being of all—oneself included. It needs to be made to take seriously the absolutely un-American idea that you can run out of things . . . and not everything is possible." (Meg Greenfield.)

"Two hundred years of living in a cornucopia is over." (Representative Floyd Fithian.)

Not all cornucopia fallout has been bad—the federal government isn't a let-'em-eat-cake outfit—and during the last ten years, through government-financed feeding programs, says Dr. Jean Mayer, we've eliminated rickets in the North, pellagra in the South.

And nobody's dying of hunger. But what about cold? ask the pessimists. Already, there are stories of old people freezing to death because they can't afford to buy both oil and food.

For everyone, the prices of food, housing, heat, and medical care rise and rise again. Only satirists get anything good from inflation. (Russell Baker has observed that $24,000 isn't so much, "basically, it's just 12,000 boxes of Grape-Nuts.")

"Oil Increase Will Be Felt All Along the Food Chain" reads a headline, and the story underneath talks of the swelling cost of shipping wheat, of fuel, of fertilizers and insecticides.

Americans are compared unfavorably to the Chinese, who use bikes where we use oil—no twenty-year-old Chinese keels over with hardened arteries—and we're told that famine is the mother of great cooking. In China, they say, a chef can make fish lips taste good.

Pope John Paul II hears the clanking of chains on people "enslaved by appetites."

But Americans are adaptable. We adapted to abundance—too wholeheartedly, perhaps—and we can probably adapt to the idea that less is more. Somewhere this side of the fish lips solution, we can get out of our cars, land on our feet, and set them to walking. We can turn down our thermostats, turn off the lights in empty rooms, and quit eating like pigs.

In fact, we may have to.

INDEX